Introduction to Splinting

A Critical-Thinking & Problem-Solving Approach

Introduction to Splinting

A Critical-Thinking & Problem-Solving Approach

BRENDA M. COPPARD, MS, OTR/L
Assistant Professor
Department of Occupational Therapy
Creighton University
Omaha, Nebraska

HELENE LOHMAN, MA, OTR/L
Assistant Professor
Department of Occupational Therapy
Creighton University
Omaha, Nebraska

EDITORIAL CONSULTANT
JUDY C. COLDITZ, OTR/L, CHT

WITH ILLUSTRATIONS BY MICHAEL TURNER
AND CHAPTER AND COVER PHOTOS BY THOMAS M. HERBERT

with 7 contributors
with 170 illustrations

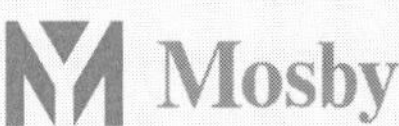

St. Louis Baltimore Boston Carlsbad Chicago Naples New York Philadelphia Portland
London Madrid Mexico City Singapore Sydney Tokyo Toronto Wiesbaden

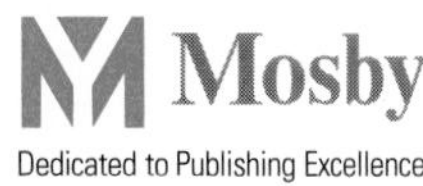

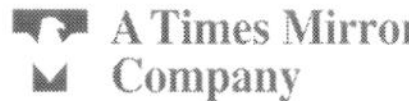

Publisher: Don Ladig
Editor: Martha Sasser
Associate Developmental Editor: Amy Dubin
Project Manager: Linda McKinley
Associate Production Editor: Paul Stoecklein
Designer: Elizabeth Fett
Manufacturing Supervisor: Linda Ierardi

Printed in the United States of America
Composition by Graphic World, Inc.
Printing/binding by World Color

Mosby-Year Book, Inc.
11830 Westline Industrial Drive
St. Louis, Missouri 63146

Library of Congress Cataloging in Publication Data
Coppard, Brenda M.
Introduction to splinting : a critical-thinking & problem-solving approach / Brenda M. Coppard, Helene Lohman ; editorial consultant, Judy C. Colditz ; with illustrations by Michael Turner and photos by Thomas M. Herbert ; with 7 contributors.
p. cm.
Includes bibliographical references and index.
ISBN 0-8151-7126-9
1. Hand—Wounds and injuries—Treatment. 2. Splints (Surgery)
I. Lohman, Helene. II. Title.
[DNLM: 1. Splints. WE 26 C785i 1996]
RD559.C68 1996
617.5'75044—dc20
DNLM/DLC
for Library of Congress 95-42842
CIP

98 99 00 / 9 8 7 6 5 4 3

Contributors

SERENA M. BERGER, MA, OTR
Clinical Instructor,
Department of Occupational Therapy,
New York University;
Technical Service Representative,
Smith and Nephew Rolyan,
New York, New York

MAUREEN T. CAVANAUGH, MS, OTR
Clinical Instructor,
Department of Occupational Therapy,
New York University;
Private Practitioner,
New York, New York

BRENDA M. COPPARD, MS, OTR/L
Assistant Professor,
Department of Occupational Therapy,
Creighton University,
Omaha, Nebraska

LINDA GABRIEL, MA, OTR/L
Assistant Professor,
Department of Occupational Therapy,
Creighton University,
Omaha, Nebraska

HELENE LOHMAN, MA, OTR/L
Assistant Professor,
Department of Occupational Therapy,
Creighton University,
Omaha, Nebraska

MICHAEL LOHMAN, MEd, OTR/L, CO
Adjunct Clinical Professor,
Department of Occupational Therapy,
Creighton University;
Staff Orthotist,
Novacare Orthotics and Prosthetics,
Omaha, Nebraska

SALLY E. POOLE, MA, OTR, CHT
Clinical Assistant Professor,
Department of Occupational Therapy,
New York University,
New York, New York;
Co-Owner,
Hands-On Rehab,
Valhalla, New York

JOAN L. SULLIVAN, MA, OTR, CHT
Co-Owner,
Hands-On Rehab,
Valhalla, New York;
Professional Associate,
Occupational Therapy Department,
Mercy College,
Dobbs Ferry, New York

JEAN WILWERDING-PECK, OTR/L, CHT
Clinical Coordinator,
Department of Occupational Therapy,
Saint Joseph Hospital,
Omaha, Nebraska

To my husband and family for their support and to my students who inspire by their curiosity.

Brenda M. Coppard, ms, otr/l

To my parents, husband, family, friends, and colleagues for their support and patience during the writing of this book and to my students, who taught me what was valuable to include.

Helene Lohman, ma, otr/l

Foreword

Sophistication in hand splinting has grown considerably over the last 2 decades. Some of the factors that have contributed to this trend are the emergence of hand rehabilitation as a specialty in occupational therapy, increased knowledge of the biomechanics, theory, and principles of hand splinting, and the technological advances in thermoplastics and splinting accessories. The entry-level occupational therapy practitioner is expected to have fundamental skills in splinting theory, design, and fabrication.

Introduction to Splinting: A Critical-Thinking & Problem-Solving Approach, is designed primarily for use in education programs that prepare students for entry-level practice in occupational therapy. Occupational therapy practitioners who need to develop skills in splinting and those reentering the field will also find this text essential to independent study. Several books on splinting are available, but none specifically address the educational needs of this student population. Instructors will enthusiastically welcome this text because it is the most appropriate book on the market for the occupational therapy student who is a novice to splinting theory, design, and fabrication. Students will love the book because it facilitates the mastery of basic theory, principles, and techniques of splinting that entry-level clinicians need for competence.

Self-quizzes and review questions throughout the book provide the reader with excellent tools to test immediate recall of basic facts. Well-illustrated and clearly described instructions guide students through splint fabrication in the classroom. Instructions for fabricating splints encountered most frequently in clinical practice are included. Forms are provided for student self-evaluation and instructor evaluation of completed splints. Case studies, splint analyses, and documentation exercises are some of the learning activities designed to stimulate critical thinking and problem solving. The learning exercises and laboratory experiences provide opportunities to test clinical reasoning and the technical skills of splint pattern design and splint fabrication.

This text fits neatly into a course on splinting or for units on splinting in more than one course. It is generously illustrated and moves through a logical progression from general theory and principles to splint design and fabrication for specific patient populations. The experience of the authors as educators is apparent in a writing style and level that addresses the unique learning needs of the occupational therapy student or clinician who may be a novice to splinting. Occupational therapy educators and novice clinicians will applaud this comprehensive textbook on splinting.

Lorraine Williams Pedretti, MS, OTR
Professor Emeritus
San José State University
San José, California

Preface

As instructors in a professional occupational therapy program, we have not found an introductory splinting textbook that addresses the development of splint fabrication skills from a critical-thinking and problem-solving approach. *Introduction to Splinting: A Critical-Thinking & Problem-Solving Approach* was inspired by students, who over the years have requested such a book to supplement their coursework and serve as a resource.

This book provides the reader with a fundamental basis of theory and skills necessary to design and fabricate splints. The book is intended for students in baccalaureate and entry-level master's degree occupational therapy programs, students in Certified Occupational Therapy Assistant programs, and therapists who need to develop basic splinting skills because of lack of experience or reentry into the field of study. Physicians that prescribe splints and physical therapists and orthotists involved in fabricating splints may also find this book to be a valuable resource. Readers can use this book as a complement to *Hand Splinting: Principles and Methods* by Elaine Fess, Cynthia Philips, and Karan Gettle-Harmon.

Introduction to Splinting is unique because of its focus on education. The book can be used in one course or throughout many courses in a curriculum and can serve as a workbook for laboratory experiences. In this book, critical-thinking and problem-solving skills are promoted through various case studies, self-quizzes, splint analyses, documentation exercises, laboratory exercises, and self-evaluation forms. Each chapter begins with chapter objectives and most end with review questions. After reading this book and completing its quizzes, laboratory exercises, and other items, the reader should be able to construct splints based on theory and skill, critically analyze splints for strengths and weaknesses, and problem solve case studies about the clinical application of splints.

Introduction to Splinting consists of 12 chapters. The first 3 chapters are an introduction to splinting, a review of anatomical and biomechanical principles, and a review of the hand examination process. These chapters present the fundamentals that are applied throughout the remaining chapters.

Chapter 4 teaches approaches to a thorough clinical problem-solving process that can be employed from the moment a splint referral is obtained until the patient's discharge. The material presented in this chapter helps to answer questions about case studies presented in later chapters.

Chapters 5 through **8** present the theory, design, and fabrication of splints that general practitioners commonly use. The specific splints included are the wrist cock-up, resting hand, thumb spica, and dynamic splints. Step-by-step instructions are provided, showing the reader the way to create the pattern, fabricate the splint, and make necessary adjustments.

The remaining chapters in the book are geared toward specialized and advanced splinting. Topics for these chapters include splinting for nerve injuries, antispasticity splinting, geriatric splinting, and pediatric splinting.

The reader has access to a glossary of terms that are used throughout the text. This book also contains three appendixes. Appendix A provides answers to quizzes, laboratory exercises, and case studies. Appendix B contains copies of self-evaluation forms that appear in the chapters. Readers can complete these forms based on the splints they fabricate. Appendix C contains copies of classroom grading sheets that appear in the chapters. Instructors can use these grading sheets to grade students' splints. Appendixes B and C have perforated pages.

Although many therapists (including Judy C. Colditz, OTR/L, CHT) reviewed this book, each experienced therapist and physician may have a personal view on splinting approaches and techniques. This book represents the authors' perspectives and is not intended to present the only correct approach.

Brenda M. Coppard, MS, OTR/L
Helene Lohman, MA, OTR/L

Acknowledgments

We are grateful to many people who made contributions for this book, especially the following:

- Judy C. Colditz, OTR/L, CHT for her editorial consultant work
- The contributors for sharing their expertise and knowledge
- The Creighton University Occupational Therapy Department faculty and staff members for their support
- The students for inspiring us to write this book
- The editorial staff members at Mosby-Year Book, Inc., for their professional guidance and assistance
- The many therapists and students for reviewing chapters of the manuscript and making contributions

Brenda M. Coppard, MS, OTR/L
Helene Lohman, MA, OTR/L

Contents

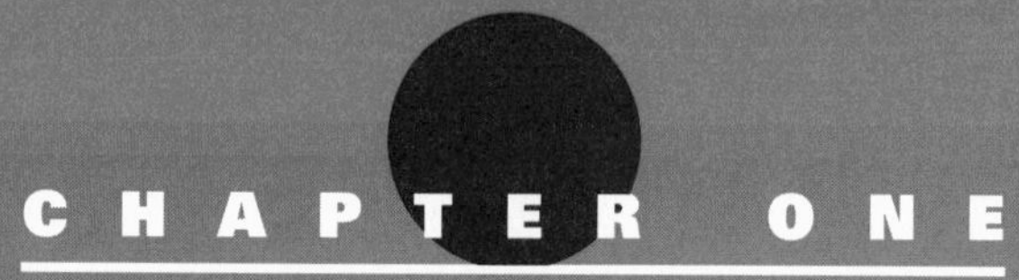

Introduction to Splinting

BRENDA M. COPPARD, MS, OTR/L

CHAPTER OBJECTIVES

1. Define the terms *splint* and *orthosis.*
2. Identify the health professionals who provide splinting services.
3. Describe how frame-of-reference approaches are applied to splinting.
4. List the purposes of static (immobilization) splints.
5. List the purposes of dynamic (mobilization) splints.
6. Identify splint material properties.
7. Describe the pattern-making process for a splint.
8. Explain the process of cutting and molding a splint.
9. Explain what should be documented with any splint provision.

Determining splint design and fabricating hand splints are extremely important aspects in providing optimal care for patients suffering from upper extremity injuries and functional deficits. Splint fabrication is a combination of science and art. Therapists must apply knowledge of pathology, physiology, kinesiology, anatomy, and biomechanics to best design splints for patients. Additionally, therapists must consider and appreciate the aesthetic value of splints. Beginning splintmakers should be aware that each patient is different, requiring a customized splint.

Therapists must also develop critical-thinking skills to splint effectively. This book emphasizes and fosters such skills for beginning splintmakers in general practice areas. After therapists are knowledgeable in the science of splint design, fabrication, and provision, practice is essential to become comfortable and competent.

What is a Splint?

Mosby's Medical, Nursing, and Allied Health Dictionary (1990, p. 1108) defines a *splint* as "an orthopedic device for immobilization, restraint, or support of any part of the body." The text (p. 850) also defines *orthosis* as "a force system designed to control, correct, or compensate for a bone deformity, deforming forces, or forces absent from the body."

Today in the health care field these terms are often used synonymously. Technically, the term *splint* refers to a temporary device that is part of a treatment program, whereas the term *orthosis* refers to a permanent device to replace or substitute for loss of muscle function. Usually, splints are made by therapists and orthoses are made by orthotists.

Splints and orthoses not only immobilize but also mobilize, position, and protect a joint or a specific body part. Design and fabrication of splints ranges from simple to complex depending on the goals established for a particular condition.

What is the Historical Synopsis of Splinting?

Years ago when splints were first available, they were made by blacksmiths and carpenters. Materials used to make the splints were limited to wood, leather, and metal.

Hand splinting became an important aspect of physical rehabilitation during World War II. Survival rates of injured troops dramatically increased because of medical, pharmacological (e.g., the use of penicillin), and technological advances. During this period, occupational and physical therapists collaborated with orthotic technicians and physicians to provide splints for patients. "Sterling Bunnell, MD, was designated to organize and to oversee hand services at nine army hospitals in the Unites States" (Rossi, 1987, p. 53). In the mid 1940s, under the guidance of Dr. Bunnell, many splints were made and sold commercially. During the 1950s, many children and adults needed splints to assist them in carrying out activities of daily living secondary to poliomyelitis (Rossi, 1987). During this time, many splints were made from high-temperature plastics by orthotists. With the advent of low-temperature thermoplastics, hand splinting became a common practice in clinics by occupational therapists.

Who Fabricates Splints?

Traditionally a variety of health care professionals have fabricated splints. Occupational therapists constitute a large population of health care providers whose services include splint design and fabrication. Along with physical therapists, occupational therapists specializing in hand rehabilitation often fabricate splints for their hand-injured patients. With supervision, certified Occupational Therapy Assistants also assist with splint fabrication. In addition, certified orthotists are trained and skilled in the designing, constructing, fitting of braces and orthoses prescribed by physicians.

Splint design must be based on scientific principles, and splint fabrication requires creative problem solving because each patient and splint may be different. Health care professionals who make splints must allow themselves to be creative and take risks. Splintmaking requires practice for the clinician to be at ease with the fabrication process. Students or therapists beginning to design and fabricate splints should be aware of personal expectations and realize that their skills will likely evolve with practice.

Occupational Therapy Frame-of-Reference Approaches for Splinting

A *frame of reference* is defined as "a conceptual structure around which a program, organization, or project is developed and organized" (Pedretti & Pasquinelli, 1990, p. 1). Frames of reference help therapists determine which evaluations and treatments to choose for a particular patient.

Occupational performance is one frame of reference used in occupational therapy for physical dysfunction and involves several approaches, including the following: biomechanical, sensorimotor, and rehabilitative. The biomechanical approach uses biomechanical principles of kinetics and forces acting on the body. The sensorimotor approach is used with patients having damaged central nervous systems to inhibit or facilitate normal motor responses. The rehabilitation approach focuses on abilities rather than disabilities and facilitates returning persons to maximal function using their capabilities (Pedretti & Pasquinelli, 1990).

Each approach can incorporate splinting as a treatment intervention depending on the rationale for using a splint with a patient. For example, if a patient is wearing a tenodesis splint to re-create grasp and release to maximize function in activities of daily living, the therapist is using the rehabilitation approach (Hill & Presperin, 1986). If the therapist is using the biomechanical approach, a dynamic hand splint may be chosen to apply kinetic forces to the patient's body. If the therapist chooses the sensorimotor approach, an antispasticity splint may be used to inhibit or reduce tone.

Splinting Materials

Low-temperature thermoplastic materials are those most commonly used to fabricate splints. The materials are low temperature because they soften in water heated between 135° and 180° F. When the plastic is heated, it becomes pliable and then hardens to its original rigidity after cooling.

The first commonly available, low-temperature thermoplastic material was

SELF-QUIZ 1-1*

Match the approach that was used in each of the following scenarios.

a. Biomechanical approach
b. Sensorimotor approach
c. Rehabilitation approach

1. _____ This approach was used on a patient who has cerebral palsy. The goal of the splint was to decrease the amount of tone present.
2. _____ This approach allowed a patient suffering from a stroke to grasp the walker by using splints that were adapted to assist with grasp.
3. _____ This approach helped a patient who had a tendon repair that resulted in flexor contractures of the metacarpophalangeal (MCP) joint to regain full range of motion.

*See Appendix A for the answer key.

Orthoplast. Currently, many types of thermoplastic materials are available from several companies. Types of materials used in clinics vary based on patient diagnoses, therapists' preferences, and availability.

Many decisions must be made regarding the best type of thermoplastic material to use for splint fabrication. Decisions are based on factors such as cost, properties of the thermoplastic material, and familiarity with the splinting materials. One type of thermoplastic material is not the best choice for every type or size of splint. If a therapist has not had experience with a certain type of thermoplastic, it is best to practice before using it to fabricate a splint and to read the manufacturer's technical literature describing the material's contents and properties.

Thermoplastic Material Content and Properties

Thermoplastic materials are elastic, plastic, plastic and rubberlike, and rubberlike (North Coast Medical, Inc, 1992). Each piece of thermoplastic material has unique properties defined by handling and performance characteristics. *Handling characteristics* refer to the thermoplastic material properties when softened (heated), and *performance characteristics* refer to the thermoplastic material properties after the material has hardened.

Thermoplastic materials described as rubbery or rubberlike tend to be more resistant to stretching and finger printing. These materials may be less conforming than their drapier counterparts. Therapists should not confuse resistance to stretch during the molding process with the rigidity of the splint on completion. Materials that are quite drapey may be extremely rigid, and the opposite may also be true. In addition, the more contours a splint contains, the more rigid it will be.

HANDLING CHARACTERISTICS

Memory

Memory is a property of thermoplastic material that describes the material's ability to return to its preheated (original) shape and size when reheated (Berger, 1995). This property allows therapists to reheat and reshape splints several times without the material stretching excessively. Materials with memory must be constantly molded throughout the cooling process to sustain maximal conformability to patients.

Drapability

Drapability is the degree of ease a material conforms to the underlying shape without assistance (Berger, 1995). Material with high drapability is difficult to use for large splints and is most successful on a cooperative patient who can place the body part in a gravity-assisted position. Thermoplastic materials with high drapability may be more difficult for beginning splinters because the materials must be handled gently. Successful molding requires therapists to refrain from pushing the material during shaping. Instead, the material should be lightly stroked into place. Light touch and constant movement of therapists' hands will result in splints that are cosmetically appealing.

Elasticity

Elasticity is a material's resistance to stretching and its tendency to return to its original shape after stretch (Berger, 1995). Materials with memory have a slight tendency to rebound to their original shapes during molding. Materials with a high resistance to stretch can be worked more aggressively than materials that stretch easily. As a result, resistance to stretch is a helpful property when working with uncooperative patients.

Bonding

Self-bonding or self-adherence is the degree to which material will stick to itself when properly heated (Berger, 1995). Material that is coated always requires surface preparation with a bonding agent. Self-bonding materials may not require surface preparation, but some thermoplastic materials have a coating that must be removed for bonding to occur. Coated material tacks at the edges but can be pried apart after the material is cool. However, after a coated material is stretched, it becomes tackier and more likely to bond.

All thermoplastic material, whether coated or uncoated, forms stronger bonds if surfaces are prepared with solvent. Bonding agent or solvent is a chemical that can be brushed onto both pieces of the plastic to be bonded. In some cases, therapists should roughen the two surfaces that will have contact with each other. This procedure, called *scoring,* can be carefully done with the end of a scissors or a utility knife. After surfaces have been scored, they can be softened, brushed with a bonding agent, and adhered together. Self-adherence is an important characteristic of dynamic splinting (see Chapter 8).

Self-Finishing Edges

A self-finishing edge is a handling characteristic that allows any cut edge to have a smooth texture if the material is cut when warm. This handling characteristic saves time for therapists because they do not have to manually roll or smooth the edges.

Other Considerations

Other handling characteristics to be considered are heating time, working time, and shrinkage. Time is required to heat thermoplastic materials to a working temperature because material left too long in hot water may become excessively soft and stretchy. After the material is sufficiently heated, it is usually pliable for 3 to 5 minutes depending on the specific type of material (Berger, 1995).

Thinner materials and perforated materials cool faster, and some plastics shrink slightly when cooling. This is an important consideration when therapists are properly fitting a circumferential splint.

Performance Characteristics

Conformability

Conformability is a performance characteristic that refers to the ability of thermoplastic material to fit intimately into contoured areas (Berger, 1995). Material that is extremely drapey and has a high degree of conformability can pick up patients' fingerprints and crease marks (as well as therapists' fingerprints). Splints that are intimately conformed to patients are more comfortable and reduce the likelihood of the splint migrating on the extremity.

Flexibility

A thermoplastic material with a high degree of flexibility can take stresses repeatedly (Berger, 1995). Flexibility is an important characteristic for circumferential splints because these splints must be pulled open for application and removal.

Durability

Durability is the length of time splint material will last (Berger, 1995). Rubber-based materials are more apt to become brittle with age.

Rigidity

Materials having a high degree of rigidity are strong and resistant to repeated stress (Berger, 1995). Rigidity is important when therapists make medium-to-large splints (such as splints for elbows or forearms). Large splints require rigid material to support the weight at larger joints.

Moisture Permeability and Air Exchange

Moisture permeability relates to perforations in the material (Berger, 1995). Various perforation patterns are available. Super-perforated materials allow air exchange to the underlying skin surface and reduce the weight of splints.

Finish, Colors, and Thickness

Finish refers to the texture of the end product. Some thermoplastics have a smooth finish, whereas others have a grainy texture. Generally, coated materials are easier to keep clean.

The color of the thermoplastic material may affect patient compliance to the wearing schedule. Brightly colored splints tend to be popular with children. In addition, colored splints are easily seen and therefore useful in preventing loss in institutional settings. For example, seeing a blue splint in white bed linen is easier than seeing a white splint in white bed linen.

The common thickness for thermoplastic material is ⅛ inch. However, if the weight of the material over a joint is a concern, a thinner plastic may be used, reducing the bulkiness of the splint and possibly increasing the patient's comfort and improving compliance to the wearing schedule. Thinner thermoplastic material is commonly used for arthritis and pediatric splints (Smith & Nephew Rolyan, 1995).

Table 1-1 lists property guidelines for thermoplastic materials.

Splint Patterns

A pattern should be made for each patient needing a splint because generic patterns rarely fit patients correctly. Therapists should trace the outline of the patient's hand on paper, making certain that the hand is flat and in a neutral position. If the patient's hand is unable to flatten on the paper, the contralateral hand may be used to draw the pattern. If the contralateral hand cannot be used, the therapist should hold the paper curved to fit the hand position. The therapist should mark on the paper any hand landmarks needed for the pattern before the

TABLE 1-1* **Thermoplastic Property Guideline**

Thermoplastic name	Degree of heating temperature(°F)
MEMORY	
Aquaplast®-T	160-170
Watercolors™	160-170
Aquaplast® Pro Drape™	160-170
Aquaplast® Resilient™	160-170
NCM Spectrum™	140-145
Orfit® Soft	135
Orfit® Stiff	135
Omega™ Plus	140-170
Encore™	140-170
RIGIDITY	
Ezeform®	160-170
NCM Clinic®	160
NCM Clinic D®	160
NCM Preferred®	160
Polyform®	150-160
CONFORMABILITY, DRAPABILITY	
Aquaplast® Pro Drape™	160-170
Ezeform®	160-170
NCM Clinic®	160
NCM Clinic D®	160
Polyform®	150-160
Polyform Light®	150-160
Polyflex® II	150-160
Polyflex® Light™	150-160
Orfit® Soft	135
Orthoplast® II	150-160
Encore™	140-170
MODERATE DRAPABILITY	
Aquaplast®-T	160-170
Ezeform®	160-170
Ezeform® Light™	150-160
RESISTANCE TO DRAPE	
Aquaplast® Resilient™	160-170
Synergy®	160-170
Omega™ Max	140-170
SELF-ADHERENCE	
Aquaplast®	160-170
Ezeform®	160
NCM Preferred®	160
NCM Spectrum™	160
Orfit® Soft	135
Orfit® Stiff	135
Synergy®	160-170
Omega™ Plus	140-170

Courtesy Serena Berger, Smith and Nephew Rolyan, Inc., Germantown, WI and North Coast Medical, Inc., San Jose, CA.

*Not all inclusive.

hand is removed. The therapist then draws the splint pattern over the outline of the hand, cuts out the pattern with scissors, and completes final sizing.

As shown in Figure 1-1, moistening the paper and applying it to the patient's hand helps the therapist determine which adjustments are required. If the pattern is too large in areas, the therapist can make adjustments by cutting or fold-

Laboratory Exercise 1-1

Low–Temperature Thermoplastics

Cut small squares of different thermoplastics. Soften them in water, and experiment with the plastics so that you can answer the following questions for each type of thermoplastic.

Name of thermoplastic: ______________________

1. Does it contour and drape to the hand? Yes ❍ No ❍
2. Does it appear to be strong when cool? Yes ❍ No ❍
3. Can its edges be rolled easily? Yes ❍ No ❍
4. Does it discolor on heating? Yes ❍ No ❍
5. Does it take fingerprints easily? Yes ❍ No ❍
6. Does it bond to itself? Yes ❍ No ❍
7. Can it be reheated several times and change back to its original shape? Yes ❍ No ❍

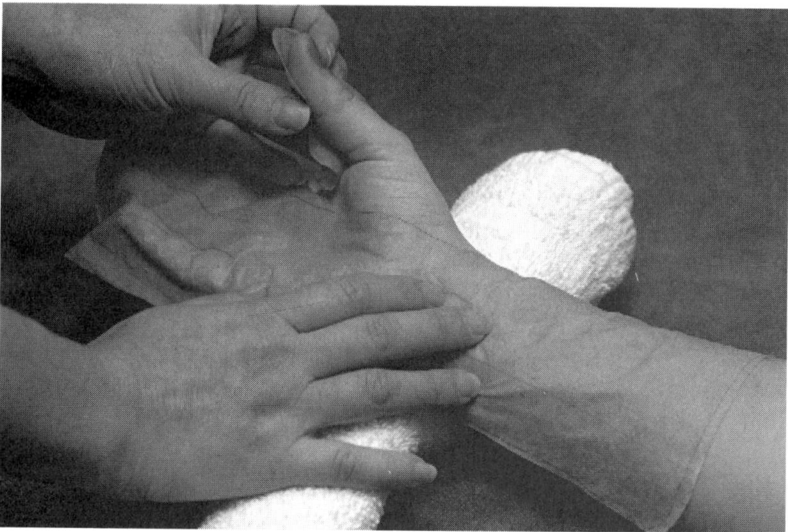

FIGURE 1-1

To make adjustments on the splint pattern, moisten the paper and apply it to the patient.

FORM 1-1* Hints for Drawing and Fitting a Splint Pattern

- ❍ Explain the pattern-making process to the patient.
- ❍ Ask and/or assist the patient in removing any jewelry from the area that is splinted.
- ❍ Position the affected extremity on a paper towel in a natural, resting position. The wrist should be in a neutral position with a slight ulnar deviation. The fingers should be extended and slightly abducted.
- ❍ To trace the outline of the patient's extremity, keep the pencil at a 90-degree angle to the paper.
- ❍ Mark the landmarks needed to draw the pattern *before* the patient removes the extremity from the paper.
- ❍ For a more accurate pattern, the paper towel can be wet and placed on the area for evaluation of the pattern.
- ❍ Folding the paper towel to mark adjustments in the pattern can help with evaluation of the pattern.
- ❍ When evaluating the pattern fit of a forearm-based splint on the patient, look for the following[†]:
  1. Half the circumference of the forearm
  2. Two-thirds the length of the forearm
  3. The length and width of metacarpal or palmar bars
  4. The correct use of hand creases for landmarks
  5. The amount of support to the wrist, fingers, and thenar and hypothenar eminencies
- ❍ When tracing the pattern onto the thermoplastic material, do not use an ink pen because the ink may smear when the material is placed in the hot water to soften.

*See Appendix B for a perforated copy of this form.
[†]These biomechanical principles and anatomical structures are discussed in Chapters 2 and 3.

ing it. Sometimes retracing a pattern is necessary if it is too small or requires major adjustments. The therapist should make certain that the pattern fits the patient before tracing it onto and cutting it out of the thermoplastic material.

Form 1-1 lists suggestions helpful to a beginning splintmaker when drawing and fitting patterns.

Tracing, Heating, and Cutting

After making the pattern, the therapist should place it on the sheet of thermoplastic material in such a way to conserve material and then trace it with a pencil. If the therapist uses an ink pen, the ink may smear onto the plastic; however,

A

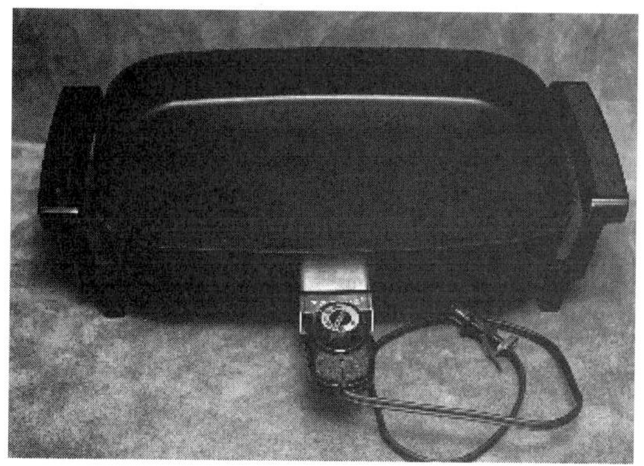

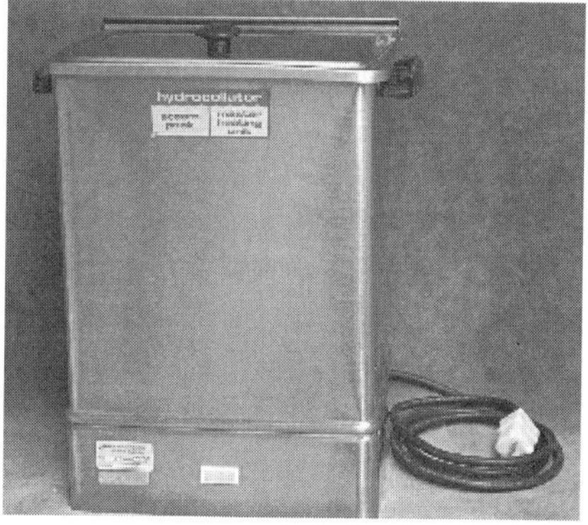

B

FIGURE 1-2
Soften thermoplastic material in an electric fry pan **(A)** or a hydrocollator **(B)**.

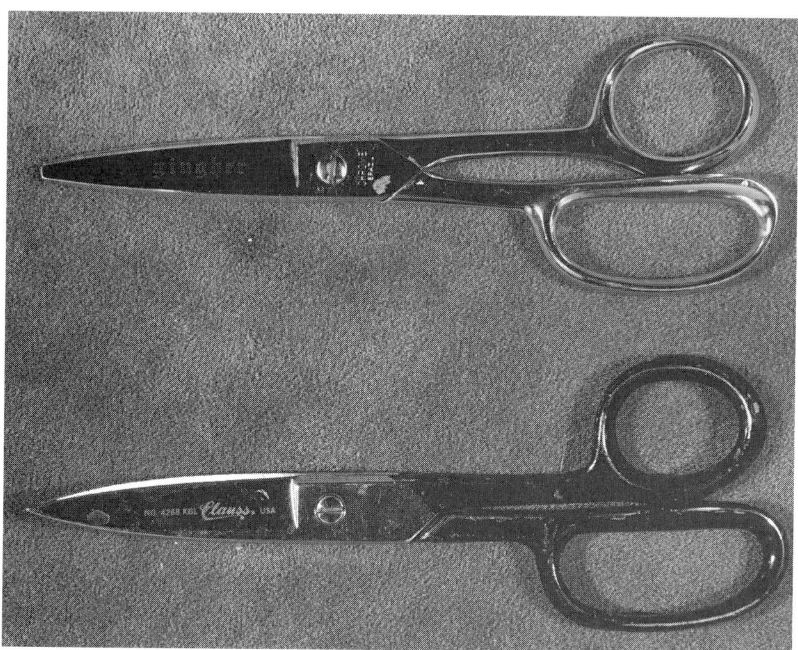

FIGURE 1-3
Round- or flat-edge scissors work well for cutting thermoplastic.

the ink can be removed with chlorine. The therapist cuts the portion of material needed with a utility knife and then softens it in an electric fry pan or a hydrocollator filled with water heated to approximately 180° F (Figure 1-2). After removing the thermoplastic material from the water, the therapist cuts out the material with either round- or flat-edged scissors (Figure 1-3). Unless the therapist is able to cut quickly, the material may require reheating. Finally, the therapist applies the thermoplastic material to the patient's extremity.

The thermoplastic material is extremely warm, so the therapist should use caution to prevent skin burn. Some thermoplastic materials will stick to the patient's hair on the skin, but this situation can be avoided by using stockinette or lotion on the skin before applying the splinting material.

Adjustments

Therapists can make adjustments to splints while the thermoplastic material is still warm, such as marking a trim line with their fingernails or a pencil or stretching small areas of the splint. The amount of allowable stretch depends on the property of the material and the cooling time that has elapsed. If the plastic is too cool to cut with scissors, the therapist can quickly dip the area in the hot water. Because heat guns warm unevenly, therapists should not use them for major trimming. However, heat guns are helpful for warming small areas for finishing touches.

Strapping

After achieving a correct fit, the therapist uses strapping materials to secure the splint onto the patient's extremity. Velcro hook and loop, which are available commercially with an adhesive backing, are commonly used for the strapping mechanism. Briefly heating the adhesive backing and the site for attachment on the splint with a heat gun increases the bond of the hook or loop to the thermoplastic material. To prevent the patient from losing the straps, the therapist may choose to attach one end of the strap to the splint with a rivet or strong adhesive glue. The therapist may also cut extra straps and give them to the patient to take home if necessary.

Padding

The therapist can use a heat gun to push out areas of the thermoplastic that may irritate bony prominences. The therapist can also use padding over these areas or to line the entire splint. Sufficient space must be available for the padding or the pressure may actually increase over the area. Also, any bony prominences should be padded before splint formation. If an entire splint is to be lined with padding, the therapist can use the splint pattern to cut out the padding needed. The therapist can trace the pattern ¼ to ½ inch larger on the padding if the intention is to overlap onto the splint's edges.

Various padding systems are commercially available, and most include an adhesive backing for easy application. Padding has either closed or open cells. Closed-cell padding resists absorption of odors, perspiration, and bacteria, and therapists can easily wipe it clean. Open-cell padding allows for absorption. Because of low durability and soiling, padding used in a splint may require periodic replacement.

Edge Finishing

Edges of a splint should be smooth and rolled or flared to prevent a pressure area on the patient's extremity. The therapist can use a heat gun or heated water in a fry pan or hydrocollator to heat, soften, and smooth edges. Fingertips moistened with water or lotion help avoid finger imprints on the plastic. Most of the newer thermoplastic materials are self-finishing. When the warm plastic is cut, it does not require detailed finishing other than that which is necessary to flare the edges.

Reinforcement

If an area of a splint requires reinforcement, an additional piece of material bonded to the top of the splint will increase the strength. A ridge molded in the reinforcement piece provides additional strength (Figure 1-4). This technique is useful when the thermoplastic material is too thin or flexible to provide support to an area such as the wrist.

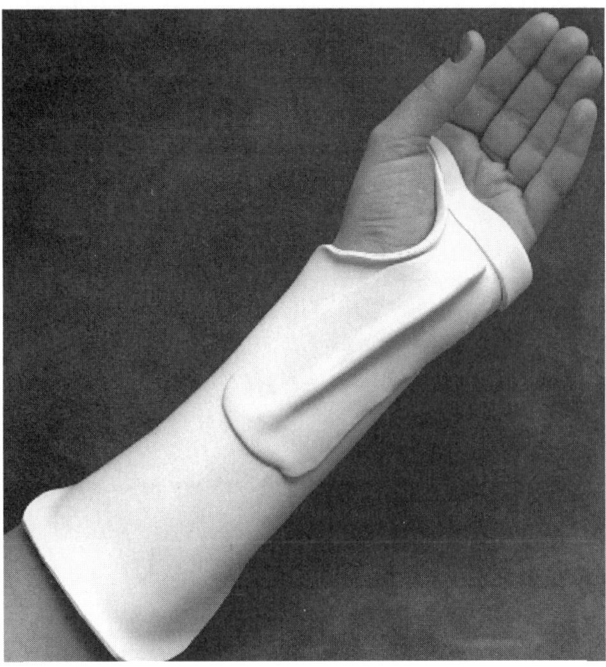

FIGURE 1-4 Splint reinforcement
This ridge on the reinforcement piece adds strength.

Purpose of Splinting

Splints are usually classified as static or dynamic. Static splints are designed to provide support to areas of the body and have no movable parts (Cailliet, 1994). Dynamic splints are designed to mobilize areas of the body and have one or more movable parts (Malick, 1982).

According to the American Society of Hand Therapists (ASHT) (1992), splints are classified as (1) mobilization, (2) immobilization, or (3) restrictive. Mobilization splints are designed to move or mobilize primary and secondary joints. Immobilization splints are designed to immobilize primary and secondary joints. Restrictive splints "limit a specific aspect of joint range of motion for the primary joints" (ASHT, 1992, p. 9).

The purpose of static (immobilization or restrictive) splints is threefold: to immobilize, to help prevent further deformity, and to prevent a soft-tissue contracture (Cannon, et al., 1985; Barr & Swan, 1988). Static splints provide rest to a joint or several joints. A common static splint is a resting hand splint (Figure 1-5). Therapists commonly use splints that immobilize with diagnoses such as rheumatoid arthritis, carpal tunnel syndrome, fractures, and soft-tissue repairs. Static splints also provide support for joint laxity and ligament injury.

Static (immobilization) splints help prevent further deformity by maintaining stretch on soft tissue to increase range of motion and help correct joint alignment. An example of this type of splint is an ulnar deviation splint (Figure 1-6), which therapists commonly use with patients suffering from rheumatoid arthritis to help prevent further ulnar deviation deformity.

Static splints can also help prevent soft-tissue contractures by maintaining joints in their most functional positions. An example of a splint used to help pre-

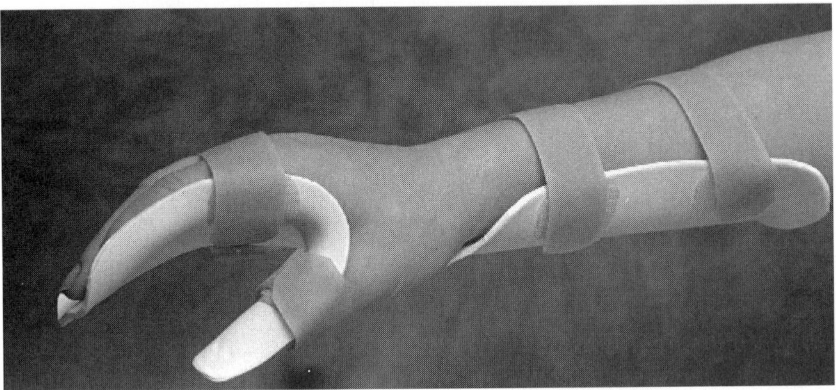

FIGURE 1-5 Resting hand splint
This static splint immobilizes the thumb, fingers, and wrist.

vent contractures is a resting hand splint for a burn patient (Figure 1-7).

Dynamic (mobilization) splints may have many purposes, including the following: (1) to substitute for loss of motor function, (2) to correct an existing deformity, (3) to provide controlled motion, and (4) to aid in fracture alignment and wound healing (Barr & Swan, 1988). An example of a splint that substitutes for

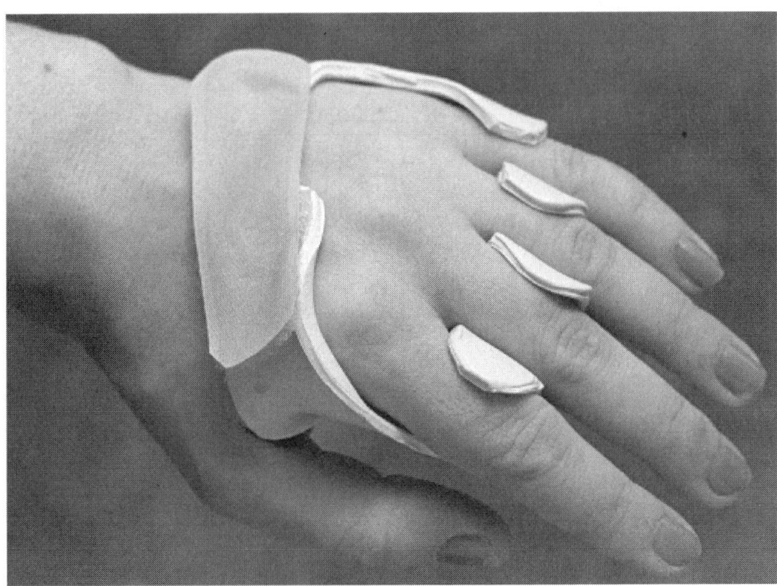

FIGURE 1-6 Ulnar deviation correction splint
This static splint helps prevent ulnar deviation for arthritic patients.

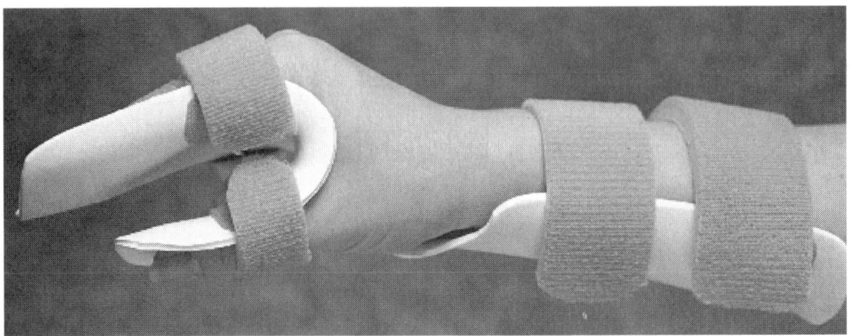

FIGURE 1-7 Burn resting hand splint
This static splint helps prevent contractures of a burned hand.

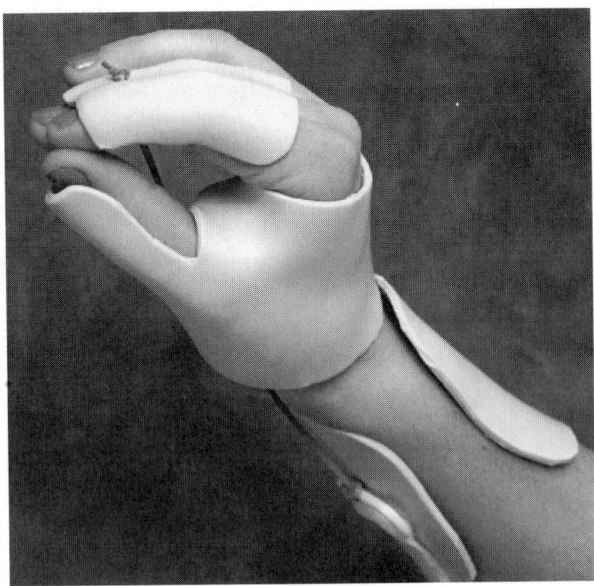

FIGURE 1-8 Tenodesis splint
This dynamic splint helps a patient with a spinal cord injury affecting the area of C6 to C7 functionally use the tenodesis grasp.

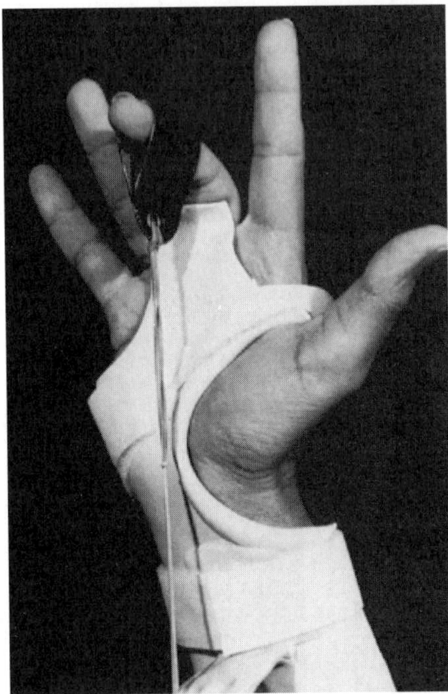

FIGURE 1-9 PIP flexion assist splint
This dynamic splint prevents the formation of a contracture by maintaining range of motion. (From Hunter, J. M., Schneider, L. H., Mackin, E. J., & Callahan, A. D. [Eds.]. [1990]. Rehabilitation of the hand: Surgery and therapy [3rd ed., p. 497]. St. Louis: Mosby.)

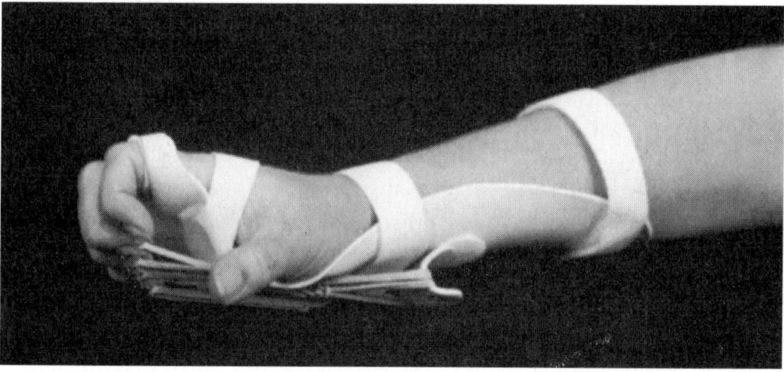

FIGURE 1-10 Dynamic flextion splint
This dynamic splint prevents the formation of a contracture by maintaining range of motion. (From Fess, E. E., & Philips C. A. [1987]. Hand splinting: principles and methods [2nd ed., p. 286]. St. Louis: Mosby.)

loss of motor function is a tenodesis splint. This splint helps persons with spinal cord injuries at the cervical level of six or seven grasp objects (Figure 1-8).

Therapists may use dynamic splints to correct contractures by applying force to soft-tissue contractures to mobilize affected joints. An example of this may be a proximal interphalangeal (PIP) joint flexion mobilization splint, which assists the PIP joint to gradually regain maximal flexion (Figure 1-9).

A dynamic (mobilization) splint with a flexor tendon repair provides controlled motion. As shown in Figure 1-10, a dynamic flexion splint protects the healing flexor tendon from stress while allowing limited glide to prevent adherence of the tendon. This prevents a contracture in later stages of the healing process.

Dynamic (mobilization) splints aid in fracture alignment and wound healing. An example of the need for dynamic splinting is the treatment of intraarticular finger fractures. By providing constant traction at various joint angles, the splint allows the fracture to heal while maintaining joint motion. This decreases soft-tissue adherence, which is a frequent complication of immobilized fractures.

Many possibilities exist for static and dynamic splint design and fabrication. Splint design is limited only by a person's creativity. Therapists must stay updated on splinting techniques and materials, which change rapidly. Reading professional literature and manufacturers' technical information helps therapists maintain knowledge about materials and techniques. A personal collection of reference books is also beneficial, and continuing-education courses provide ongoing updates on the latest theories and techniques.

Documentation

Splint application must be well documented. Documentation assists in third-party reimbursement, communication to other health care providers, and demonstration of efficacy of the intervention.

Splint documentation should include several elements, such as the type, purpose, and anatomical location of the splint. Therapists should also document that they have communicated an oral and written schedule and discussed precautions with patients.

In follow-up visits, documentation should include any changes in the splint's design and wearing schedule. In addition, the therapist should note whether problems with compliance are apparent. For example, the therapist should determine whether the range of motion is increasing with splint wearing time or whether the patient can perform independently some type of function as a result of wearing the splint.

The therapist should perform splint reassessments regularly until completion of the patient's weaning from the splint or discharge from services. Facilities use different methods to document, and the therapist should be familiar with the routine method of the facility.

Case Study*

Read the following scenario and answer the questions based on information in this chapter:

Greta is a new therapist working in an outpatient care setting. She has an order to make a static splint for a patient. Her patient is diagnosed with carpal tunnel syndrome and needs a splint to provide rest and protection.

1. What two properties listed below should be present in the thermoplastic material Greta chooses?
   a. Durability
   b. Rigidity
   c. Flexibility
2. If Greta is focusing on the patient's ability to perform activities of daily living with the splint, what is the guiding theory approach?
   a. Biomechanical
   b. Sensorimotor
   c. Rehabilitation
3. When fabricating the splint, which of the following should Greta *not* do?
   a. Flare the proximal end of the splint
   b. Keep pressure on the radial and ulnar styloids to ensure a proper fit
   c. Use light touch while the thermoplastic material is soft to avoid fingerprints
4. When making the pattern, which of the following should Greta do?
   a. Keep the pen at a 45-degree angle to the paper
   b. Mark the locations of landmarks before the patient's hand lifts off the paper
   c. Use an ink pen to trace the pattern onto the thermoplastic material because an ink pen is more visible than a pencil

*See Appendix A for answer key.

Review Questions

1. What health care professionals provide splinting services to patients?
2. What are the three theory approaches used in physical dysfunction? Give an example of how splinting could be used as a therapeutic intervention for each of the three approaches.
3. What are six handling characteristics of thermoplastics?
4. What are six performance characteristics of thermoplastics?
5. At what temperature range are low-temperature thermoplastics softened?
6. What steps are involved in making a splint pattern?
7. What equipment can be used to soften thermoplastic materials?
8. How can a therapist prevent a tacky thermoplastic from sticking to the hair on a patient's arms?
9. What are the purposes of using a heat gun?
10. Why should a therapist use a bonding agent?
11. Why should the edges of a splint be rolled or flared?
12. What are the purposes of static (immobilization) splints and of dynamic (mobilization) splints?
13. Why is documentation important with any splint provision?
14. What should be included in the documentation of any splint provision?

References

American Society of Hand Therapists. (1992). Splint classification system. Garner, NC: The American Society of Hand Therapists.

Barr, N. R., & Swan, D. (1988). The hand: Principles and techniques of splintmaking (2nd ed.). Boston: Butterworth Publishers.

Berger, S. (1995). Personal communication.

Cailliet, R. (1994). Hand pain and impairment (4th ed.). Philadelphia: F. A. Davis Co.

Cannon, N. M., et al. (1985). Manual of hand splinting. New York: Churchill Livingstone Inc.

Glance, W. D., Anderson, K. N., & Anderson, L. E. (Eds.). Mosby's medical, nursing, and allied health dictionary (3rd ed.). St. Louis: Mosby.

Hill, J., & Presperin, J. (1986). Deformity control. In S. Intagliata (Ed.), Spinal cord injury: A guide to functional outcomes in occupational therapy (pp. 49-81). Rockville, MD: Aspen Publishers Inc.

Malick, M. H. (1982). Manual on dynamic hand splinting with thermoplastic material (2nd ed.). Pittsburgh: Harmarville Rehabilitation Center.

North Coast Medical, Inc. (1992). Hand therapy catalog. San Jose, CA.

Pedretti, L. W., & Pasquinelli, S. (1990). A frame of reference for occupational therapy in physical dysfunction. In L. W. Pedretti, & B. Zoltan (Eds.), Occupational therapy: Practice skills for physical dysfunction (3rd ed., pp. 18-39). St. Louis: Mosby.

Rossi, J. (1987). Concepts and current trends in hand splinting. Occupational Therapy in Health Care, 53-68.

Smith & Nephew Rolyan. (1995). Rehabilitation products catalog. Germantown, WI.

CHAPTER TWO

Anatomical and Biomechanical Principles of Splinting

BRENDA M. COPPARD, MS, OTR/L

Chapter Objectives

1. Understand the terminology used in splint prescriptions.
2. Identify arches of the hand.
3. Identify creases of the hand.
4. Understand the importance of the hand's arches and creases on splinting.
5. Recall actions and nerve innervations of hand muscles.
6. Differentiate prehensile and grasp patterns of the hand.
7. Explain the rationale for increasing the surface area of a splint's force application.
8. Describe the correct width and length for a forearm splint.
9. Describe uses of padding on a splint.
10. Explain the reason splint edges should be rolled or flared.

Basic Anatomical Review for Splinting

Splinting requires sound knowledge of anatomical structures and the way in which pathological conditions impair function. The following is an overview of anatomical terminology, structures, and landmarks of the forearm and hand.

Terminology

Knowing anatomical location terms is extremely important when a therapist receives a splint prescription. The terms *palmar* and *volar* are used interchangeably and refer to the front of the hand and forearm in relationship to the anatomical position. The term *dorsal* refers to the back of the hand and forearm in relationship to the anatomical position. *Radial* indicates the thumb side, and *ulnar* refers to the side of the fifth digit, or the little finger. Therefore if a therapist receives an order for a dorsal wrist splint, the physician has ordered a splint that is to be applied on the back of the hand and wrist. Another example of location terminology in a splint prescription is a radial gutter thumb spica splint. The therapist applies this type of splint to the thumb side of the hand and forearm.

Arches of the Hand

To have a strong functional grasp, the hand uses the following three arches: (1) the longitudinal arch, (2) the distal transverse arch, and (3) the proximal transverse arch (Figure 2-1). Because of the functional significance of these arches, they require care during the splinting process for their preservation. The therapist should never splint a hand in a flat position because doing so compromises function. Especially in cases of muscle atrophy (such as with a tendon or nerve injury), the splint should maintain mobility of the arches.

The proximal transverse arch consists of the distal row of carpal bones and is a rigid arch acting as a stable pivot point for the wrist and long-finger flexor muscles (Chase, 1990). The transverse carpal ligament and the bones of the proximal transverse arch form the carpal tunnel.

The distal transverse arch, which deepens with flexion of the fingers, is mobile and passes through the metacarpal heads (Malick, 1972). A splint must allow for the functional movement of the distal arch to maintain or increase normal hand function (Chase, 1990).

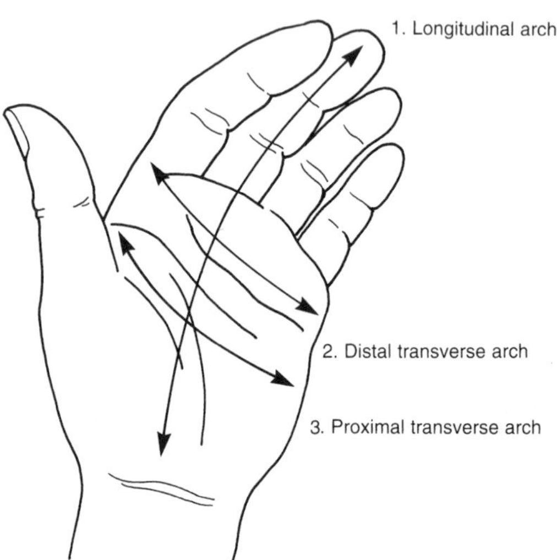

FIGURE 2-1 Arches of the hand
1, Longitudinal arch; *2*, distal transverse arch; *3*, proximal transverse arch.

The longitudinal arch allows the distal interphalangeal (DIP), the proximal interphalangeal (PIP), and the metacarpophalangeal (MCP) joints to flex (Fess & Philips, 1987). This arch follows the longitudinal axes of each finger. The second, fourth, and fifth metacarpals move in relationship to the shape and size of an object placed in the palm because of the mobility of their base. Grasp is the result of holding an object against the rigid portion that the second and third digits provide. The flattening and cupping motions of the palm allow the hand to pick up and handle objects of various sizes.

Creases of the Hand

The creases of the hand are critical landmarks for splint-pattern making and molding. Therefore knowing the creases and their functional implications is important. Three flexion creases are on the palmar surface of the hand, and additional creases are on the palmar surface of the digits and wrist (Figure 2-2).

The three primary palmar creases are the distal, proximal, and thenar creases. As shown in Figure 2-2, the distal palmar crease extends transversely from the fifth MCP joint to a point midway between the third and second MCP joints (Cailliet, 1994). This crease is the landmark for the distal edge of the palmar portion of a splint. By positioning the splint proximal to this crease, the therapist makes full MCP joint flexion possible. Below the distal palmar crease is the proximal palmar crease. This crease is not a significant landmark for splinting.

The thenar crease begins at the proximal palmar crease and curves around the

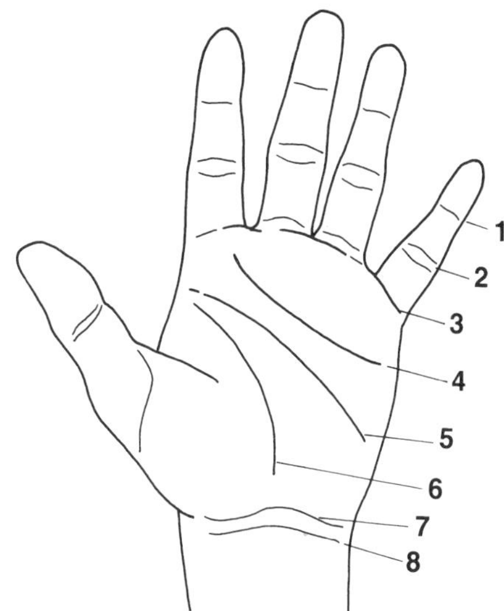

FIGURE 2-2 Creases of the hand

1, Distal digital crease; *2*, middle digital crease; *3*, proximal digital crease; *4*, distal palmar crease; *5*, proximal palmar crease; *6*, thenar crease; *7*, distal wrist crease; *8*, proximal wrist crease.

base of the thenar eminence (see Figure 2-2) (Cailliet, 1994). To allow thumb motion, this crease should define the limit of the splint's edge. If the splint extends beyond the thenar crease toward the thumb, the inhibition of thumb opposition and palmar abduction results.

The two palmar (or volar) wrist creases are the distal and proximal wrist creases. The distal wrist crease extends from the pisiform bone to the tubercle of the trapezium (see Figure 2-2) and forms a line that separates the proximal and distal rows of the carpal bones. The proximal wrist crease corresponds to the radiocarpal joint and delineates the proximal border of the carpal bones, which articulates with the distal radius (Cailliet, 1994). The distal and proximal wrist creases assist in locating the axis of the wrist motion (Clarkson & Gilewich, 1989).

The three digital palmar flexion creases are on the palmar aspect of each finger (see Figure 2-2). The distal digital crease marks the DIP joint axis, and the middle digital crease marks the PIP joint axis. The proximal digital crease is distal to the MCP joint axis at the base of the proximal phalanx. The creation of the proximal and distal palmar creases results from the thick palmar skin folding because of force to allow full MCP flexion (Malick, 1972). The flexion axis of the interphalangeal (IP) joint of the thumb corresponds to the IP crease of the thumb. Similarly, the MCP crease describes the axis of thumb MCP joint flexion.

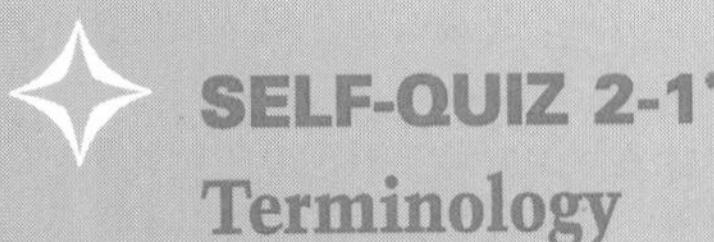

SELF-QUIZ 2-1*

Terminology

Match the following with the correct splints.

Part I

a. Based on the front of the hand and forearm
b. Based on the back of the hand and forearm
c. Based on the thumb side of the hand and forearm
d. Based on the little finger side of the hand and forearm

1. _____ Ulnar gutter wrist cock-up splint
2. _____ Volar- or palmar-based dynamic flexion splint
3. _____ Dorsal MCP protection splint
4. _____ Palmar-based wrist cock-up splint
5. _____ Radial gutter dynamic extension splint

*See Appendix A for the answer key.

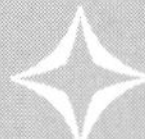

SELF-QUIZ 2-1—cont'd

Part II

On the following diagram, label the creases of the hand.

1. ______________________
2. ______________________
3. ______________________
4. ______________________
5. ______________________

Part III

On the following diagram, label the arches of the hand.

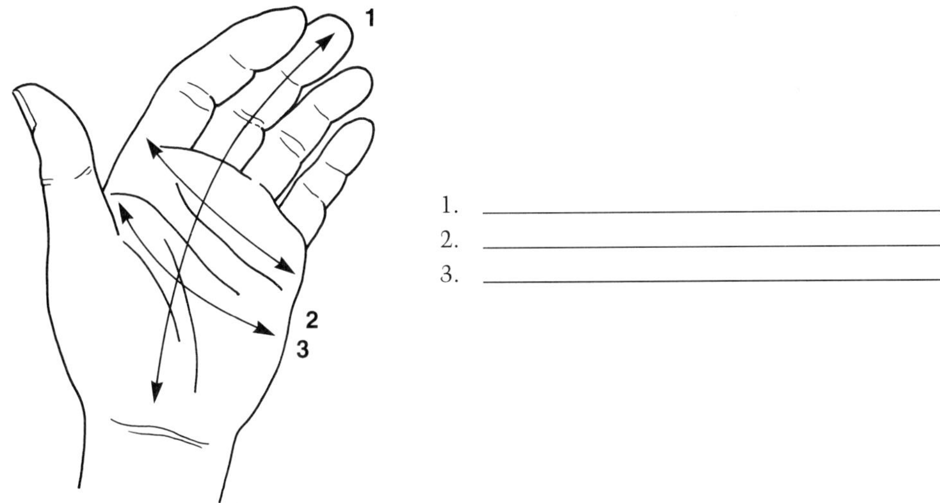

1. ______________________
2. ______________________
3. ______________________

TABLE 2-1 **Hand Musculature Actions and Nerve Supply**

Muscle	Actions	Nerve
Flexor carpi radialis	Wrist flexion Wrist radial deviation	Median
Palmaris longus	Wrist flexion Tenses palmar fascia	Median
Flexor carpi ulnaris	Wrist flexion Wrist ulnar deviation	Ulnar
Extensor carpi radialis longus	Wrist radial deviation Wrist extension	Radial
Extensor carpi radialis brevis	Wrist extension Wrist radial deviation	Radial
Extensor carpi ulnaris	Wrist ulnar deviation Wrist extension	Radial
Flexor digitorum superficialis	Finger PIP flexion	Median Ulnar
Flexor digitorum profundus	Finger DIP flexion	Median
Extensor digitorum communis	Finger MCP extension	Radial
Extensor indicis proprius	Index finger MCP extension	Radial
Extensor digiti minimi	Little finger MCP extension	Radial
Interosseous		
a. dorsal	Finger MCP abduction	Ulnar
b. palmar	Finger MCP adduction	Ulnar
Lumbricales	Finger MCP flexion and IP extension	Ulnar Median
Abductor digiti minimi	Little finger MCP abduction	Ulnar
Opponens digiti minimi	Little finger opposition	Ulnar
Flexor digiti minimi	Little finger MCP flexion	Ulnar
Flexor pollicus longus	Thumb IP flexion	Median
Flexor pollicus brevis	Thumb MCP flexion	Median Ulnar
Extensor pollicis longus	Thumb IP extension	Radial
Extensor pollicis brevis	Thumb MCP extension	Radial
Abductor pollicis longus	Thumb radial abduction	Radial
Abductor pollicis brevis	Thumb palmar abduction	Median
Adductor pollicis	Thumb adduction	Ulnar
Opponens pollicis	Thumb opposition	Median

The creases are close to but not always directly over bony joints (Chase, 1990). When splinting to immobilize a particular joint, the therapist must be sure to include the corresponding joint flexion crease within the splint in order to provide adequate support for immobilization. Conversely, when attempting to mobilize a specific joint, the therapist must not incorporate the corresponding flexion crease in the splint in order to allow for full range of motion (Fess & Philips, 1987).

Muscle Actions and Nerve Supply

When treating a patient with a hand injury, the therapist must understand which anatomical structures are relevant. Knowledge of anatomical structures is necessary in the choice and fabrication of a splint. This knowledge also influences the therapeutic regimen and home program. Table 2-1 provides a review of muscle actions and nerve supply of the wrist and hand (Clarkson & Gilewich, 1989).

PREHENSILE PATTERNS

The normal hand can perform many prehensile patterns in which the thumb is a crucial factor. Therapists must be knowledgeable about prehensile patterns, especialy when splinting to assist one of the prehensile patterns.

Even though hand movements are extremely complex, they can be categorized into several basic prehensile and grasp patterns, including the following: fingertip prehension, palmar prehension, lateral prehension, cylindrical prehension, cylindrical grasp, spherical grasp, and hook grasp (Lehmkuhl & Smith, 1983). Therapists should keep in mind that finer prehensile movements require less strength than grasp movements. Pedretti (1990) remarked, "The grasp and prehension patterns that may be provided by hand splinting are determined by the muscles that are functioning, potential and present deformities, and how the hand is to be used" (p. 405).

Fingertip prehension is the contact of the pad of the index or middle finger to the pad of the thumb (Lehmkuhl & Smith, 1983). This movement, which patients use to pick up small objects such as beads and pins, is the weakest of the pinch patterns and requires fine motor coordination.

Palmar prehension, also known as the *tripod* pinch (Clarkson & Gilewich, 1989), is the contact of the thumb pad to the pads of the middle and index fingers. Patients use palmar prehension for holding pencils and picking up small, spherical objects.

Lateral prehension, the strongest of the pinch patterns, is the contact between the thumb pad to the lateral aspect of the index finger (Lehmkuhl & Smith, 1983). Patients typically use this pattern for holding keys.

Patients use cylinderical grasp for holding cylindrical-shaped objects such as soda cans (Lehmkuhl & Smith, 1983). The object rests against the palm of the hand, and the fingers flex around the object to maintain a grasp.

Patients use the spherical grasp to hold round objects such as tennis balls and baseballs (Lehmkuhl & Smith, 1983). The object rests against the palm of the hand, and the abducted five digits flex around the object.

The hook grasp, which patients accomplish with their fingers only, involves the carrying of items such as briefcases and suitcases by the handles (Lehmkuhl & Smith, 1983). The PIPs and DIPs flex around the object, and thumb often remains passive in this type of grasp.

Biomechanical Principles of Splinting

Splinting involves applying external forces on the hand, so understanding basic biomechanical principles is important for the therapist when constructing and fitting a splint. Correct biomechanics of a splint design provides optimal fit and reduces risks for skin irritation and pressure areas.

Thermoplastic splints can cause pressure points over areas with minimal soft tissue or over bony prominences. To avoid this risk, the therapist should use a splint design that is wider and longer (Fess & Philips, 1987). A larger design is more comfortable because it decreases the force concentrated on the hand and arm by increasing the surface area of the splint's force application.

The length of a splint's forearm trough should be approximately two-thirds the length of the forearm. Patients wearing splints should be able to flex their elbows without the splints interfering with the full motion (Barr & Swan, 1988). The width of a thumb or forearm trough should be one-half the circumference of the thumb or forearm. The muscle bulk of an extremity gradually increases more proximal to the body, and the splint trough should widen proportionately in the proximal area. When making a splint pattern, the therapist must maintain the one-half circumference of the thumb or forearm for a correct fit.

Continuous, well-distributed pressure is the goal of a splint, but pressure over any bony prominence should be nonexistent (Cailliet, 1994). Therapists should

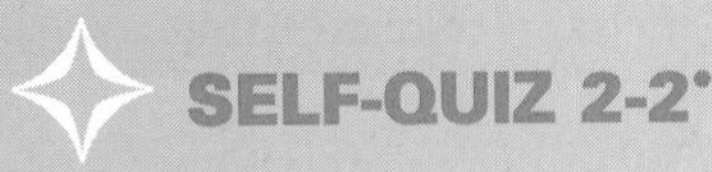

SELF-QUIZ 2-2*

Determine whether the following statements are true or false.

1. _____ The forearm trough should be two-thirds the circumference of the forearm.
2. _____ Short, narrow splints apply less pressure to the skin's surface than long, wide splints and are therefore better.
3. _____ A splint should be approximately two-thirds the length of the forearm.
4. _____ Avoidance of pressure over a bony prominence is preferable to unequal pressure.
5. _____ A patient uses a spherical grasp when holding a soda can.

*See Appendix A for the answer key.

be cautious of pressure over bony prominences such as the radial and ulnar styloids, the dorsal aspect MCPs, and the PIPs. Therapists can use heat guns to alleviate pressure by pushing out these areas and can use padding around these areas to lift off pressure. Therapists should keep in mind that padding takes up space, reducing the circumference measurement of the splint and possibly increasing the pressure over an area.

Moist substances such as perspiration and wound drainage can cause skin maceration, irritation, and breakdown. Bandages help absorb the moisture but require frequent changing for infection control (Agency for Health Care Policy and Research, 1992). Therapists can fabricate splints over bandaged extremities but should alter splints frequently as the bulk of dressings or bandages changes.

Rolled or round edges on the proximal and distal ends of splints cause less pressure than straight edges (Cailliet, 1994). Imperfect edges are potential causes of pressure areas.

Review Questions

1. To what do the terms *palmar, dorsal,* and *radial* (or *ulnar*) refer in regard to splint fabrication?
2. What are the three arches of the hand?
3. Why is support for the arches of the hand important when therapists splint a hand?
4. What is the significance of the distal palmar crease when therapists fabricate a splint?
5. If a splint's edge does not extend beyond the thenar crease toward the thumb, what thumb motions can occur?
6. What is an example of each of the following prehensile or grasp patterns: fingertip prehension, palmar prehension, lateral prehension, cylindrical grasp, spherical grasp, and hook grasp?
7. How can a therapist determine the correct length of a forearm splint?
8. What is the correct width for a splint that has a forearm or thumb trough?
9. What precautions should a therapist take when using padding on a splint?
10. What are two methods a therapist can use to prevent the edges of a splint from causing a pressure sore?

References

Agency for Health Care Policy and Research. (1992). Pressure ulcers in adults: Prediction and prevention (No. 92-0047). Rockville, MD: U.S. Department of Health and Human Services.

Barr, N. R., & Swan, D. (1988). The hand. Boston: Butterworth Publishers.

Cailliet, R. (1994). Hand pain and impairment (4th ed.). Philadelphia: F. A. Davis Co.

Chase, R. A. (1990). Anatomy and kinesiology of the hand. In J. M. Hunter, L. H. Schneider, E. J. Mackin, & A. D. Callahan (Eds.), Rehabilitation of the hand: Surgery and therapy (3rd ed.). St. Louis: Mosby.

Clarkson, H. M., & Gilewich, G. B. (1989). Musculoskeletal assessment: Joint range of motion and manual muscle strength. Baltimore: Williams & Wilkins.

Fess, E. E., & Philips, C. A. (1987). Hand splinting. St. Louis: Mosby.

Lehmkuhl, L. D., & Smith, L. K. (1983). Brunnstrom's clinical kinesiology. Philadelphia: F. A. Davis Co.

Malick, M. H. (1972). Manual on static hand splinting. Pittsburgh: Hamarville Rehabilitation Center.

Pedretti, L. W. (1990). Hand splinting. In L. W. Pedretti, & B. Zoltan (Eds.), Occupational therapy: Practice skills for physical dysfunction (3rd ed., pp. 18-39). St. Louis: Mosby.

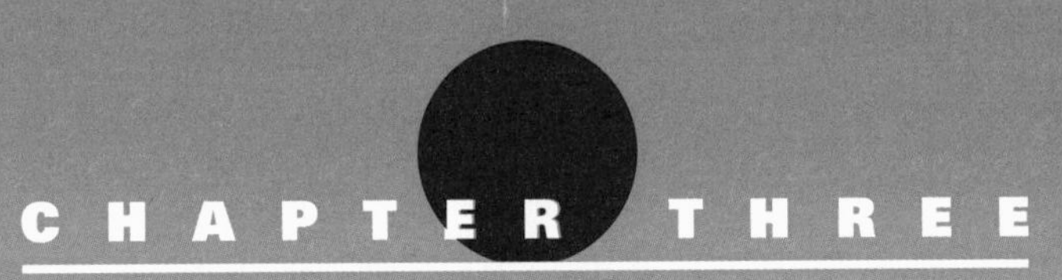

Clinical Examination of the Hand for Splinting

BRENDA M. COPPARD, MS, OTR/L

Chapter Objectives

1. List components of a clinical hand examination.
2. Identify components of a patient history.
3. Describe the resting hand posture.
4. Relate how skin, bone, joint, muscle, tendon, and nerve assessments are relevant to splinting.
5. Explain the three phases of wound healing.
6. Explain splint precautions therapists give to patients.
7. Develop a splint-wearing schedule and understand the rationales for it.
8. Explain the proper care for splints.

Clinical Examination

Clinical examinations are crucial to therapists and physicians. A thorough, organized, and clearly documented examination should be the basis for the development of a treatment plan and splint design. Form 3-1 is a check-off sheet that therapists can use in hand evaluations.

An examination requires the gathering of data from various sources, such as the physician's referral or prescription, the medical chart, a general inspection of the patient's upper extremity (including the shoulder, elbow, forearm, wrist, and hand), and precise and objective measurements from evaluations (Aulicino & DuPuy, 1990). The therapist should determine whether the hand problem is the result of neurological or orthopedic dysfunction. The answer to this question helps to determine the splinting approach that the therapist takes.

FORM 3-1* Hand Evaluation Check-Off Sheet

- ❍ Patient's history: interview, chart review, and reports
  - ❍ age
  - ❍ occupation
  - ❍ date of injury and surgery
  - ❍ method of injury
  - ❍ hand dominance
  - ❍ vocation
  - ❍ avocational interests
  - ❍ family composition
  - ❍ patient complaints
  - ❍ activities of daily living responsibilities before and after injury
  - ❍ impact of injury on family, economic status, and social well-being
- ❍ Cognition
- ❍ Reimbursement
- ❍ Motivation
- ❍ Hand posture
- ❍ Skin
- ❍ Wound healing
- ❍ Bone
- ❍ Joint
- ❍ Muscle and tendon
- ❍ Nerve
- ❍ Vascular status
- ❍ Range of motion
- ❍ Strength
- ❍ Coordination and dexterity
- ❍ Function

*See Appendix B for a perforated copy of this form.

With postoperative patients, therapists must know the anatomical structures involved and the surgical procedures performed. Therapists should be aware that physicians may prefer to follow standardized rehabilitative programs for certain postoperative diagnoses. Other physicians may prefer to follow different rehabilitative programs that they have developed for specific postoperative diagnoses. Whether standardized or nonstandardized, these programs are known as *proto-*

cols. Protocols delineate which types of splints and exercises are necessary in rehabilitation programs.

Patient History

The therapist should collect the patient's history at the time of the initial evaluation. Collecting this history includes reading the patient's chart and any documented surgical reports. The therapist should obtain information on the patient's age, occupation, date of injury, method of injury, hand dominance, functional abilities, avocation interests, family composition, and subjective complaints. During the interview the therapist should try to determine the impact of the condition on the patient's family, economic status, and social-emotional well being.

The therapist should determine the patient's motivational level for compliance with a splint-wearing schedule and a home program. In some cases the presence or absence of a third-party reimbursement source affects the patient's motivation. Whenever possible, the therapist should discuss reimbursement issues with the patient before completing the initial visit. If a third party is paying for the patient's services, the therapist should first determine whether that source intends to pay for any or all of the splint fabrication services.

Hand Posture

The therapist should note the posture of the affected extremity and look for any guarded or protective positioning. A normal hand at rest assumes a posture of 10° to 20° of wrist extension, 10° of ulnar deviation, slight flexion and abduction of the thumb, and approximately 15° to 20° flexion of the metacarpophalangeal (MCP) joints. The fingers in a resting posture exhibit a greater composite flexion to the radial side of the hand, as shown in Figure 3-1 (Aulicino & DuPuy, 1990). The thumbnail usually lies perpendicular to the index finger. These hand postures are a useful basis for splint fabrication because a patient's hand often deviates from the normal resting posture when injury or disease is present.

Skin

A thorough examination of the surface condition and contour of the extremity defines a possible pathological condition, which influences splint design. During the examination the therapist should observe and document the skin's color, temperature, and texture. The therapist should also observe the skin for muscle atrophy, scarring, edema, and abnormal masses. Persons having fragile skin, especially geriatric and diabetic patients, need careful monitoring. For these patients the therapist may need to consider carefully the splinting material to prevent harm to the already fragile skin (see Chapter 11).

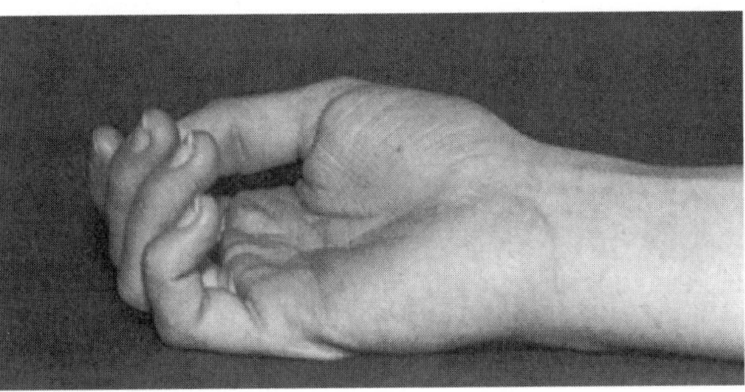

FIGURE 3-1 Normal posture of the hand in a resting position

(From Hunter, J. M., Schneider, L. H., Mackin, E. J., & Callahan, A. D. [Eds.]. [1990]. Rehabilitation of the hand: Surgery and therapy [3rd ed., p. 33]. St. Louis: Mosby.)

Wounds

The therapist should measure wounds or incisions (usually in centimeters) and assess discharge from wounds for color, amount, and odor. In addition, the therapist may need to perform debridement for some wounds before splinting and as a part of the treatment regimen. Because open wounds threaten exposure to the patient's body fluids, the therapist should follow universal precautions.

Many hand injuries include wounds, whether from trauma or surgery, so therpists must know the stages of wound healing (Figure 3-2). Experts have identified three such stages (Smith, 1990; Staley, Richard, & Falkel, 1988), which consist of the inflammatory, proliferative or fibroblastic, and maturation phases (Smith, 1990).

The first stage is the inflammatory phase (Smith, 1990; Staley, Richard, & Falkel, 1988). This phase begins immediately after trauma and lasts 3 to 6 days. Vasoconstriction occurs during the first 5 to 10 minutes of this stage, leading to platelet adhesion of the damaged vessel wall and resulting in clot formation. This activity stimulates fibroblast proliferation.

The second stage is the proliferative or fibroblastic phase, which begins 2 to 3 days after the injury and lasts about 2 to 6 weeks. During this stage, epithelial cells migrate to the wound bed. Fibroblasts begin to multiply 24 to 36 hours after the injury. The fibroblast cells produce collagen. The fibers link closely and increase tensile strength. A balanced interplay between collagen synthesis and its remodeling and reorganization prevents hypertrophic scarring.

The final stage is the maturation phase, which can last up to 1 or 2 years after the injury (Smith, 1990; Staley, Richard, & Falkel, 1988). During this stage the

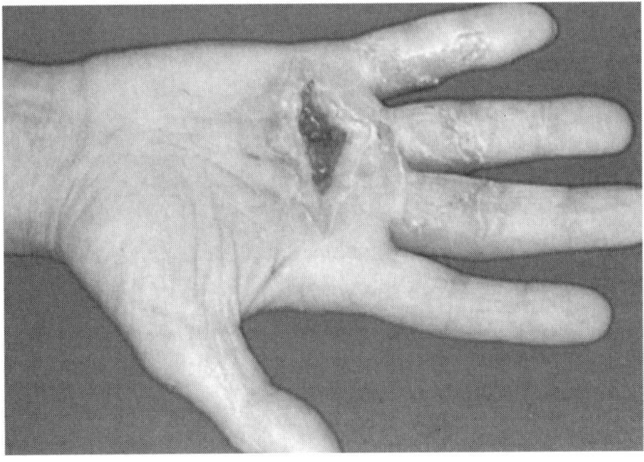

FIGURE 3-2
Dressing changes and continuous splinting in extension manage this clean wound. (From Hunter, J. M., Schneider, L. H., Mackin, E. J., & Callahan, A. D. [Eds.]. [1990]. Rehabilitation of the hand: Surgery and therapy [3rd ed., p. 179]. St. Louis: Mosby.)

tensile strength continues to increase. Initially the scar may appear red, raised, and thick, but with maturation a normal scar softens and becomes more pliable.

Bone

When splinting a patient suffering from a skeletal injury, the therapist must review the surgery and radiology reports. The therapist should place importance on knowing the stability level of the fracture reduction, the method the physician used to maintain good alignment, the amount of time since the fracture's repair, and fixation devices still present in the upper extremity. After the fracture heals a physician may request that the therapist fabricate a splint. On other occasions the therapist may follow a physician's prescription and use fracture braces to stabilize a fracture before healing is complete.

Joint

Joint stability is important to assess. Each digital articulation achieves its stability through the collateral ligaments and a dense palmar plate (Cailliet, 1994). The therapist should carefully assess the continuity, length, and glide of these ligaments. Unstable joints, subluxations, dislocations, and limited passive range of motion directly affect splint application. The therapist and patient should avoid lateral stress on joints while the patient wears the splint to prevent unequal stress on the collateral ligaments (Cannon, et al., 1985).

Muscle and Tendon

Tensile strength is the amount of force a muscle or tendon can withstand (Fess & Philips, 1987). When a tendon experiences damage or undergoes surgical repair, tensile strength directly affects the amount of force a splint should provide and which exercises or activities the patient can perform.

Therapists should also keep in mind that proximal musculature can affect distal musculature tension in patients experiencing spasticity. For example, wrist position can influence the amount of tension placed on finger musculature.

Nerve

Sensory evaluations are important to determine areas of diminished or absent sensibility. Tests for protective sensibility can include the sharp-dull and hot-cold assessment. Discriminatory sensibilities can include assessment for stereoagnosis, proprioception, kinesthesia, tactile location, and light touch. Aulicino and DuPuy (1990) have recommended two-point discrimination testing (Figure 3-3) as a quick screening for sensibility. The Semmes-Weinstein Monofilaments (Figure 3-4) provide useful, detailed mapping of the level of functional sensibility. This mapping is useful to physicians, therapists, patients, and employers (Tomancik, 1987).

During the fitting process the hand splint may cause pressure and friction on vulnerable areas having impaired sensibility. If a patient has decreased sensibility, the therapist should use a splint design with long, well-molded components. The reason for using such a splint is to distribute the forces of the splint over as much surface area as possible, thereby decreasing the potential for pressure areas.

When splinting occurs across the wrist the superficial branch of the radial nerve is at risk for compression. According to Cannon, et al. (1985), "If the radial edge of the forearm splint stops beyond the midlateral forearm, near the dorsum of the thumb, the superficial branch of the radial nerve can be compressed."

Vascular Status

To understand the vascular status of a diseased or injured hand, the therapist should monitor the skin's color and check for edema. The therapist should clearly define areas of questionable tissue viability and adapt splints to prevent obstruction of venous circulation. To assess radial and ulnar artery patency, the therapist can use Allen's test (American Society for Surgery of the Hand, 1983).

A therapist can take circumferential measurements proximal and distal to the location of the circumferential splint's application. Then after applying the splint to the extremity, the therapist measures the same areas and compares them with the previous measurements. An increase in measurements taken while the splint is on indicates too much force from the splint. This situation poses a risk for circulation. When fluctuating edema is present, the therapist should make the splint design larger.

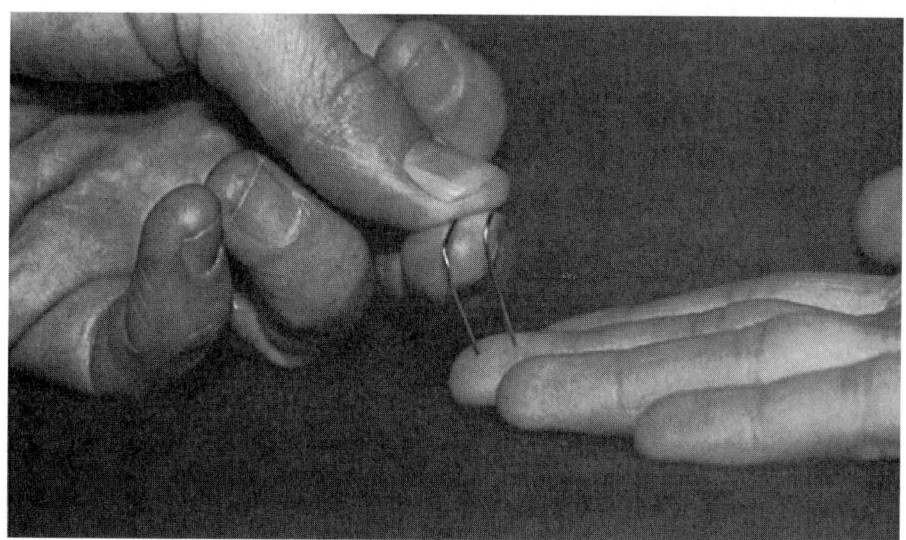

FIGURE 3-3 Two-point discrimination test using a paper clip
(From Hunter, J. M., Schneider, L. H., Mackin, E. J., & Callahan, A. D. [Eds.]. [1990]. Rehabilitation of the hand: Surgery and therapy [3rd ed., p. 50]. St. Louis: Mosby.)

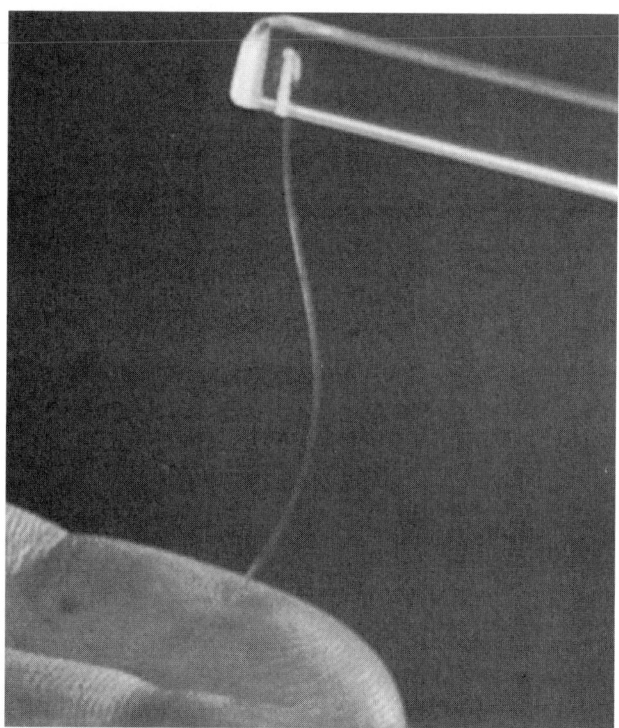

FIGURE 3-4
The monofilament collapses when a force dependent on filament diameter and length is reached, controlling the magnitude of the applied touch pressure. (From Hunter, J. M., Schneider, L. H., Mackin, E. J., & Callahan, A. D. [Eds.]. [1990]. Rehabilitation of the hand: Surgery and therapy [3rd ed., p. 76]. St. Louis: Mosby.)

The therapist can also use the fingernail Blanch Test to assess circulation (Aulicino & DuPuy, 1990). Long-lasting blanched areas of the fingertips indicate restricted circulation.

When a therapist applies a splint to the upper extremity, the skin should maintain its natural color. Red or purple areas indicate obstructed circulation.

Range of Motion and Strength

The therapist should record active and passive motions when no contraindications are present (Figure 3-5) and take measurements on both extremities for a baseline data comparison. The therapist should also record total active motion and total passive motion (American Society for Surgery of the Hand, 1983) but test grasp and pinch strengths only when no contraindications are present (Figures 3-6 and 3-7).

Coordination and Dexterity

Hand coordination and dexterity are important to evaluate. Many standardized tests for coordination and dexterity exist, including the Nine Hole Peg Test (Figure 3-8), the Minnesota Rate of Manipulation Test, and the Purdue Peg Board. Normative data are available for all these tests.

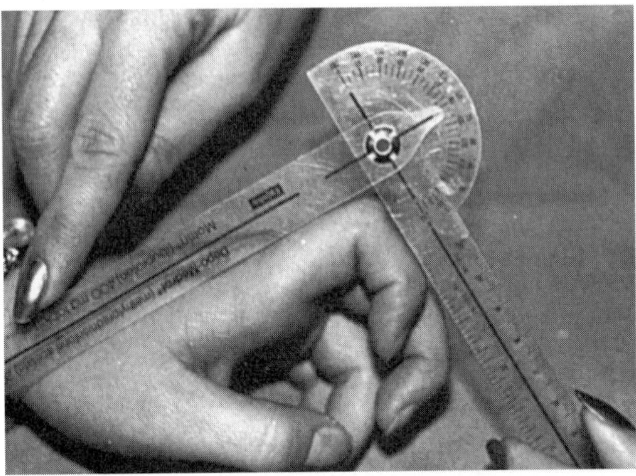

FIGURE 3-5

Goniometric measurements of active and passive motion are taken regularly when no contraindications are present. (From Hunter, J. M., Schneider, L. H., Mackin, E. J., & Callahan, A. D. [Eds.]. [1990]. Rehabilitation of the hand: Surgery and therapy [3rd ed., p. 34]. St. Louis: Mosby.)

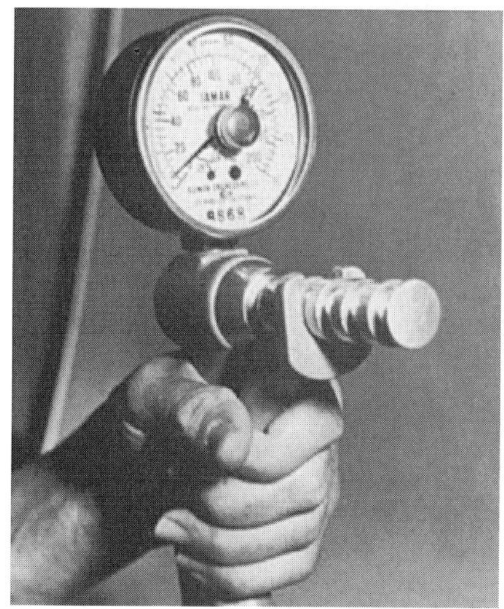

FIGURE 3-6

Therapists use the Jamar dynamometer to obtain reliable and accurate grip strength measurements. (From Hunter, J. M., Schneider, L. H., Mackin, E. J., & Callahan, A. D. [Eds.]. [1990]. Rehabilitation of the hand: Surgery and therapy [3rd ed., p. 333]. St. Louis: Mosby.)

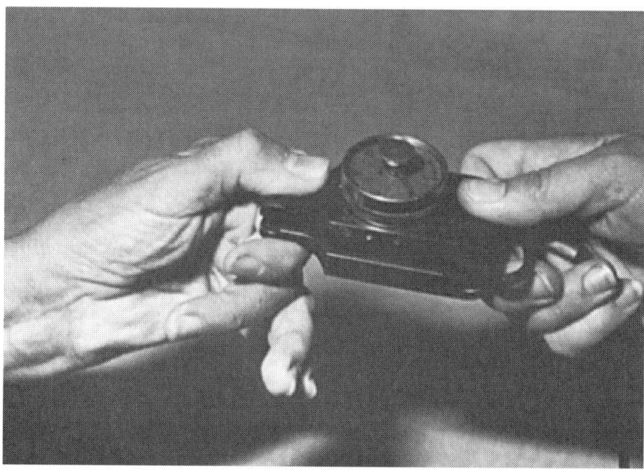

FIGURE 3-7

The pinch meter measures lateral, tip, and pulp pinches. (From Hunter, J. M., Schneider, L. H., Mackin, E. J., & Callahan, A. D. [Eds.]. [1990]. Rehabilitation of the hand: Surgery and therapy [3rd ed., p. 333]. St. Louis: Mosby.)

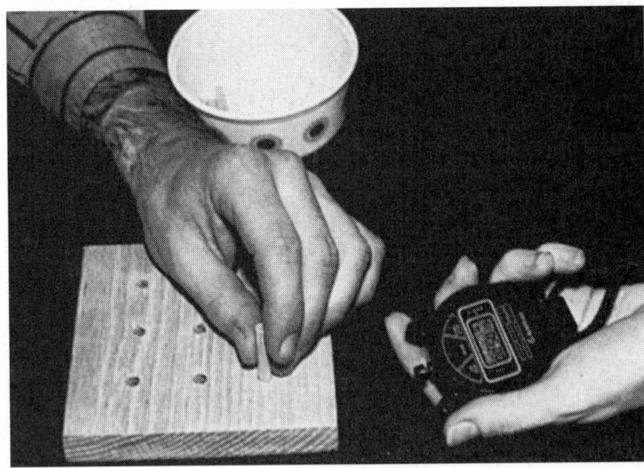

FIGURE 3-8

The Nine Hole Peg Test is a quick test for coordination. (From Hunter, J. M., Schneider, L. H., Mackin, E. J., & Callahan, A. D. [Eds.]. [1990]. Rehabilitation of the hand: Surgery and therapy [3rd ed., p. 1158]. St. Louis: Mosby.)

Function

Close observation during the interview and splint fabrication gives the therapist information regarding the patient's views of the injury and disability. The therapist also observes the patient for the following: protected or guarded positioning, abnormal hand movements, muscle substitutions, and pain involvement. The therapist notes the patient's willingness for the therapist to touch and move the affected extremity.

During the initial interview the therapist questions the patient about the status of activities of daily living and avocational and vocational activities. The therapist notes problem areas.

The therapist may use standardized hand function assessments. The Jebsen-Taylor Hand Function Test (Figure 3-9) is helpful by giving objective measurements of standardized tasks with norms that the therapist uses for comparison (Jebsen, Taylor, Trieschmann, Trotter, & Howard, 1969). The Dellon modification of the Moberg Pick-up Test evaluates hand function when the person grasps common objects (Figure 3-10) (Moberg, 1958). Similar objects in the test require the patient to have sensory discrimination ability and prehensile ability (Callahan, 1990).

Other Considerations

The patient's motivation, ability to understand and carry out instructions, and compliance may affect the type of splint the therapist chooses. With an increase

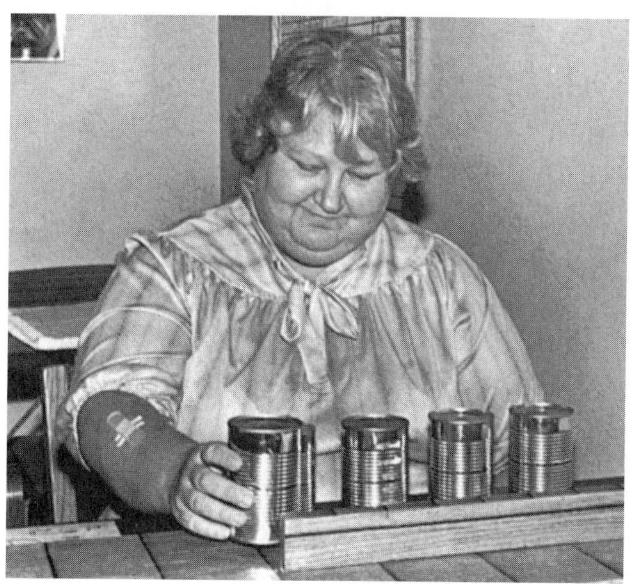

FIGURE 3-9

The Jebsen-Taylor Hand Test assesses the ability to perform prehension tasks. (From Hunter, J. M., Schneider, L. H., Mackin, E. J., & Callahan, A. D. [Eds.]. [1990]. Rehabilitation of the hand: Surgery and therapy [3rd ed., p. 98]. St. Louis: Mosby.)

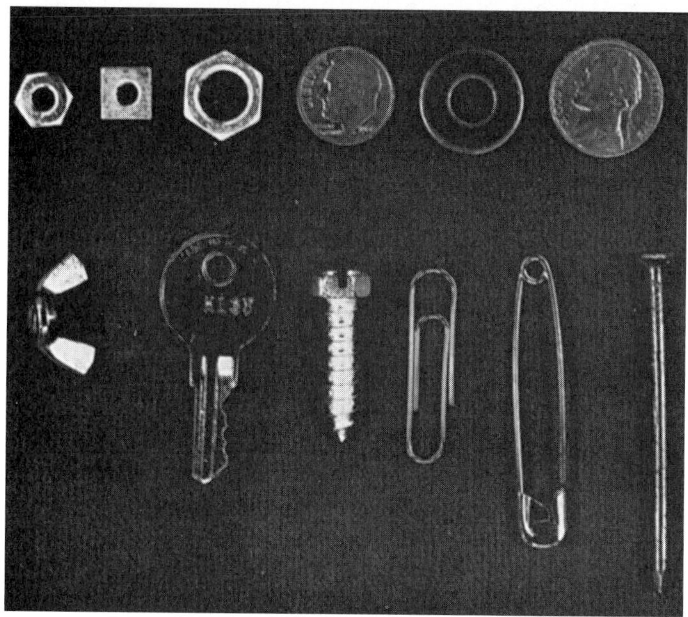

FIGURE 3-10 Items used in the Dellon modification of the Moberg Pick-up Test

(From Hunter, J. M., Schneider, L. H., Mackin, E. J., & Callahan, A. D. [Eds.]. [1990]. Rehabilitation of the hand: Surgery and therapy [3rd ed., p. 608]. St. Louis: Mosby.)

in the prevalence of cumulative trauma injuries, the fabrication of splints that can be worn at work is common, although some consider this controversial (Pascerelli & Quilter, 1994). The therapist should consider a patient's vocational and avocational interests when designing a splint. Some patients wear more than one splint throughout the day to allow for completion of various activities. In addition, some patients wear one splint design during the day and a different design during the night.

Splinting Precautions

During the splint assessment the therapist must be aware of splinting precautions. An ill-fitting splint can harm a patient. Several precautions are outlined in Form 3-2, which a therapist can use as a check-off sheet. Form 3-3 lists splint-making hints.

Pressure Areas

After fabricating a splint, the therapist should not allow the patient to leave until checking the splint for problem areas. A general guideline is to have the patient wear the splint at least 20 to 30 minutes after fabrication. Red areas should not be present 20 minutes after removal of the splint. Splints often require some adjustment. After receiving assurance that no pressure areas are present, the therapist must still instruct the patient to remove the splint and call if any problems arise. Patients with fragile skin have a high risk for developing pressure areas. The therapist should provide the patient with thorough written and verbal instructions on the wear and care of the splint. The instructions should include a phone number for emergencies.

Edema

The therapist should complete an evaluation for excessive tightness of the splint or straps. If the splint is too narrow, it may inadvertently contribute to increased edema. Patients can usually wear splints over pressure garments if necessary; however, therapists should monitor circulation closely.

The therapist can assess the patient for edema by taking circumferential or volumetric measurements (Figure 3-11). When taking volumetric measurements, the therapist should compare the involved extremity reading with that of the uninvolved extremity. If the involved extremity has a reading of 25 ml or more than the uninvolved extremity, the therapist should use a wider splint design to accommodate for the edema (Cannon, et al., 1985).

Timing

Patients should never wear splints 24 hours a day without removal. Each splint requires removal for patient hygiene and exercises, if the diagnosis permits. The

FORM 3-2* Splint Precaution Check-Off Sheet

❍ Account for bony prominences such as the following:
- metacarpophalangeal (MCP), proximal interphalangeal (PIP), and distal interphalangeal (DIP) joints
- pisiform bone
- radial and ulnar styloids
- lateral and medial epicondyles of the elbow

❍ Identify fragile skin and select the splinting material carefully. Monitor the temperature of the thermoplastic closely before applying the material to the fragile skin.

❍ Identify skin areas having impaired sensation. The splint design should not impinge on these sites.

❍ If fluctuating edema is a problem, use a wider splint design.

❍ Do not compress the superficial branch of the radial nerve. If the radial edge of a forearm splint impinges beyond the middle of the forearm near the dorsal side of the thumb, the branch of the radial nerve may be compressed.

*See Appendix B for a perforated copy of this form.

therapist should provide the patient with a written splint schedule and should review the schedule with the patient, nurse, and caregiver responsible for putting on and taking off the splint. If the patient is confused, the therapist is responsible for instructing the appropriate caregiver regarding proper splint wear and care.

While sleeping at night, patients should never wear dynamic splints. Because of moving parts on dynamic splints, patients could accidentally scratch, poke, or cut themselves. Wearing dynamic splints during sleep can also impair circulation.

Patients should wear dynamic splints for a few minutes out of each hour and gradually work up to longer time periods. A therapist should never fabricate a dynamic splint without checking its effect on the patient. The therapist should also consider the diagnosis and make the splint wearing as intermittent as possible, allowing for times of rest, exercise, hygiene, and skin relief. In addition, the therapist must use clinical judgment to determine and adjust the splint-wearing schedule and should reevaluate the splint consistently to alter the treatment plan as necessary.

FORM 3-3* Hints for Splint Provision

- ❍ Give the patient *oral* and *written* instructions regarding the following:
  - ❍ wearing schedule
  - ❍ care of splint
  - ❍ purpose of splint
  - ❍ responsibility in therapy program
  - ❍ phone number of contact person if problems arise
  - ❍ actions to take if skin reactions such as the following occur:
    - rashes
    - numbness
    - reddened areas
    - pain increase because of splint application
- ❍ Evaluate the splint after the patient wears it at least 20 to 30 minutes, and make necessary adjustments.
- ❍ Position all joints incorporated into the splint at the correct therapeutic angle(s).
- ❍ Design the splint to account for bony prominences such as the following:
    - MCP, PIP, and DIP joints
    - pisiform
    - radial and ulnar styloids
    - lateral and medial epicondyles of the elbow
- ❍ If fluctuating edema is a problem, make certain the splint design can accommodate for the problem by using a wider design.
- ❍ Make certain the splint design does not mobilize or immobilize unnecessary joint(s).
- ❍ Make certain the splint does not impede or restrict motions of joints adjacent to the splint.
- ❍ Make certain the splint supports the arches of the hand.
- ❍ Take into consideration the creases of the hand for allowing immobilization or mobilization depending on the purpose of the splint.
- ❍ Make certain the splint does not restrict circulation.
- ❍ Make certain application and removal of the splint is easy.
- ❍ Secure the splint to the patient's extremity using a well-designed strapping mechanism.
- ❍ Make certain the appropriate edges of the splint are flared or rolled.

*See Appendix B for a perforated copy of this form.

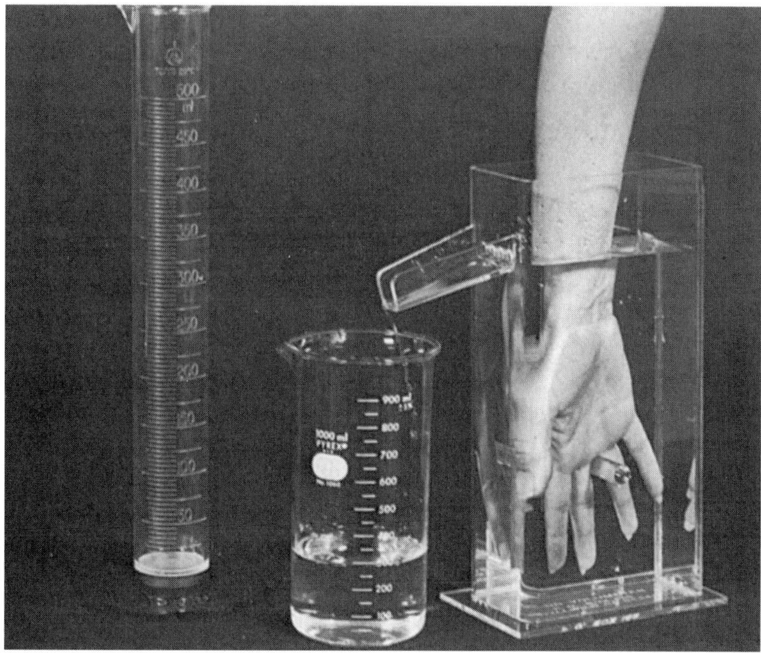

FIGURE 3-11
The volumeter measures composite hand mass via water displacement. (From Hunter, J. M., Schneider, L. H., Mackin, E. J., & Callahan, A. D. [Eds.]. [1990]. Rehabilitation of the hand: Surgery and therapy [3rd ed., p. 63]. St. Louis: Mosby.)

Compliance

Based on the initial interview and statements from conversations, the therapist should determine whether compliance to the wearing schedule is a problem. (Chapter 4 contains strategies to help patients with compliance and acceptance.)

Skin Reactions

Therapists should educate patients to report to them immediately if rashes or other skin reactions occur. Padding and strapping material on a splint may create an allergic reaction. In addition, a patient who has sensitive skin may not be able to tolerate thermoplastic material.

Splint Care

Therapists are responsible for educating patients about splint care. Washing the hand and splint with warm water and a mild soap is effective. The patient or caregiver should dry the hand and splint thoroughly before reapplying the splint. Chlorine removes ink marks on the splint. Rubbing alcohol, clorox, and hydrogen peroxide are good disinfectants to use on the splint for infection control.

Patients should be aware that heat may melt their splints and should be careful not to leave their splints in hot cars, on sunny windowsills, or on radiators. Therapists should discourage patients from making self-adjustments, including the heating of splints in microwave ovens, which cause splints to soften, fold in on themselves, and adhere. If the patient successfully softens the plastic, a burn could result from the application of hot plastic to the skin.

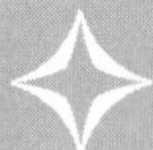

SELF-QUIZ 3-1*

Please circle either true (T) or false (F).

1. T F All physicians follow the same protocol for post-operative conditions.
2. T F Motivation may affect the patient's compliance for wearing a splint, so determining the patient's motivational level is an important task for the therapist.
3. T F The resting hand posture is 10° to 20° of wrist extension, 10° of ulnar deviation, 15° to 20° of MCP flexion, and partial flexion and abduction of the thumb.
4. T F In regard to tensile strength, proximal musculature can never affect distal musculature.
5. T F Therapists should encourage patients to carry their affected extremities in guarded or protective positions to ensure that no harm is done to the injury.
6. T F A general guideline for evaluating splint fit is to have the patient wear the splint for 20 minutes and then remove the splint. If no reddened areas are present, no adjustments are necessary.
7. T F All splints require 24 hours of wearing to be most effective.

***See Appendix A for the answer key.**

SELF-QUIZ 3-1—cont'd

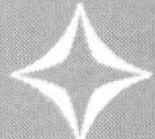

8. T F Every patient should receive a splint-wearing schedule in written and verbal forms.
9. T F For infection control purposes, patients and therapists should use extremely hot water to clean splints.

REVIEW QUESTIONS

1. What are components of a thorough hand examination before splint fabrication?
2. What is the posture of a resting hand?
3. What information should a therapist obtain about the patient's history?
4. What sources can therapists use to obtain information about patients and their conditions?
5. Why is knowing a patient's reimbursement source important before providing services?
6. What procedure can a therapist use when assessing whether a newly fabricated splint is fitting well on a patient?
7. What precautions should a therapist keep in mind when designing and fabricating a splint?
8. What are the guidelines for the duration of splint wear?
9. How can therapists and patients clean splints?
10. What instructions should every patient with a splint have before leaving a clinic?

References

American Society for Surgery of the Hand. (1983). The hand. New York: Churchill Livingstone Inc.

Aulicino, P. L., & DuPuy, T. E. (1990). Clinical examination of the hand. In J. M. Hunter, L. H. Schneider, E. J. Mackin, & A. D. Callahan (Eds.), Rehabilitation of the hand: Surgery and therapy (3rd ed.). St. Louis: Mosby.

Cailliet, R. (1994). Hand pain and impairment (4th ed.). Philadelphia: F. A. Davis Co.

Callahan, A. D. (1990). Sensibility testing: Clinical methods. In J. M. Hunters, L. H. Scheider, E. J. Macklin, & A. D. Callahan (Eds.), Rehabilitation of the hand: Surgery and therapy (3rd ed.). St. Louis: Mosby.

Cannon, N. M., Foltz, R. W., Koepfer, J. M., Lauck, M. F., Simpson, D. M., & Bromley, R. S. (1985). Manual of hand splinting. New York: Churchill Livingstone Inc.

Fess, E. E., & Philips, C. A. (1987). Hand splinting: Principles and methods (2nd ed.). St. Louis: Mosby.

Jebsen, R. H., Taylor, N., Trieschmann, R. B., Trotter, M. J., & Howard, L. A. (1969). An objective and standardized test of hand function. Archives of Physical Medicine & Rehabilitation, 311-319.

Moberg, E. (1958). Objective methods for determining the functional value of sensibility in the hand. J Bone Joint Surg 40B, 454-476.

Pascerelli, E., & Quilter, D. (1994). Repetitive strain injury. New York: John Wiley & Sons.

Smith, K. L. (1990). Wound care for the hand pateint. In J. M. Hunters, L. H. Scheider, E. J. Macklin, & A. D. Callahan (Eds.). Rehabilitation of the hand: Surgery and therapy (3rd ed.). St. Louis: Mosby.

Staley, M. J., Richard, R. L., & Falkel, J. E. (1988). Burns. In S. B. O'Sullivan & T. J. Schmidtz. Physical rehabilitation: Assessment and treatment (3rd ed.). Philadelphia: F. A. Davis Co.

Tomancik, L. (1987). Directions for using Semmes-Weinstien monofilaments. San Jose, CA: North Coast Medical, Inc.

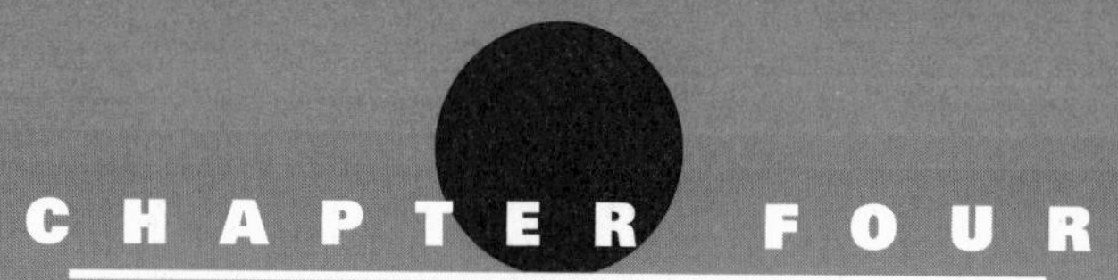

CHAPTER FOUR

Problem Solving for Splint Fabrication

SALLY E. POOLE, MA, OTR, CHT
JOAN L. SULLIVAN, MA, OTR, CHT
HELENE LOHMAN, MA, OTR/L

Chapter Objectives

1. Identify essential components of a splint referral.
2. Discuss reasons for the importance of communication with the physician about a splint referral.
3. Discuss diagnostic implications for splint provision.
4. List helpful hints regarding the hand evaluation.
5. Explain factors the therapist considers when selecting a splinting approach and design.
6. Describe problem-solving factors the therapist weighs during splint fabrication.
7. Describe areas that require monitoring after splint fabrication is completed.
8. Explain the evaluation process of a splint after fabrication and the ways the therapist makes adjustments.
9. Discuss important factors concerning a splint-wearing schedule.
10. Identify conditions that determine splint discontinuation.
11. Relate issues regarding splint cost and reimbursement.

In clinical practice no simple design or type of splint exists that applies to all patient diagnoses. Splint selection, joint positioning, and wearing protocols vary because each injury is unique. Problem solving regarding which splint to fabricate involves considering the physician's referral, the physician's surgical and rehabilitation approach, and the therapist's assessment of the patient's needs.

Instructors sometimes teach students only one way to do something. For example, this textbook emphasizes the typical methods that generalist clinicians use to fabricate common splints. Learning a foundation for splint fabrication is important. However, in clinical practice the therapist should use a problem-solving approach to address each patient who needs a splint.

The ability to problem solve is based on the following: knowledge about the patient diagnosis; awareness of the patient's motivation, compliance, and lifestyle needs; understanding of splinting protocols and techniques; and clinical experience. Splint fabrication is a trial-and-error process, requiring the therapist to be willing to take risks and experiment with techniques and materials to fabricate the most beneficial splint for the patient.

This chapter addresses approaches to clinical problem solving from the moment the therapist obtains a splint referral until the patient's discharge. This chapter also presents prime questions in problem solving that the therapist should consider during treatment planning throughout the patient's course of therapy.

Essentials of Splint Referral

The first step in the problem-solving process is consideration of the splint referral. The ideal situation is to receive the splint referral from the physician's office early to allow plenty of time for preparation. In reality, however, the first time the therapist sees the referral is often when the patient arrives for the appointment. In these situations the therapist makes quick clinical decisions.

Aside from patient demographics, Fess and Philips (1987) suggest that therapists also need the following information:

1. Diagnosis
2. Date of the condition's onset
3. Medical or surgical management
4. Purpose of the splint
5. Type of splint (static, static progressive, or dynamic)
6. Anatomical parts the therapist should immobilize or mobilize
7. Precautions
8. Wearing schedule

Therapist-Physician Communication About Splint Referral

A problem many therapists encounter is an incomplete splint referral lacking a clear diagnosis. Even an experienced therapist becomes frustrated when receiving a referral that simply states, "splint." Splint what? For what purpose? For how long? An open line of communication between the physician and therapist is essential for good splint selection and fabrication. Most physicians welcome calls from the treating therapist when those calls are specific. If the physician's splint referral does not contain the pertinent information, the therapist is responsible for requesting this information. The therapist should prepare a list of questions before calling, and if the physician is not available, the therapist should give the list to the secretary or nurse and agree on a specific time to call again. The therapist must never rely solely on the patient's perception of the diagnosis and splint requirements.

In some cases the physician expects the therapist to have the clinical problem-solving skills to decide on the appropriate splint choice for the specific clinical diagnosis. The therapist should make successful independent decisions with a knowledge base about the fundamentals of splinting and with the ability to locate additional information.

Diagnostic Implications for Splint Provision

The therapist identifies the patient diagnosis after reviewing the splint order. Usually the therapist can use a categorical splinting approach by knowing the patient diagnosis. The first category involves chronic conditions such as hemiplegia. In such a situation a splint may prevent skin maceration or contracture. The second category involves a traumatic or acute condition that may encompass surgical or nonsurgical intervention. For example, the patient may have tendinitis and require a nonsurgical splint intervention for the affected extremity.

Helpful Hints Regarding Hand Evaluation

The following are specific hints that elaborate on areas of the splinting evaluation and problem solving. (See Chapter 3 for essential components to include in a thorough hand evaluation.)

Age

The patient's age, which the therapist obtains from the patient history, is important information for many reasons. Barring other problems, most children, adolescents, and adults can wear splints according to the particular treatment programs. An infant or toddler, however, can usually get out of any splint at any time or place. Extraordinary and creative methods are often necessary to keep splints on these patients (Byron, 1990). Older patients, especially those with diminished functional capacities, may require careful monitoring by the caregiver to ensure a proper fit and compliance to the wearing schedule.

Occupation

From the interview with the patient, family, and caregiver and from the chart review, the therapist obtains information about the impact a splint may have on occupational function, economic status, and social well-being. When choosing the splint design and material, the therapist should consider the patient's lifestyle needs. The following are some specific questions to consider when determining lifestyle needs:

1. Will the patient use the splint for functional activities?
2. If so, what are the specific activities?
3. Will the patient wear the splint during work or sports?
4. Do special considerations exist due to rules and regulations for work or sports?
5. In what kind of environment will the patient wear the splint? For example, will the patient use the splint in extreme temperatures? Will the splint get wet?
6. Will the splint impede a necessary hand function for the patient's job?

If a physician refers a patient for a wrist cock-up splint because of wrist strain, the therapist might contemplate the following question: Is the patient a construction worker who does heavy manual work or a computer operator who does light, repetitious work? A construction worker may require a splint with stronger material and extremely secure strapping. The computer operator may use a lighter, thinner splint material with soft velfoam straps.

The therapist should determine the patient's activity status even when the patient is wearing a splint that does not allow function or movement, such as a positioning splint. If the patient must return to work immediately, albeit in a limited capacity, the splint must be secure. Proper instructions regarding appropriate care of the limb and splint are necessary. This care may involve elevation of the affected extremity, wound management, and periodic range-of-motion exercises while the patient is working.

When the patient plans to continue in a sports program (professional, school, or community based), the therapist must check the rules and regulations governing that particular sport. Rules and regulations usually prevent athletes from wearing hard splint material during participation in the sport, unless the splint's design accommodates interior and exterior padding. School-based athletics may not allow hard splint materials under any circumstances, so the therapist must consider other options, such as a splint fabricated from soft neoprene material or an elastic-prefabricated splint.

Expected Environment

The therapist must consider the patient's discharge environment. Some patients return to their own homes and have families and friends who can lend assistance if necessary. For those patients returning to inpatient units or nursing homes, therapists should consider the staff instruction in the care and use of the splints. If patients return to psychiatric units or prison wards, therapists should consider whether supervision is necessary so that patients cannot use their splints as potential weapons to harm themselves or others.

Activities of Daily Living Responsibilities Before and After Injury

The splintmaker should consider the following question: Is the patient physically able to apply and remove the splint, or are staff members or other caregivers responsible? Not only is patient education important, but the education of those caring for the patient is also essential. This is especially true for parents of extremely young children and caregivers of emotionally or physically challenged patients of any age.

Patient Motivation and Compliance

A limited amount of research investigating compliance issues with splint provision exists. Only recently have experts considered this issue as it relates to hand patients. Groth and Wilder (1994) found in their study on compliance that "splint use and exercise was clearly an important factor in determining the result of treatment for mallet finger injuries" (p. 23).

Many considerations affect patient compliance with a treatment regimen, including external factors such as socioeconomic status and family support and internal factors such as the patient's perception of the severity, knowledge, and beliefs and attitudes about the injury (Groth and Wulf, 1995; Bower, 1985). Another commonly discussed factor in research is the psychosocial construct of locus of control, which proposes a relationship between an individual's perception of control over treatment outcomes and the individual's likelihood of taking responsibility in treatment. This perception of control can be internally or externally based (Bower, 1985).

The therapist can positively influence the patient's compliance and motivation to wear a splint. The therapist should perceive the patient as a whole person with a lifestyle beyond the clinic, not just as a patient with a hand injury. Paramount to patient cooperation is education about the medical necessity of wearing splints, in which therapists should consider patients' perspectives on the ways splints affect their lifestyles. Education should be repetitive throughout the time the patient wears the splint (Southam & Dunbar, 1987; Groth & Wulf, 1995). When the therapist and physician communicate clearly about the type of splint necessary, the patient receives consistent information regarding the rationale for wearing the splint. Showing the patient the way the splint works and explaining the goal of the splint helps with patient compliance.

Rather than labeling the patient as noncompliant or uncooperative, trained personnel must make a serious attempt to help the patient better cope with the injury. The therapist should be an empathetic listener as the patient learns to adjust to the diagnosis and splint. In addition, therapists should convey that success with splints involves shared responsibility between themselves and patients. To attain the purpose of splints, therapists must clarify patients' responsibilities in the treatment plans. Sometimes a peer wearing a splint can be a role model to help a noncompliant patient.

Selection of an appropriate design may alleviate a patient's difficulty in adjusting to the injury and wearing a splint. Therapists should ask themselves the following questions: Will a static splint accomplish the purpose of the program? If a dynamic splint is necessary, will a low-profile splint be less cumbersome than a high-profile one?

Making the splint aesthetically pleasing helps with patient compliance. A patient is less likely to wear a splint that is messy or sloppy. This is especially true for children and adolescents, for whom personal appearance is often an important issue.

Splint and strapping materials are now available in a variety of colors. Patients, both children and adults, who are coping successfully with the injury may want to have fun with the splint and select one or more colors. However, a patient who is having a difficult time adjusting to the injury may not want to wear a splint in public at all, let alone a splint with a color that draws more attention.

Finally, fabricating a correct-fitting splint on the first attempt eases a patient's anxiety. The therapist is responsible for listening to patient complaints and adjusting the splint. Encouraging effective communication with the patient facilitates understanding and satisfaction about splint provision.

Cognitive Status

When the patient's cognitive status renders an inability to attend the therapy program and follow the splinting regimen, the therapist must train the patient's family, a caregiver, or staff members. Educating the family and caregiver about medical reasons for the splint provision leads to better cooperation.

Splinting Approach and Design Considerations

The four approaches to splint design are as follows: dorsal, volar, radial, and ulnar. The therapist must determine whether to fabricate a dynamic or static splint, or both. Understanding the purpose of the splint clarifies these decisions. For example, when dealing with a radial nerve injury, the therapist may choose to fabricate a dynamic metacarpophalangeal (MCP) extension splint to substitute for the loss of motor function in the wrist extensors and MCP extensors.

In addition to the information the therapist obtains from a thorough evaluation, certain suggestions should dictate splint choice. To determine the most efficient and effective splint choice, the therapist must consider the physician's orders, diagnosis, therapist's judgment, and patient function.

Physician's Orders

Physicians often predetermine the splint-application approach based on their training, surgical technique, and success with certain designs. For example, for an ulnar nerve injury the physician may order a static ulnar gutter splint with the ring and little fingers in the anticlaw position of MCP flexion. The physician may also order a dynamic splint in the same position if the need exists for stronger traction to the soft tissues.

Diagnosis

The diagnosis determines the number of joints the therapist must splint, their positions, and whether the splint should be dynamic or static. Frequently the diagnosis mandates the splint design approach. For example, for a flexor tendon repair using an early mobilization protocol the therapist must place the static base of the splint on the dorsum of the forearm and hand to protect the tendon and to allow for rubber band traction. The wrist and MCPs should be in a flexed position to block extension. This splint protects the repair, allows early tendon glide into flexion, and avoids placement of the thermoplastic material over the surgical site. In this example, the repaired structures and the need to begin tendon gliding dictate the design (von Strien, 1990).

Therapist's Judgment

The therapist can also determine the splint design and type. For example, when dealing with elective carpal tunnel release, the therapist can place a wrist cock-up splint dorsally or volarly directly over the surgical site. As an advocate of early-scar management, the therapist chooses a volar splint and adds silicone elastomer or Otoform to the splint.

Patient Function

The patient's primary task responsibilities may influence the splint choice. As previously stated, a construction worker's wrist has different demands placed on it than the wrist of a computer operator with the same diagnosis. Not only does the therapist choose different materials for each scenario, but the design approach may be different. A thumb hole volar wrist cock-up splint decreases the risk of the splint migrating up the arm during the construction worker's activities. The computer operator may prefer a dorsal wrist splint to allow adequate sensory feedback and unimpeded flexibility of the digits during keyboard use. (See Chapter 5 for a pattern for a volar thumb hole wrist cock-up splint.)

TABLE 4-1 Common Positioning Choices in Splint Design

Splint	Volar	Dorsal	Radial	Ulnar
Resting hand splint	X	X		
Wrist cock-up splint	X	X		X
Thumb splint	X	X	X	
Ulnar nerve splint (anticlaw)		X		X
Radial nerve splint (dynamic)		X		
Median nerve splint (thumb involvement)	X	X	X	
Elbow positioning splint	X	X		
Dynamic hand extension splint		X		
Dynamic hand flexion splint	X			

Table 4-1 illustrates a variety of positioning choices for splint design. However, therapists should not view these suggestions as strict rules. For example, a skin condition may necessitate that a dynamic extension splint be volarly based rather than dorsally based.

Finally, the therapist should keep the design simple and make the splint easy for the patient to wear. Splints should restrict the least number of joints possible, allowing the splint to accomplish its purpose. A simple design also enhances the cosmetic appeal of the splint. Splints that look great in a supply catalog may require hours to make and may impair the patient's ability to apply and remove them independently.

Problem-Solving Considerations during Splint Fabrication

The splint-fabrication process involves many clinical decisions about materials and techniques that the therapist can use. The therapist should consider issues related to infection-control procedures and time allotment for splint fabrication and patient education.

Infection-Control Procedures

The therapist should consider whether dressing changes are necessary. If so, the therapist should follow universal precautions and maintain a sterile environment. Also, the therapist should be aware that macerated skin under a splint can more easily occur with the presence of a draining wound. The therapist must carefully first apply a dressing that absorbs the fluid.

Splint fabrication should take place over the dressing, and the therapist should instruct the patient to apply new dressings at appropriate intervals (Skotak & Stockdell, 1988). Before the application of the splinting material, the therapist can place a moist paper towel over the patient's bandages. This action prevents the thermoplastic material from sticking to the bandages.

If the patient has a draining or infected wound, the therapist should not use regular strapping material to hold the splint in place. Strapping material can absorb bodily bacteria. Instead, the therapist should use gauze bandages that are replaceable at each dressing change. If a patient is unwilling or unable to change a dressing, the therapist can instruct a family member or friend to do so. If this is not possible, the patient may need to visit the therapist more frequently.

Time Allotment for Splint Fabrication and Patient Education

If possible, a beginning therapist should schedule a large block of time for splint fabrication. As therapists gain clinical experience, they require less time to fabricate splints. With any splint application the therapist should allow enough time for educating the patient, family and caregiver. As discussed, education helps with patient compliance. In addition, education alerts patients and others of precautions.

Postfabrication Monitoring

Several areas involve problem solving after splint fabrication. In particular, the splintmaker must be aware of pressure areas, edema, and the patient's physical status.

Monitoring Pressure

Regardless of its purpose or design, the splint requires monitoring to determine the effect on the skin. The therapist must remember that a patient wearing a splint is superimposing a hard lever system on an existing lever system that is covered by fragile skin. The therapist must therefore follow mechanical principles during splint fabrication to avoid excessive pressure on the skin. To reduce pressure, the therapist should design a splint that increases its surface area (Fess & Philips, 1987). Splint designs that use circumferential components may jeopardize vascular circulation, especially in conditions with fluctuating edema (Malick, 1972). Warning signs of an ill-fitting splint are red marks, white macerated skin, and skin ulcerations.

A well-fitting splint, after its removal, may leave a red area on the patient's skin. This normal response to the pressure of the splint disappears within seconds. When a splint has applied too much pressure on one area, which usually occurs over a bony prominence, the redness may last longer. For patients with dark skin in whom redness is not easily visible, the therapist can lightly touch the skin to determine the presence of hot spots, which are areas of pressure warmer than the rest of the covered skin. The therapist checks the skin after 20 to 30 minutes of wearing time.

Wet and white macerated skin can occur when the skin under a splint holds too much moisture. When this problem happens to a patient with intact skin who has simply forgotten to remove the splint, the therapist can easily correct the problem by washing and drying the area. Educating the patient about proper care of the hand and providing a stockinette to absorb moisture should resolve this situation.

An ill-fitting splint may cause skin ulceration. A patient with intact sensibility who has an ill-fitting splint usually requests an adjustment or simply discards the splint because it is not comfortable. For a condition in which sensation is absent, vigorous splint monitoring is critical (Brand, 1993). The therapist teaches the patient and family to remove the splint every 1 to 2 hours to check the skin and avoid a disastrous situation.

Monitoring Edema

A therapist often needs to splint an edematous extremity. The patient may have recently undergone surgery, may have an infection, may have an injury that causes severe edema (e.g., from a burn), or may have an injury involving vascular compromise. A well-designed, well-fitting splint can reduce edema and prevent the sequelae of tissue damage and joint contracture. A poorly designed or ill-fitting splint can contribute to or increase the damaging results of persistent edema. Generally, the design and fit principles already discussed in this text apply.

The therapist must also consider the method used to hold the splint in place. Soft, wide straps accommodate increases in edema and are better able to disperse pressure than rigid, nonyielding Velcro straps (Cannon, et al., 1985). For severe edema the therapist may use an ace bandage to keep the splint in place and thus reduce edema rather than circumferential straps, which may further restrict circulation. When using ace wraps or compressive gauzes, the therapist must apply them in a figure 8 and use gradient pressure distal to proximal. The therapist must properly monitor the splint and wrap to ensure that the wrap does not roll or bunch (Hunter & Mackin, 1990). Pressure created by rolling or bunching could cause constriction and further edema and could thus mean disaster for both the patient and the therapist.

Edema reduction begins relatively quickly with appropriate wound healing (i.e., no infection), proper elevation, and gentle, active exercises as permitted. When this activity occurs, the therapist must remold the splint to fit the new configuration of the extremity. The therapist asks the patient suffering from severe edema to return to the clinic daily for monitoring and treatment. When the edema appears to be of the normal postoperative amount, the therapist asks the patient to return to the clinic in 3 to 5 days for a splint check. Again, patient education is an important part of the edema reduction regime (Hunter & Mackin, 1990). Helping the patient understand the time and purpose of the splint adjustment is also important.

Monitoring Physical Status

When a patient's physical or functional status changes, a splint adjustment is often necessary. If a patient is receiving treatment for a specific injury and treatment is effective, the splint requires adjustments according to improvement. For example, a patient suffering from a Colles' fracture may need a splint to help support the wrist in the early phase of rehabilitation. On day one, when the therapist makes the splint, the patient may only be able to place the wrist in a neutral position. As treatment progresses and wrist extension increases, the therapist adjusts the splint to accommodate the gains made in wrist range of motion. The therapist monitors the range of motion at least weekly, if not every 2 to 3 days (Hunter, et al., 1990).

Another example is a patient suffering from rheumatoid arthritis who has a resting hand splint fabricated during an acute flare-up of the disease. While in remission the patient does not need the splint and therefore does not wear it until another inflammatory period occurs.

Evaluation and Adjustment of Splints

After fabricating the splint, the splintmaker carefully evaluates the design to determine fit and necessary adjustments. The therapist looks carefully at the splint when the patient is and is not wearing it and considers whether the splint serves its purpose. The splint should be functional for the patient and should accomplish the goals for which it was intended. It should also have a design that uses correct biomechanical principles and should be cosmetically appealing. (Refer to specific chapters in this book for hints and splint-evaluation forms.)

If major adjustments are required, the therapist should avoid using a heat gun except to smooth splint edges. If the therapist has selected the appropriate simple splint design and has used a thermoplastic product that is easily reheatable and remoldable, the water immersion method is the best way to adjust the splint. Years of experience demonstrate that reheating the entire splint in water and reshaping it is more efficient than spot heating. The activity of the therapist reheating and adjusting one spot often affects the adjacent area, thereby producing another area requiring adjustment. This cycle may not end until the splint is useless. When possible, the therapist should use a splint product that is reheatable in water and easily reshapeable on the patient for a proper fit.

Splint-Wearing Schedule Factors

Developing a splint-wearing schedule for a patient is sometimes extremely frustrating for a beginning splintmaker because no magical numbers or formulas exist for each type of splint or diagnostic population. The therapist must tailor and customize the wearing schedule to the individual and exercise clinical judgment. Only general guidelines for splint-wearing schedules exist.

If joint limitation decreases motion, the therapist should increase the wearing frequency and time as much as the patient can tolerate or adjust the treatment plan to try a different splint. If motion is increasing steadily, the therapist may decrease the splint-wearing time, allowing the patient to functionally use the limited joint or joints. If the splint improves function or the extremity requires protection, the patient should wear the splint when necessary.

The following are questions to consider when determining a wearing schedule:

1. What is the purpose of the splint?
2. Does the therapist anticipate patient compliance with a splint-wearing schedule?
3. Does the patient have any medical contraindications or precautions for removing the splint?
4. Which variables may affect the patient's tolerance of the splint?
5. Does the patient need assistance to apply or remove the splint?
6. Is the splint for day or night use, or both?
7. Does the patient need to apply or remove the splint for any functions?
8. How often does the patient need to perform exercises and hygiene tasks?

Sample Wearing Schedule

Patient's name: ____________________
Name of splint: ____________________

The purpose of this splint is to maintain the hand in a functional position.

Prescribed wearing schedule:

8:00 AM-12:00 PM	On*	
12:00 PM- 2:00 PM	Off	Provide PROM
2:00 PM- 6:00 PM	On*	
6:00 PM- 8:00 PM	Off	Provide PROM
8:00 PM-12:00 AM	On*	
12:00 AM- 2:00 AM	Off	Provide PROM
2:00 AM- 6:00 AM	On*	
6:00 AM- 8:00 AM	Off	Provide PROM

Wear the splint on the right upper extremity. Please contact J. Smith at (phone number) in the Occupational Therapy Department if any of the following occur:

- Pink or reddened areas
- Complaints of increased pain because of the splint
- Increased swelling with splint wear
- Skin rash
- Complaints of decreased sensation because of the splint

PROM, Passive Range of Motion
*Skin check to be performed.

Answers to these questions should guide the development of a wearing schedule. The therapist should keep in mind that the wearing schedule may require adjustment as progress occurs with the patient's condition. In any situation the therapist should discuss the wearing schedule with the patient and caregiver. The box on the opposite page is a sample wearing schedule that the therapist can post in a patient's room or give to the patient to take home.

Discontinuation of a Splint

No distinct rules exist concerning a splint's discontinuation. Sometimes the physician makes the decision to discontinue a splint. Other times the physician defers to the clinical judgment of the therapist to determine when a splint is no longer beneficial. The therapist should then contact the physician for a splint-discharge order.

The following are questions to consider when making the clinical decision to discontinue a splint:

1. Have the patient and caregivers been compliant with the splint-wearing schedule? If not, why?
2. What are the original objectives for the splint's provision, and has the patient accomplished them?
3. Will the same objectives be compromised or accomplished without a splint?

Patient and caregiver compliance is essential for success with a splint-wearing regimen. If the patient is not wearing the splint, the therapist should first use clinical reasoning to identify the reasons for noncompliance. For example, the noncompliance of an older patient in an institutional setting could be the result of one or more of the following factors: (1) poor communication among the staff about the splint-wearing schedule, (2) poor staff follow through with the splint-wearing schedule, (3) lack of patient understanding about the splint's purpose, (4) uncomfortableness of the splint, (5) the patient's fear of hidden costs associated with the splint, and (6) the patient's dislike of the splint's cosmetic appearance. After identifying the reason or reasons for noncompliance, the therapist can work on possible solutions.

An important factor in determining the discontinuation of the splint is a careful review of the splint's objectives. For example, a therapist fabricates a dynamic splint for a patient suffering from a proximal interphalangeal (PIP) soft-tissue flexion contracture of the middle finger with the objective of mobilizing the PIP joint to help correct the flexion deformity. Gradually, the splint pulls the PIP joint out of the flexion deformity. From monitoring range of motion (ROM) and evaluating the traction pull of the splint, the therapist determines that the splint has maximally helped the patient and the original treatment objectives were accomplished. Thus the therapist calls the physician for an order to discontinue the dynamic splint.

The therapist must consider whether the accomplishment of the objectives is possible without the splint. Timely discontinuation of any splint is important. The therapist should keep in mind that inappropriately provided or poorly fabricated splints can restrict movement, make postural compromises by causing atrophy in one muscle group and overuse in another, and can injure other parts of the anatomy. Also, preventing patient dependence on a splint is important. When the patient has the functional capabilities, the therapist should adjust the splint-wearing schedule to wean the patient gradually from wearing the splint (Pascarelli & Quilter, 1994).

Cost and Reimbursement Issues

Two sides exist regarding the cost of splints. First, how does the therapist arrive at the price of a splint? Second, how does the therapist receive payment for a splint?

To calculate the price of a splint, the therapist totals the direct and indirect costs. Direct costs include items such as the thermoplastic material, strapping material, stockinette, and rivets. Because the hospital or clinic purchases supplies at wholesale cost, a percentage markup may appear on the cost. Indirect costs include nondisposable supplies such as scissors and fry pans, the time required for the average therapist to make the splint, and overhead costs such as rent and electricity.

Because of tighter control of the health-care dollar with managed care and health maintenance organizations (HMOs), many therapists are finding that reimbursement for splints is becoming increasingly difficult. Taking an active role in helping the patient determine the reimbursement policy of an insurance plan regarding splints may be necessary; however, the therapist must remember that the plan belongs to the patient, not to the therapist. If a particular insurance plan reimburses partially or not at all, the patient is responsible for paying the balance of the cost. Some facilities make accomodations for patients who are uninsured or underinsured and need splint provision. Additionally, documentation for insurance companies should be specific about the affected extremity and the type and purpose of the splint (Evans, 1995).

Some insurance companies simply refuse to pay for splints, and others ask for so much documentation that more time is required to prepare the bill than to make the splint. For example, some insurance companies ask therapists for original invoices for the purchase of thermoplastic and strapping materials. The American Society of Hand Therapists recently published *Splint Classification Systems,* a book on naming and designing splints. This book may result in terminology becoming uniform and thus help with some reimbursement questions (American Society of Hand Therapists, 1992).

SELF QUIZ 4-1*

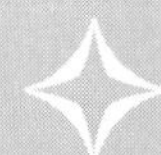

Please circle either true (T) or false (F).

1. T F An infant can follow a splint-wearing program without extraordinary methods.
2. T F Determining a person's lifestyle needs for splint design and material is important.
3. T F Paramount to a patient's cooperation is education about the medical necessity for wearing a splint.
4. T F If a patient has a wound that requires dressing, the therapist should fabricate the splint over the dressing and instruct the patient to apply new dressings at appropriate intervals.
5. T F The only sign of an ill-fitting splint is red marks.
6. T F A well-fitting splint, on removal, may leave a red area on the patient's skin.
7. T F In the presence of severe edema the therapist should use circumferential straps.
8. T F The therapist should use a heat gun for all necessary adjustments.
9. T F If motion is decreased because of joint limitation, the therapist should decrease the frequency and/or time that the patient wears the splint.
10. T F When deciding to discontinue a splint, the therapist must consider the original objectives of the splint's fabrication.
11. T F To calculate the cost of a splint, the therapist should consider the direct and indirect costs.

*See Appendix A for the answer key.

Case Study*

Read the following scenario and answer the questions based on information in this chapter:

Pete is a 34-year-old man employed as a roofer who sustained a right-sided Colles' fracture to his dominant upper extremity while on the job. Several weeks after the bone healed and the physician removed the cast, Pete returned to his physician complaining of pain and swelling in not only the wrist but the entire extremity. The physician ordered Pete to receive therapy. Pete arrives at the clinic with two prescriptions. The first prescription states, "Evaluate and treat patient," and the second prescription reads, "Fabricate a right wrist splint."

You are a new therapist at the outpatient clinic where Pete has already completed his initial evaluation by a more experienced therapist. The plan is to fabricate the splint on the subsequent visit. On that day, Pete's therapist is absent and you are asked to fabricate the splint on the patient. You have only a few minutes to prepare to see the patient. You quickly scan the patient's initial evaluation report, which highlights the following problems: severely decreased active range of motion (AROM) in wrist flexion, extension, and radial and ulnar deviation; edema over the fracture site and all fingers limiting finger AROM; and pain during AROM and while attempting even light activities.

When you meet Pete, he appears distraught and you have difficulty engaging him in conversation. He is with his wife, who has been crying and is now hovering over her husband.

1. How might you better prepare yourself to understand the diagnosis?

___

___

___

2. Discuss the way you will approach Pete and his wife about the need to fabricate the splint, taking into consideration his distraught state.

___

___

___

***See Appendix A for some suggested approaches to these questions. You may have different answers that are also appropriate.**

Case Study—cont'd

3. How do you clarify the physician order if you are unsure about it?

4. Would you fabricate a dorsal or volar wrist splint? Explain your choice.

5. Considering the patient's occupation and other diagnostic factors, which qualities of thermoplastic material would you choose to fabricate the splint?

6. Considering that the patient has edema, which splint-fabrication factors do you need to keep in mind to help reduce and manage it?

7. After the completion of the splint fabrication, how long will Pete remain in the clinic? Why?

8. Which type of patient education and splint-wearing schedule will you provide? Why?

Review Questions

1. What does a splint referral include?
2. How can the therapist facilitate communication with the physician's office about the splint referral?
3. Why is knowing the patient's age important for the therapist when fabricating a splint?
4. Which lifestyle needs of the patient must the therapist consider with splint provision?
5. How can the therapist enhance the compliance of a patient wearing a splint?
6. What are the infection control procedures a therapist should follow with splint provision?
7. What should the therapist monitor when providing a splint for a patient during the following conditions: pressure, edema, and physical status of a patient?
8. What are the four directions of splint design?
9. What are some helpful hints for making adjustments after splint fabrication?
10. What are the factors the therapist should consider when establishing a patient on a splint-wearing schedule?
11. What are the factors that a therapist should consider for splint discontinuation?
12. What are the cost and reimbursement issues that the therapist must keep in mind?

References

American Society of Hand Therapists. (1992). Splint classification systems. Garner, NJ: The American Society of Hand Therapists.

Bower, K. A. (1985). Compliance as a patient education issue. In K. M. Woldum, V. Ryan-Morrell, M. C. Towson, K. A. Bower, & K. Zander (Eds.), Patient education: Foundations of practice (pp. 45-111). Rockville, MD: Aspen Publication.

Brand, P. W., & Hollister, A. (1993). Clinical mechanics of the hand (2nd ed.). St. Louis: Mosby.

Byron, P. M. (1990). Splinting the hand of a child. In J. M. Hunter, L. H. Schneider, E. J. Mackin, & A. D. Callahan (Eds.). Rehabilitation of the hand (pp. 1147-1152). St. Louis: Mosby.

Cannon, N. M., Foltz, R. W., Koepfer, J. M., Lauck, M. R., Simpson, D. M., & Bromley R. S. (1985). Manual of hand splinting. New York: Churchill Livingstone Inc.

Evans, R. B. (February 7, 1995). Personal communication.

Fess, E. E., & Philips, C. A. (1987). Hand splinting principles and methods (3rd ed.). St. Louis: Mosby.

Groth, G. N., & Wilder, D. M. (1994). The impact of compliance of rehabilitation of patients with mallet finger injuries. J Hand Ther, 7(1), 21-24.

Groth, G. N., & Wulf, M.B. (1995). Compliance with hand rehabilitation: Health beliefs and strategies. J Hand Ther, 8(1), 18-22

Hunter J. M., Schneider, L. M., Mackin, E. J., & Callahan, A. D. (1990). Rehabilitation of the hand: Surgery and therapy. St. Louis: Mosby.

Malick, M. H. (1972). Manual on static splinting. Hamarville, PA: Harmarville Rehabilitation Center.

Pascarelli, E., & Quilter, D. (1994). Repetitive strain injury. New York: John Wiley & Sons Inc.

Skotak, C. H., & Stockdell, S. M. (1988). Wound management in hand therapy. In F. S. Cromwell, & J. Bear-Lehman (Eds.). Hand rehabilitation in occupational therapy (pp. 17-35). Binghamton, NY: Haworth Press Inc.

Southam, M. A., & Dunbar, J. M. (1987). Integration of adherence problems. In D. Meichenbaum & D. C. Turk (Eds.), Facilitating treatment adherence. New York: Plenum Publishing Corp.

von Strien, G. (1990). Postoperative management of flexor tendon injuries. In J. M. Hunter, L. H. Schneider, E. J. Mackin, & A. D. Callahan (Eds.), Rehabilitation of the hand (pp. 390-409). St. Louis: Mosby.

CHAPTER FIVE

Wrist Cock-Up Splints (Wrist Immobilization Splints)

HELENE LOHMAN, MA, OTR/L

Chapter Objectives

1. Discuss diagnostic indications for wrist cock-up splints.
2. Identify major features of wrist cock-up splints.
3. Understand the fabrication process for a volar or dorsal wrist splint.
4. Relate hints for a proper fit to a wrist cock-up splint.
5. Review precautions for wrist cock-up splinting.
6. Use clinical judgment to evaluate a problematic wrist cock-up splint.
7. Use clinical judgment to evaluate a fabricated wrist cock-up splint.
8. Apply knowledge about the application of wrist cock-up splints to a case study.

In general practice, one of the most common wrist splints is a wrist cock-up splint, or a wrist immobilization splint (American Society of Hand Therapists, 1992). This type of splint maintains the wrist in either a neutral or mildly extended position depending on the protocol for a particular diagnostic condition and the patient's treatment goals. A wrist cock-up splint immobilizes the wrist while allowing full metacarpophalangeal (MCP) flexion and thumb mobility. Thus the patient can continue to perform functional activities with the added support and proper positioning of the wrist that the splint provides. Therapists can fabricate wrist cock-up splints to provide volar or dorsal forearm, wrist, and hand support (Figures 5-1 and 5-2). Therapists can also use wrist cock-up splints as bases for dynamic splinting. Wrist cock-up splints are commercially available, though they cannot provide the exact form fit of custom-made splints. However,

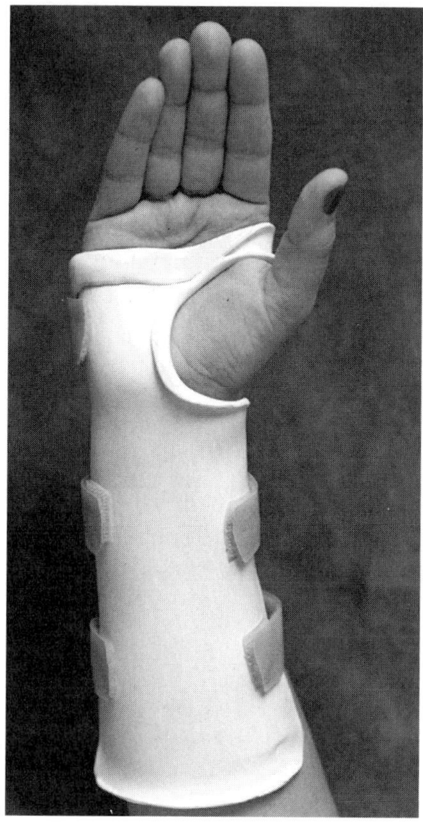
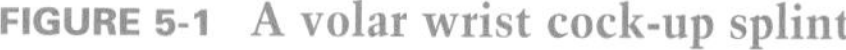

FIGURE 5-1 A volar wrist cock-up splint

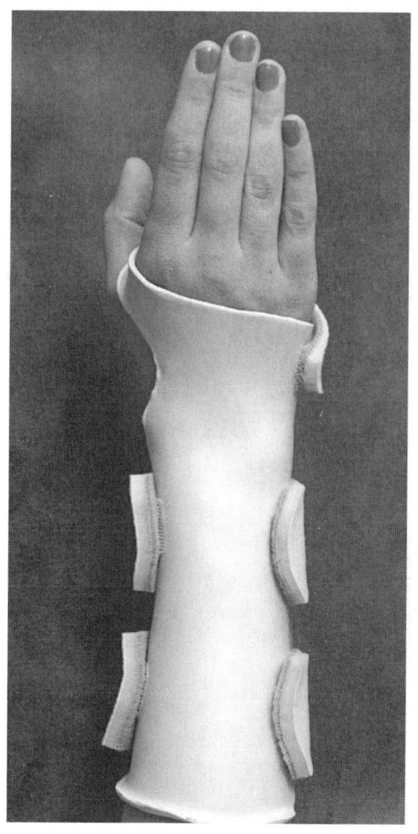

FIGURE 5-2 A dorsal wrist cock-up splint

commercially available splints made from cloth material may be more comfortable for certain patients, especially in a work setting, because these splints allow some wrist movement.

Diagnostic Indications

The clinical indications for wrist cock-up splints vary according to the diagnoses. Application of this splint usually decreases wrist pain or inflammation, provides support, enhances digital function, and prevents wrist deformity. Specific diagnostic conditions that may require a wrist cock-up splint can include but are not limited to cumulative trauma disorder, post-Colles' fracture, wrist sprain, radial nerve palsy, carpal ganglion, ligamentous injuries of the wrist, stable wrist fracture, and wrist arthroplasty. The therapist can apply the wrist cock-up splint for any upper extremity condition that requires the wrist to be in a resting position.

The specific wrist positioning depends on the diagnostic protocol, physician referral, and patient-treatment goals. The therapist must avoid extreme wrist flexion or extension because either position disrupts the normal functional position of the hand. These positions could contribute to the development of carpal tunnel syndrome (Fess & Philips, 1987). For carpal tunnel syndrome, splinting as close as possible to 0° helps avoid added pressure on the median nerve (Cailliet, 1994). For some conditions, therapists fabricate wrist cock-up splints in functional positions of 0° to 30° wrist extension, thus promoting synergistic wrist-extension and finger-flexion patterns. This position allows the greatest level of function with grip activities (Melvin, 1989).

The therapist should perform a thorough hand evaluation before fitting a patient with a wrist cock-up splint and should provide the patient with a wearing schedule, instructions about precautions, and an exercise program based on particular needs. Physicians and experienced therapists may have developed detailed guidelines for positioning and wearing schedules. Every hand is slightly different, so splint positioning and wearing protocols vary. Table 5-1 lists suggested wearing schedules and positioning protocols of common hand conditions that may require wrist cock-up splints.

TABLE 5-1 **Conditions that May Require a Wrist Cock-Up Splint**

Hand condition	Suggested wearing schedule	Type of splint and wrist position
NERVE COMPRESSION		
Carpal tunnel syndrome (median nerve compression)	During an acute flare-up the patient wears the wrist cock-up splint continuously for 4 to 6 weeks except for removal for hygiene and range of motion (ROM) exercises. The splint-wearing schedule gradually decreases. Some physicians advocate nighttime wear only during an acute flare-up.	Volar, dorsal, or ulnar gutter splint with the wrist in a neutral position
Carpal tunnel release surgery	A therapist may fit a patient with a wrist cock-up splint 1 week after surgery and include a splint-wearing schedule that applies during sleep, during strenuous activities, and for support throughout the healing phase.	A volar splint with the wrist in a neutral or slightly extended position

TABLE 5-1 **Conditions that May Require a Wrist Cock-Up Splint—cont'd**

Hand condition	Suggested wearing schedule	Type of splint and wrist position
NERVE COMPRESSION—CONT'D		
Radial nerve palsy	Some physicians may advocate a wrist cock-up splint that maintains the wrist in a functional position and substitutes for the loss of the radial nerve by placing the wrist in extension.*	Volar or dorsal, 0° to 30° extension
Wrist extensor tendonitis	A patient wears a wrist cock-up splint continuously, followed by gradual weaning of the splint.	Volar, 20° to 30° wrist extension
FRACTURES		
Colles' fracture (closed reduction)	After removal of the cast and healing of the fracture, the therapist may fabricate a wrist cock-up splint. Usually the therapist discontinues the splint use as soon as possible to encourage functional hand movement.	Volar, maximum passive extension that the patient can tolerate up to 30°
RHEUMATOID ARTHRITIS		
Periods of swelling and joint inflammation	The therapist fabricates a wrist cock-up splint that the patient wears continuously with established periods for ROM exercises between the splint-wearing schedule.	Volar, in extension up to 30° based on patient comfort level
OTHER		
Reflex sympathetic dystrophy	The therapist fabricates a wrist cock-up splint that the patient wears primarily at night.	Volar, in extension as patient tolerates
Wrist joint synovitis or tenosynovitis	A patient wears a wrist cock-up splint continuously during acute flare-ups.	Volar, 0° to 15° extension

*The diganosis may require additional types of splinting.

Volar and Dorsal Wrist Immobilization Splints

In clinical practice the therapist may need to decide whether to make a volar or dorsal wrist cock-up splint. Each has advantages and disadvantages (Colditz, 1995).

The volar wrist cock-up splint (Figure 5-3) depends on a dorsal strap to hold the wrist in extension in the splint. The design furnishes adequate support for the weight of the wrist and hand. "In cases where the weight of the hand (flaccidity) must be held by the splint, or when the patient is pulling against it (spasticity), the strap is not adequate to hold the wrist in the splint. The volar design is best suited for circumstances requiring rest and/or immobilization of the wrist when the patient still has muscle control of the wrist" (Colditz, 1995). This splint's greatest disadvantage is interference with tactile sensibility on the palmar surface of the hand. "In the presence of edema one must use this design carefully, as the dorsal strap can impede lymphatic and venous flow" (Colditz, 1995).

The dorsal wrist cock-up splint (Figure 5-4) has the advantage of providing stronger mechanical support of the wrist and freeing up some of the palmar sur-

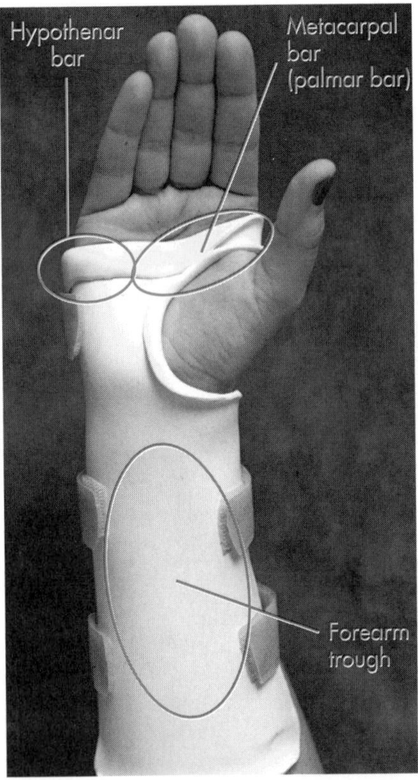

FIGURE 5-3 A volar wrist cock-up splint with identified components

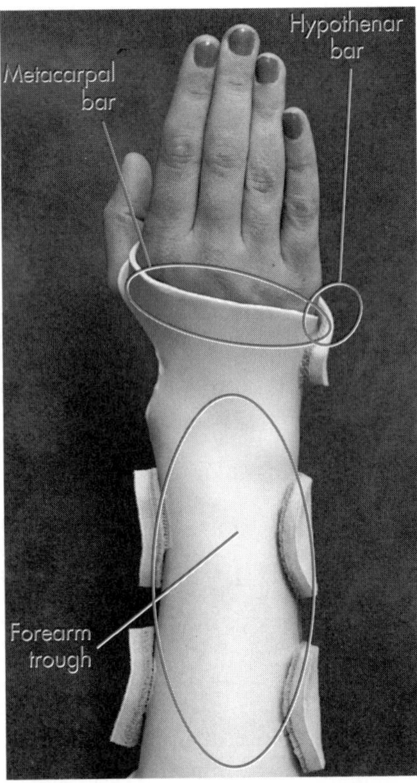

FIGURE 5-4 A dorsal wrist cock-up splint with identified components

face for sensory imput. Rather than depending on the small surface area of the dorsal strap as the point of counter force, the dorsal design distributes pressure over the larger dorsal wrist surface area. "This design is better tolerated by edematous hands because of the pressure distribution. Either design may be used as a base for dynamic splinting, but the dorsal design stabilizes the wrist more effectively when splinting for dynamic finger flexion" (Colditz, 1995).

Features of the Wrist Cock-Up Splint

The static wrist cock-up splint maintains the wrist in proper alignment and provides support for the hand by stabilizing the wrist. When serving as a base for a dynamic splint, a wrist cock-up splint properly positions the wrist to provide an attachment site for the outrigger.

When fabricating a volar or dorsal wrist cock-up splint, the therapist must be aware of certain features of the various components (Fess & Philips, 1987). For example, the forearm trough should be two-thirds the length of the forearm and one-half the width of the forearm for a proper biomechanical fit. The hypothenar bar helps to place the hand in a neutral resting position by preventing extreme

SELF QUIZ 5-1*

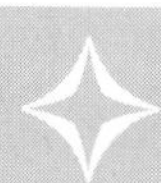

Please circle either true (T) or false (F).

1. T F Wrist cock-up splints can be volar or dorsal.
2. T F A wrist cock-up splint usually decreases wrist pain or inflammation, provides support, enhances digital function, and prevents wrist deformity.
3. T F The therapist must follow standard treatment protocols *exactly* for any diagnosis that requires a wrist cock-up splint application.
4. T F With a wrist cock-up splint the therapist usually splints the wrist in extreme extension, which promotes functional movement.
5. T F The hypothenar bar on a wrist cock-up splint helps to position the hand in a neutral resting position by preventing extreme ulnar deviation.
6. T F The therapist should position the volar wrist cock-up splint distal to the distal palmar crease.

***See Appendix A for the answer key.**

ulnar deviation. The hypothenar bar should not inhibit the motions of the ring and little fingers. The metacarpal (MP) bar supports the transverse MP arch. When supporting the palmar surface of the hand, the MP bar is sometimes called a *palmar bar.* With a volar wrist cock-up splint the therapist should position this bar proximal to the distal palmar crease and distal to the thenar crease to ensure full MCP flexion. On a dorsal wrist cock-up splint the therapist should position this bar slightly below the MP heads.

Fabrication of a Wrist Cock-Up Splint

The initial step in the fabrication of a wrist cock-up splint (after evaluation of the patient's hand) is the drawing of a pattern. Every patient's hand is different in shape and size and requires a specific pattern.

A common mistake of a beginning splintmaker during fabrication of a wrist cock-up pattern is drawing the forearm trough narrower than the natural curve of the forearm muscle-bulk contour. This mistake is common with a patient who

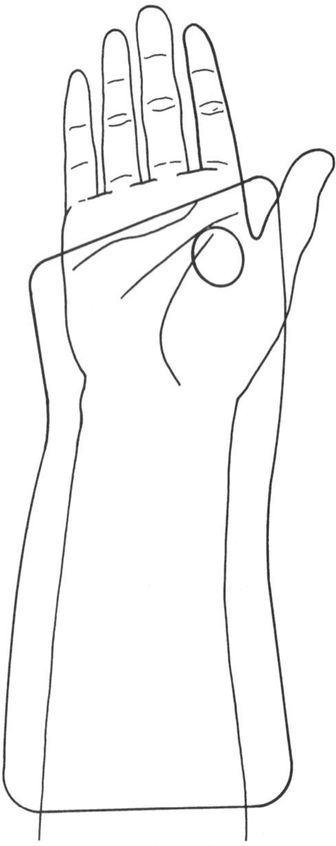

FIGURE 5-5 A volar wrist cock-up splint pattern

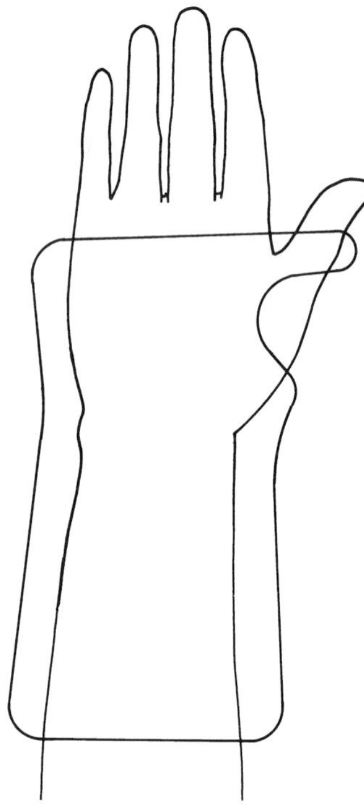

FIGURE 5-6 A dorsal wrist cock-up splint pattern

has a large forearm. If the forearm trough is not one-half the circumference of the forearm, the splint does not provide adequate support. To avoid lack of wrist support, the therapist must begin drawing the forearm aspect of the pattern on the radial side just proximal to the thumb carpometacarpal (CMC) joint (Figure 5-7). This guideline is important because some thermoplastic splinting materials tend to stretch. If the therapist leaves too much space at the wrist joint, the patient will not have enough wrist support. In addition, the therapist must follow the angle of the MP heads with the pattern to allow adequate hand support.

This volar wrist cock-up pattern presents another splinting option (Figure 5-5). The therapist constructs the splint by punching a hole in the heated thermoplastic material and pushing the thumb through the hole. The therapist rolls the material away from the thumb and thenar eminence far enough so that it does not interfere with functional thumb movement and yet allow adequate wrist support.

Beginning splintmakers may learn to fabricate splint patterns by following detailed written instructions and looking at pictures of patterns. As therapists gain experience, they can easily draw patterns without copying from pictures. (See Figures 5-1 and 5-2 for pictures of completed splint products.) The following instructions are for construction of a volar wrist cock-up splint (Figure 5-7) and are similar to instructions for a dorsal wrist cock-up splint (Figure 5-6):

1. Position the patient's hand palm down on a piece of paper. The fingers should be in a natural resting position and slightly abducted. Draw an outline of the hand and forearm to the elbow.
2. While the patient's hand is still on the paper, mark an *A* at the radial styloid and a *B* at the ulnar styloid. Mark the second and fifth MP heads *C* and *D*, respectively. Mark the CMC joint of the thumb *E*, and mark the olecranon process of the elbow *F*. Remove the hand from the pattern. Mark two-thirds the length of the forearm on each side with an *X*. Place another *X* on each side of the pattern about 1 to 1½ inches outside and parallel to the 2 previous *X* markings for two-thirds the length of the forearm and label each *G*.
3. Draw an angled line connecting the marks of the second and fifth metacarpal heads (*C* to *D*). Extend this line approximately 1 to 1½ inches from the ulnar side of the hand and mark it *H*. On the radial side of the hand, extend the line straight out approximately 2 inches and mark it *I*.
4. On the ulnar side of the splint, extend the metacarpal line from the *H* down the hand and forearm of the splint pattern, and make sure that the pattern follows the patient's forearm muscle bulk. End this line at *G*.
5. Measure and place a *J* approximately ¾ inch below the mark for the head of the index finger *(C)*. Extend a line parallel from *J* to the line between *C* and *I*. Curve this line to meet *I*. This area represents the extension of the MP bar and usually measures approximately ¾ inch down from *C* to the outline on the other side of the MP bar. Draw a curved line that simulates

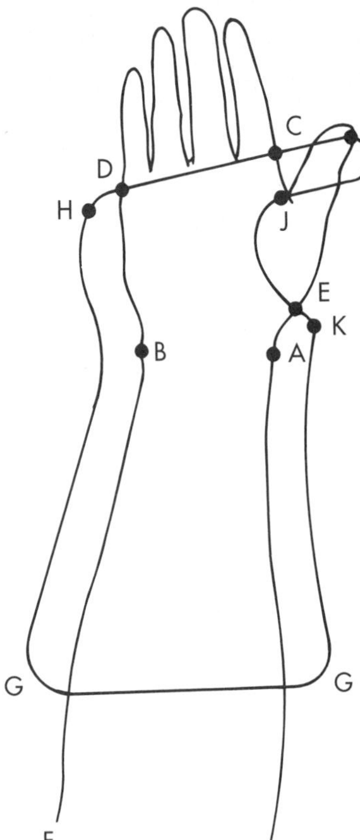

FIGURE 5-7 A detailed pattern for a volar wrist cock-up splint

the thenar crease from *J* to *E*. Extend the line past *E* about 1 inch and mark it *K*.

6. Draw a line from *K* down the radial side of the forearm, and make sure that the line follows the increasing size of the forearm. To ensure that the splint is two-thirds the length of the forearm, end the line at *G*.
7. For the bottom of the splint, draw a straight line connecting both *G* marks.
8. Make sure that the pattern lines are rounded at *I, H, K,* and the two *G*s.
9. Cut out the pattern.
10. Position the patient's upper extremity with the elbow resting on the table and the forearm in a neutral position. Make sure the fingers are relaxed and the thumb is lightly touching the index finger. Place the wrist cock-up pattern on the patient as Figure 5-8 demonstrates. Check that the wrist has adequate support. On the dorsal surface of the hand, check whether the hypothenar bar ends just proximal to the fifth metacarpal head and whether the metacarpal bar on the radial side of the hand ends just proximal to the third

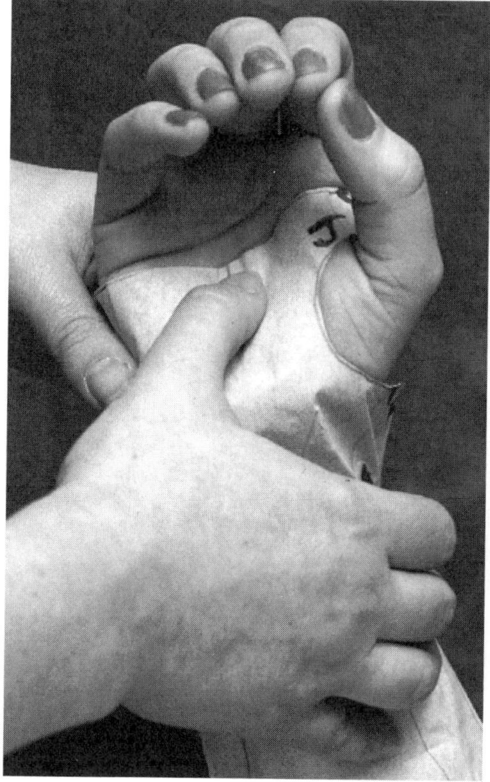

FIGURE 5-8 Placing of the wrist cock-up pattern on the patient

metacarpal head. On the volar surface of the hand, check below the thumb CMC joint to determine whether the pattern provides enough support at the wrist joint. Make sure that the forearm trough is two-thirds the length and one-half the width of the forearm. Make necessary adjustments (i.e., additions or deletions) on the pattern.

11. Trace the pattern onto the sheet of thermoplastic material.
12. Heat the thermoplastic material.
13. Cut the pattern out of the thermoplastic material.
14. Measure the wrist of the patient by using a goniometer to determine whether the wrist has been placed in the correct degree of extension (Figure 5-9).
15. Reheat the thermoplastic material.
16. Mold the form onto the patient's hand. One way to fit the splint is to place the patient's elbow in a resting position on the table with the forearm in a neutral position. Make sure the fingers are relaxed and the thumb is lightly

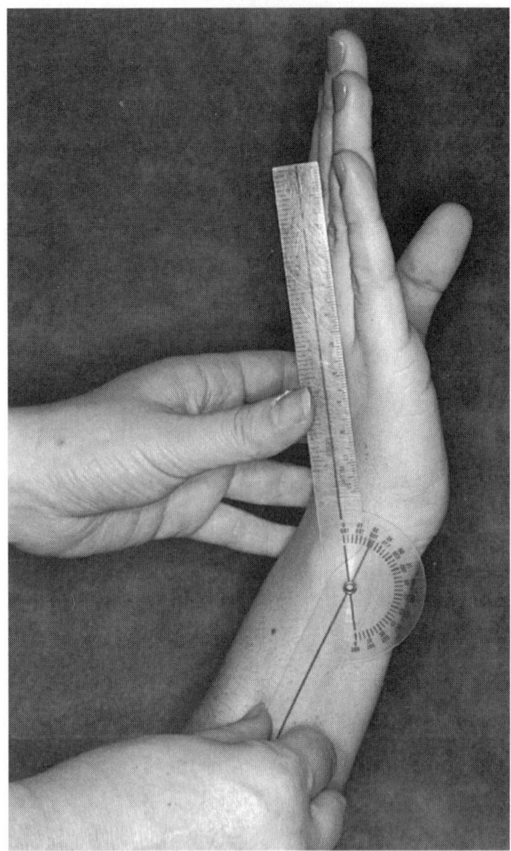

FIGURE 5-9
Before forming the splint, the therapist should measure the patient's wrist with a goniometer to obtain the correct amount of extension.

touching the index finger (Figure 5-10). The advantage of this approach is that the therapist can better monitor the wrist position visually during splint formation. Another way to fit a volar wrist cock-up splint is to position the patient's upper extremity with the shoulder adducted, the elbow flexed, and the forearm supinated over a towel roll (Figure 5-11). For a dorsal wrist cock-up splint, use the same positions but pronate the forearm. The advantage of positioning the patient's upper extremity in this gravity-eliminated position is that the theromoplastic material is less likely to stretch.

17. Make sure the wrist remains correctly positioned as the thermoplastic material hardens. During the formation phase, roll the metacarpal bar just proximal to the distal palmar crease and roll the thermoplastic material to the thenar crease (Figure 5-12). Flair the distal end of the splint on a flat surface (Figure 5-13).
18. Make necessary adjustments on the splint (Figures 5-14 and 5-15).

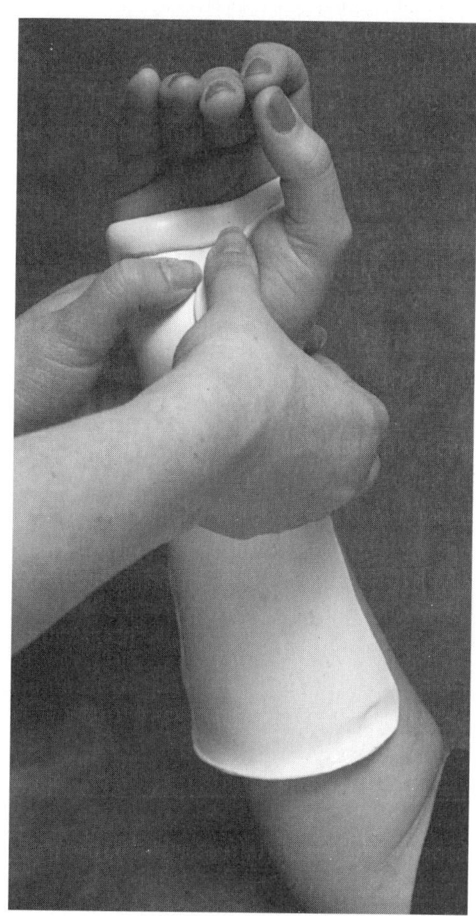

FIGURE 5-10 A position for molding the wrist cock-up splint

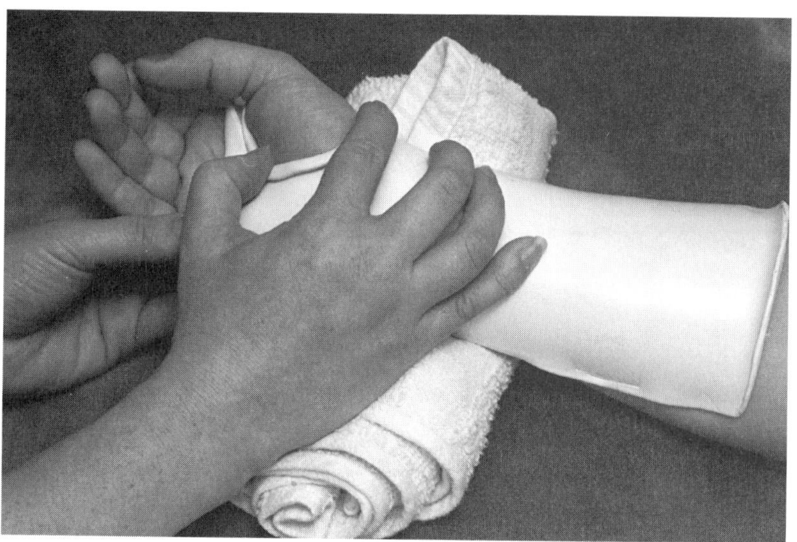

FIGURE 5-11 A position for molding the wrist cock-up splint

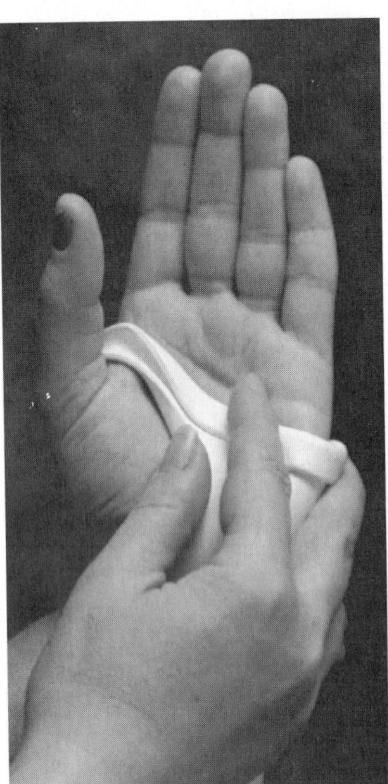

FIGURE 5-12
The therapist should roll the metacarpal bar just proximal to the distal palmar crease and roll the thermoplastic material to the thenar crease.

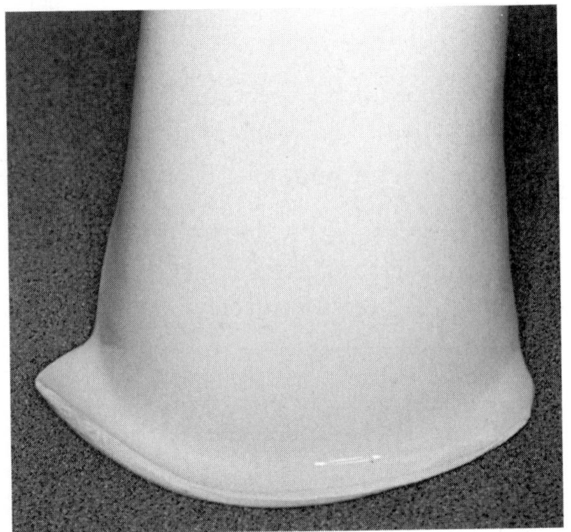

FIGURE 5-13 Flaring of the distal end of the splint on a flat surface

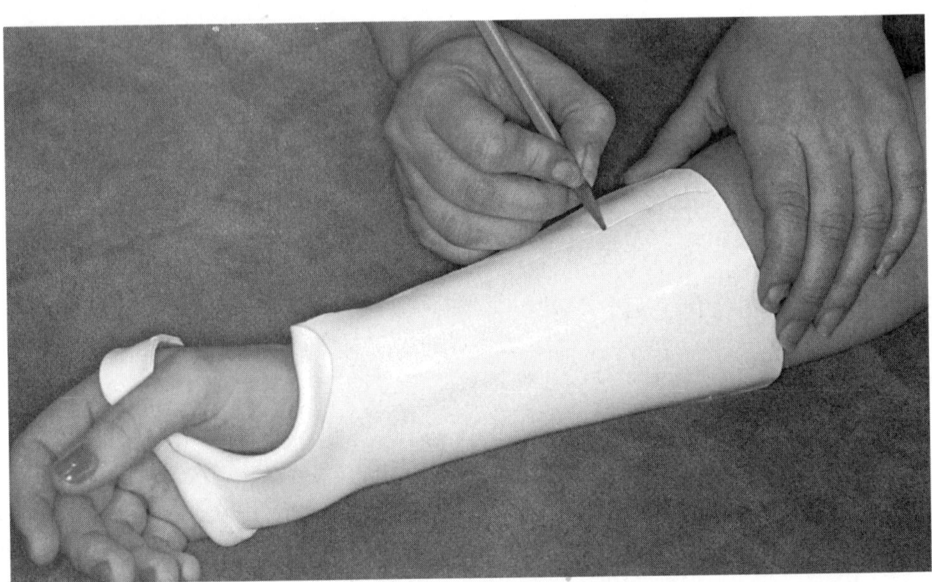

FIGURE 5-14 Marking of the splint to make an adjustment

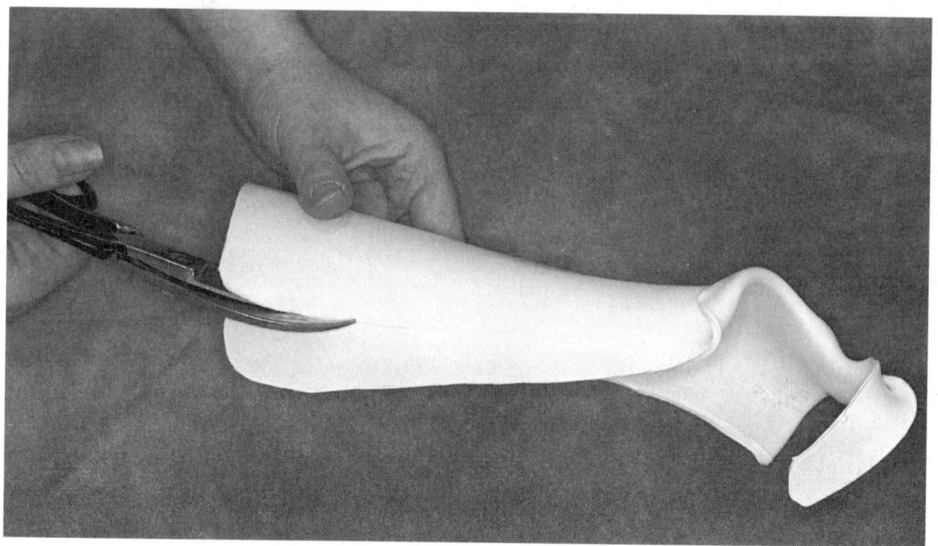

FIGURE 5-15 Cutting of excess warm thermoplastic material to make an adjustment

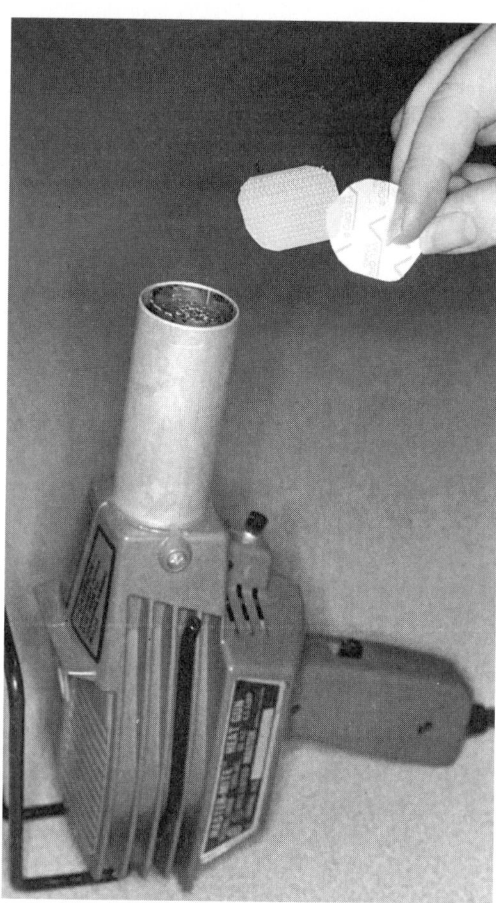

FIGURE 5-16 Heating of the velcro tabs with a heat gun to help them adhere to the splint

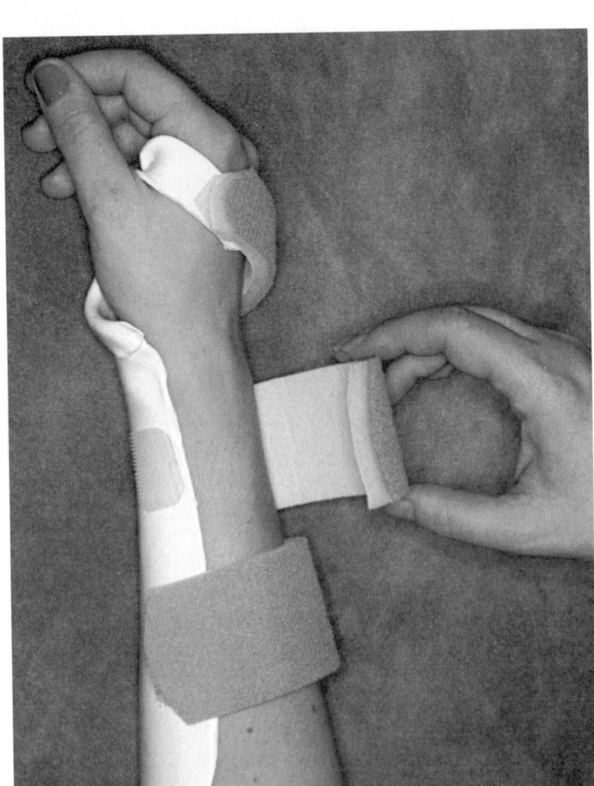

FIGURE 5-17
The therapist should place two straps on the forearm trough and one strap on the dorsal surface of the hand that connects the metacarpal bar to the hypothenar bar.

19. Cut the velcro tabs and heat them with a heat gun to encourage adherence before putting them on the splint (Figure 5-16). Add two straps on the forearm trough and one strap on the dorsal surface of the hand, thus connecting the metacarpal bar on the radial side to the hypothenar bar on the ulnar side of the hand (Figure 5-17).

Technical Tips for a Proper Fit

1. Use caution when cutting a pattern out of thermoplastic material that stretches easily. Leave stretchable thermoplastic material flat on the table when cutting to prevent the material from stretching and the splint from losing the original shape.

Laboratory Exercise 5-1

1. Practice making a wrist cock-up splint pattern on another person. Use the detailed instructions provided to draw the pattern.
2. Using the outline for the left hand below, draw a wrist cock-up pattern without the detailed instructions.

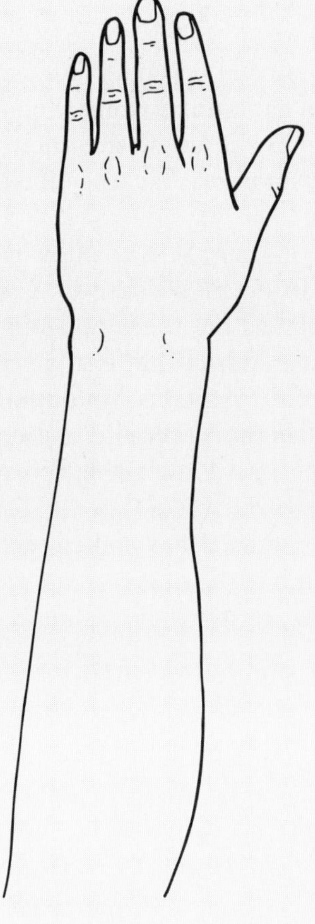

2. Make sure the splint follows the natural curves of the longitudinal, distal, and proximal arches. Choose a thermoplastic splinting material that has a high degree of conformability. To maintain the natural curves and arches when fabricating the splint, mold the thermoplastic material in the center of the palm.

3. For a volar wrist cock-up splint, position the metacarpal bar on the volar surface just proximal to the distal palmar crease. This position allows adequate wrist support and full MCP flexion. Always determine whether the patient has full finger flexion when wearing the splint. In addition, make sure the metacarpal bar follows the natural angle of the distal transverse arch (Figure 5-18).
4. Roll the thermoplastic material around the thumb-web section to help prevent skin irritation (Figure 5-18).
5. Make sure the hand and wrist are positioned correctly by taking into consideration the position of a normal resting hand. On volar and dorsal wrist cock-up splints the metacarpal bar (which wraps around the radial side of the hand) and the hypothenar bar (on the ulnar side) help position and hold the wrist (Figure 5-19). If adequate support is lacking on either side, the wrist may be in an incorrect position.

   A frequent fabrication mistake is to allow the wrist to deviate radially or ulnarly. This mistake can occur because of a lack of careful monitoring of the patient's wrist position as the thermoplastic material is cooling. If a mistake occurs with a splint material that easily stretches, be extremely careful with adjustments to avoid further compromising of wrist positioning. For splinting material with memory, remold the entire splint rather than spot heating the wrist area because doing the latter tends to cause the material to buckle.
6. After the thermoplastic material has cooled, determine whether the patient can fully oppose the thumb to all fingers. The thenar eminence should not be restricted or flattened. Yet, wrist support should be adequate.

Precautions for a Wrist Cock-Up Splint

A careful splintmaker must continuously think of precautions. The therapist must instruct the patient to remove the splint for an ROM program to prevent joint stiffness and limitations (Pedretti & Zoltan, 1990). Precautions for making a wrist cock-up splint include the following:

1. Be aware of and make adjustments for potential pressure points on the ulnar styloid, at the first web space, and over the dorsal aspects of the metacarpals. The thumb-web space is a prime area for skin irritation. Instruct the patient to monitor the skin for reddened areas and to communicate immediately about any irritation that occurs.
2. Try to control edema before splint provision. For patients with sustained edema, avoid using constricting wrist splints. Instead, fabricate a wider forearm trough with wide strapping material (Cannon, et al., 1985). Dorsal splints are better for edematous hands (Colditz, 1995). Carefully monitor patients

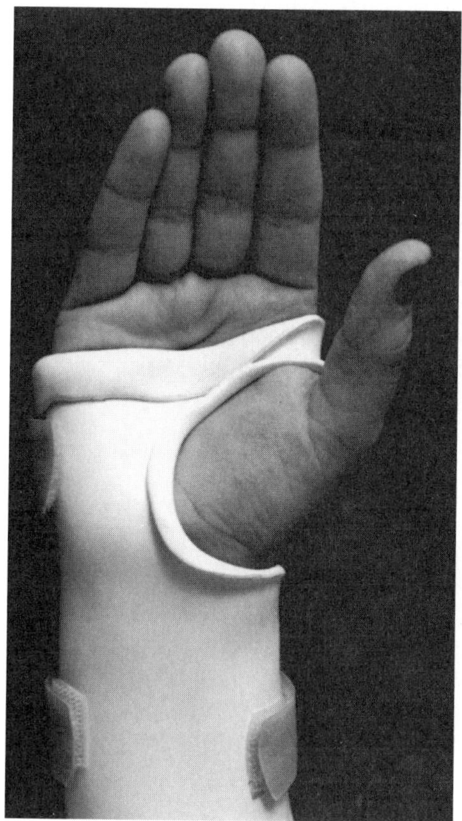

FIGURE 5-18
The therapist should position the metacarpal bar just proximal to the distal palmar crease and follow the natural angle of the distal transverse arch. Note the rolled thermoplastic material around the thenar eminence.

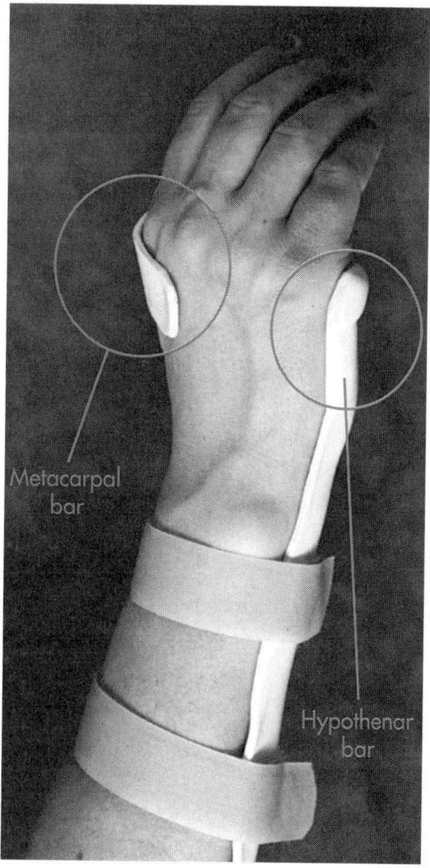

FIGURE 5-19
The metacarpal bar and hypothenar bar help position and hold the wrist.

who have the potential for edematous hands and make necessary splint adjustments.

3. For patients with thin skin, carefully monitor the skin for pressure areas. Lining the splint with padding may help, but several adjustments may be necessary for a proper fit.
4. Make sure the splint provides adequate support for functional activities.
5. Wrist cock-up splints are contraindicated for patients suffering from active MCP synovitis and proximal interphalangeal synovitis (Melvin, 1989). These conditions often occur with rheumatoid arthritic hands.

6. For a patient with rheumatoid arthritis, pressure increases on the MCP joints during wrist immobilization with a splint. Joint inflammation can contribute to "stretching of the periarticular structures and resultant volar subluxation or ulnar deviation" (Geisser, 1984, p. 37).

Laboratory Exercise 5-2* Splint Problem Identification and Evaluation

Splinting involves critical evaluation skills. The beginning splintmaker must be able to identify splint problems by looking at the splint on the patient. For the following patient scenarios, determine problems by looking at the pictures. In addition, problem solve consequences of splinting a patient in the wrong positions.

SPLINT A

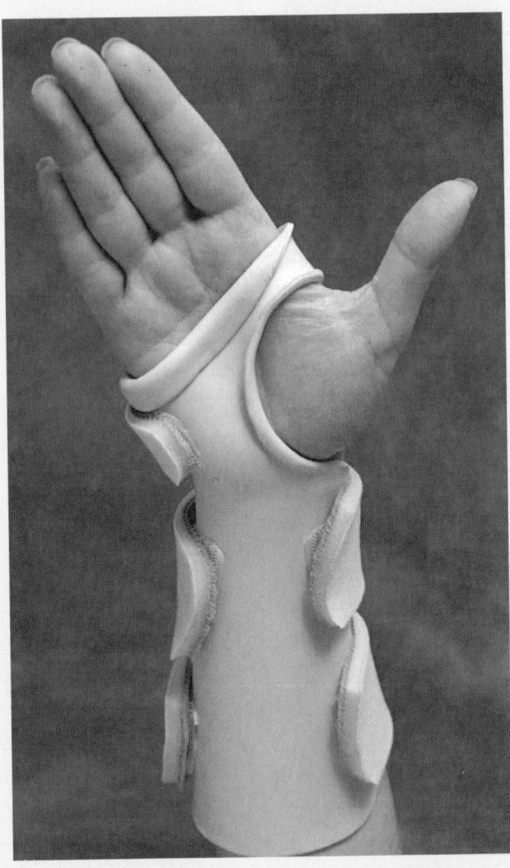

*See Appendix A for the answer key.

Laboratory Exercise 5-2 Splint Problem Identification and Evaluation—cont'd

Splint A was made for a 33-year-old woman suffering from carpal tunnel syndrome. She works 40 hours weekly as a checkout clerk in a grocery store.

1. What problems can you identify regarding this splint?

____

____

____

2. What problems may arise from continual splint wear?

____

____

____

SPLINT B

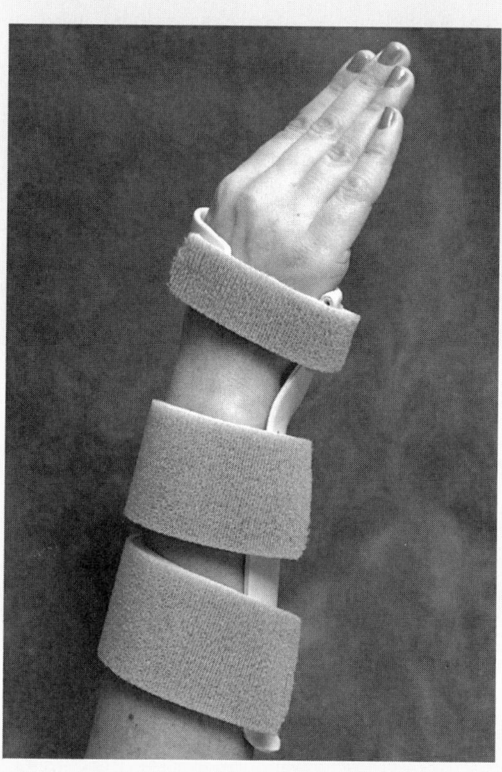

Continued.

Laboratory Exercise 5-2 Splint Problem Identification and Evaluation—cont'd

You are supervising a student in clinical practice. You ask the student to practice making a wrist cock-up splint before actually fabricating a splint on a patient. Splint B is a picture of the student's splint.

1. What problems should you address with the student regarding the splint?

____

____

____

SPLINT C

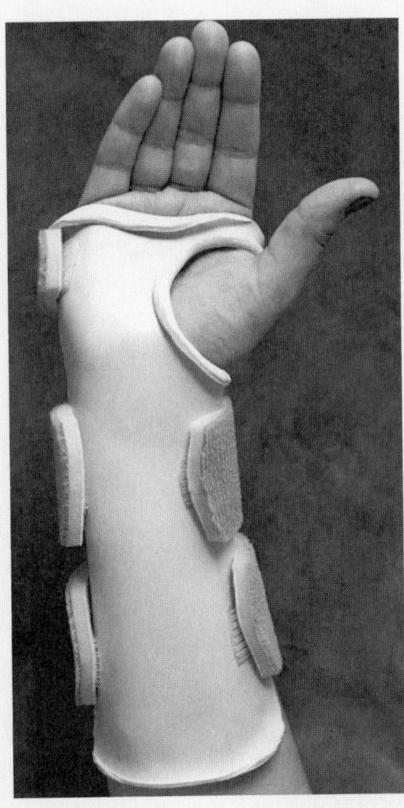

Laboratory Exercise 5-2 Splint Problem Identification and Evaluation—cont'd

Splint C was made for a 54-year-old man working as a bus driver. The patient works full time and suffers from wrist extensor tendinitis.

1. What problems can you identify regarding this splint?

   ____

   ____

   ____

2. What problems may arise from continual splint wear?

   ____

   ____

   ____

Laboratory Exercise 5-3

Practice fabricating a wrist cock-up splint on a partner.

Before starting, determine the correct position for your partner's hand. Measure the angle of wrist extension with a goniometer to ensure a correct position. After fitting your splint and making all adjustments, use Form 5-1 as a self-evaluation of the wrist cock-up splint, and use Grading Sheet 5-1 as a classroom grading sheet.

FORM 5-1* Wrist Cock-Up Splint

Name: ____________________

Date: ____________________

Type of wrist cock-up splint:

Volar Dorsal

Wrist position: ____________________

After the person wears the splint for 30 minutes, answer the following questions. (Mark *NA* for nonapplicable situations.)

Evaluation Areas		Comments
Design		
1. The wrist position is at the correct angle.	Yes ❍ No ❍ NA ❍	
2. The wrist has adequate support.	Yes ❍ No ❍ NA ❍	
3. The sides of the thenar and hypothenar eminences have support in the correct position.	Yes ❍ No ❍ NA ❍	
4. The thenar and hypothenar eminences are not restricted or flattened.	Yes ❍ No ❍ NA ❍	
5. The splint is two-thirds the length of the forearm.	Yes ❍ No ❍ NA ❍	
6. The splint is one-half the width of the forearm.	Yes ❍ No ❍ NA ❍	
Function		
1. The splint allows full thumb motions.	Yes ❍ No ❍ NA ❍	
2. The splint allows full MCP joint flexion of the fingers.	Yes ❍ No ❍ NA ❍	
3. The splint provides wrist support that allows functional activities.	Yes ❍ No ❍ NA ❍	

*See Appendix B for a perforated copy of this form.

FORM 5-1 Wrist Cock-Up Splint—cont'd

Evaluation Areas				Comments
Straps				
1. The straps avoid bony prominences.	Yes ❍	No ❍	NA ❍	
2. The straps are secure and rounded.	Yes ❍	No ❍	NA ❍	
Comfort				
1. The splint edges are smooth with rounded corners.	Yes ❍	No ❍	NA ❍	
2. The proximal end is flared.	Yes ❍	No ❍	NA ❍	
3. Impingements or pressure areas are not present.	Yes ❍	No ❍	NA ❍	
Cosmetic Appearance				
1. The splint is free of fingerprints, dirt, and pencil and pen marks.	Yes ❍	No ❍	NA ❍	
2. The splinting material is not buckled.	Yes ❍	No ❍	NA ❍	

Discuss possible splint adjustments or changes you should make based on the self-evaluation:

___

___

___

___

___

___

___

___

___

___

___

___

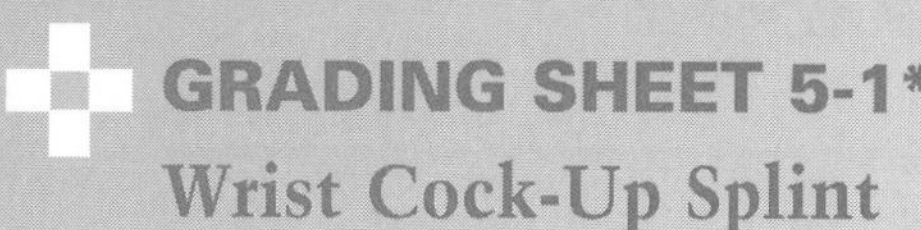

GRADING SHEET 5-1*
Wrist Cock-Up Splint

Name: ______________________________

Date: ______________________________

Type of wrist cock-up splint:
Volar Dorsal

Wrist position: ______________

Grade: ______________

1 = beyond improvement, not acceptable
2 = requires maximal improvement
3 = requires moderate improvement
4 = requires minimal improvement
5 = requires no improvement

Evaluation Areas		**Comments**
Design		
1. The wrist position is at the correct angle.	1 2 3 4 5	
2. The wrist has adequate support.	1 2 3 4 5	
3. The sides of the thenar and hypothenar eminences have support in the correct position.	1 2 3 4 5	
4. The thenar and hypothenar eminences are not restricted or flattened.	1 2 3 4 5	
5. The splint is two-thirds the length of the forearm.	1 2 3 4 5	
6. The splint is one-half the width of the forearm.	1 2 3 4 5	

*See Appendix C for a perforated copy of this grading sheet.

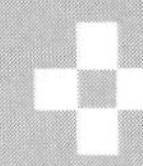

GRADING SHEET 5-1
Wrist Cock-Up Splint—cont'd

Evaluation Areas		Comments
Function		
1. The splint allows full thumb motion.	1 2 3 4 5	
2. The splint allows full MCP joint flexion of the fingers.	1 2 3 4 5	
3. The splint provides wrist support that allows functional activities.	1 2 3 4 5	
Straps		
1. The straps avoid bony prominences.	1 2 3 4 5	
2. The straps are secure and rounded.	1 2 3 4 5	
Comfort		
1. The splint edges are smooth with rounded corners.	1 2 3 4 5	
2. The proximal end is flared.	1 2 3 4 5	
3. Impingements or pressure areas are not present.	1 2 3 4 5	
Cosmetic Appearance		
1. The splint is free of fingerprints, dirt, and pencil and pen marks.	1 2 3 4 5	
2. The splinting material is not buckled.	1 2 3 4 5	

Case Study*

Read the following scenario and answer the questions based on information in this chapter:

Mrs. Smith is a 42-year-old woman who works in the billing department at a local hospital. Much of her work involves typing on the computer. About 2 years ago she started complaining about numbness, tingling, and pain in her right, dominant hand, including the thumb, index finger, middle finger, and half of the ring finger. Mrs. Smith ignored the symptoms until they became unbearable. She then went to her physician. The physician referred her to a neurologist who determined from testing that Mrs. Smith had substantial median nerve damage. The physician ordered the occupational therapist to fabricate a wrist splint, provide education about carpal tunnel syndrome, and establish the patient on a home ROM exercise program.

1. Which of the following is the physician's rationale for ordering the wrist splint?
   a. To provide rest and support for the involved upper extremity during the acute flare-up of the condition
   b. To help decrease wrist pain
   c. Both a and b
2. Which of the following is the best wrist cock-up splint for Mrs. Smith?
   a. A dorsal wrist cock-up splint
   b. A volar wrist cock-up splint
   c. Either a or b depending on the patient's need for support
3. Which of the following is the correct wrist position for the splint?
   a. Neutral (0°)
   b. Extension of 20°
   c. Extension of 30°
4. Which of the following most likely describes an appropriate wearing schedule for this patient?
   a. Wear the wrist cock-up splint only during sleep.
   b. Wear the wrist cock-up splint 4 to 6 weeks continuously with removal for ROM and hygiene.
   c. Either a or b is correct depending on the protocol.
5. Which of the following precautions should you include in the patient's instructions and education?
   a. Observe areas such as the ulnar styloid, the first web space, and the volar and dorsal aspect of the hand over the metacarpal bones for skin irritation.
   b. Notify the therapist immediately if irritation occurs.
   c. a and b are both correct.

*See Appendix A for the answer key.

REVIEW QUESTIONS

1. What are three main indications for use of a wrist cock-up splint?
2. What is the advantage of a volar wrist cock-up splint?
3. What is a disadvantage of a dorsal wrist cock-up splint?
4. What purpose does the hypothenar bar serve on a wrist cock-up splint?
5. What are two positions that the therapist can use for molding a static wrist splint, and what are the advantages of each?
6. Which precautions are unique to static wrist cock-up splints?

References

American Society of Hand Therapists. (1992). Splint classification system. Garner, NC: American Society of Hand Therapists.

Cailliet, R. (1994). Hand pain and impairment. Philadelphia: F. A. Davis Co.

Cannon, N. M., Foltz, R. W., Koepfer, J. M., Lauck, M. R., Simpson, D. M., & Bromley R. S. (1985) Manual of hand splinting. New York: Churchill Livingstone Inc.

Colditz, J. C. (1984). Arthritis. In M. H. Malick & M. C. Kasch (Eds.), Manual on management of specific hand problems (pp. 112-136). Pittsburgh: AREN Publications.

Colditz, J. C. (March, 1995). Personal communication.

Colditz, J. C. (October 15, 1995). Personal communication.

Fess, E. E., & Philips, C. A. (1987). Hand splinting principles and methods (2nd ed.). St. Louis: Mosby.

Geisser, R. W. (1984). Splinting the rheumatoid arthritic hand. In E. M. Ziegler (Ed.), Current concepts in orthosis (pp. 29-49). Germantown, WI: Rolyan Medical Products.

Melvin, J. L. (1989). Rheumatic disease in the adult and child (3rd ed.). Philadelphia: F. A. Davis Co.

Pedretti, L. W., & Zoltan, B. (1990). Occupational therapy practice skills for physical dysfunction. St. Louis: Mosby.

CHAPTER SIX

Resting Hand Splints (Hand Immobilization Splints)

BRENDA M. COPPARD, MS, OTR/L

Chapter Objectives

1. List diagnoses that benefit from resting hand splints.
2. Describe the functional or midjoint position of the wrist, thumb, and digits.
3. Describe the antideformity or intrinsic plus position of the wrist, thumb, and digits.
4. List the purposes of a resting hand splint.
5. Identify the components of a resting hand splint.
6. Explain the precautions to consider when fabricating a resting hand splint.
7. Determine a resting hand splint–wearing schedule for different diagnostic indications.
8. Apply knowledge about the application of the resting hand splint to a case study.
9. Use clinical judgment to evaluate a fabricated resting hand splint.

Physicians commonly order resting hand splints, also known as hand immobilization splints (American Society of Hand Therapists, 1992). A resting hand splint is a static splint that immobilizes the fingers, thumb, and wrist. Therapists can make resting hand splints from scratch or purchase them commercially. Some of the commercially sold resting hand splints are prefabricated, premolded, and ready to wear. Others are sold in kits. Each of these splints has advantages and disadvantages.

Therapists can order premolded commercial splints according to hand size (i.e., small, medium, large, and extra large) for the right or left hand. An advantage of premade splints is their quick application; usually only straps require application. A disadvantage is that the splint may not exactly fit each patient.

A resting hand splint kit typically contains strapping materials and precut thermoplastic material in the shape of a resting hand splint. Kits are available according to hand size (i.e., small, medium, large, and extra large). An advantage of using a kit is the time the therapist saves by eliminating pattern making and thermoplastic material cutting. A disadvantage is that the pattern is not customized to the patient. Therefore the splint may require many adjustments.

A therapist can customize a resting hand splint by making a pattern and fabricating the splint from thermoplastic material. The advantage is an exact fit for the patient, which increases the splint's support and comfort. A disadvantage is that customization may require more of the therapist's time to complete the splint and may be more costly.

Diagnostic Indications

Patients requiring resting hand splints commonly have arthritis (Ouellette, 1991) or burn injuries to the hand. The resting hand splint provides localized rest to the tissues of the fingers, thumb, and wrist.

For inflammatory conditions the resting hand splint positions the hand in a functional or midjoint position (Colditz, 1995) (Figure 6-1). The functional position of the splint places the wrist in 20° to 30° of extension, the thumb in palmar abduction, the metacarpophalangeal joints in 15° to 20° of flexion, and all the digits in slight flexion. Therapists use this splint with patients who have periods of acute inflammation and pain (Ziegler, 1984) and with patients who do not use their hands for activities but require support and immobilization (Leonard, 1990). The use of splints on patients who have rheumatoid arthritis for purposes of rest dur-

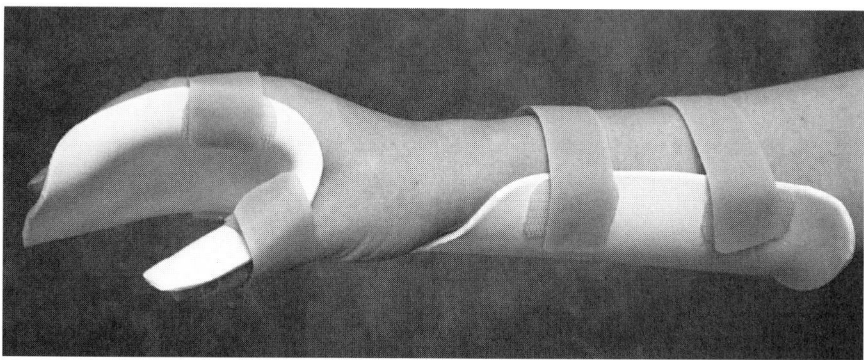

FIGURE 6-1 A resting hand splint with the hand in a functional (midjoint) position

ing pain and inflammation is controversial. Periods of rest (3 weeks or less) seem to be beneficial, but longer periods may cause loss of motion (Ouellette, 1991).

For a patient who has severe deformities or exacerbations from arthritis the resting hand splint often positions the wrist at neutral or slight extension and 5° to 10° of ulnar deviation (Marx, 1992; Geisser, 1984). The thumb may be positioned midway between radial and palmar abduction to increase comfort.

Therapists do not splint patients who have hand burns in the functional position. Instead, the therapist places the hand in the (intrinsic plus) (Colditz, 1995) antideformity position (Figure 6-2). The antideformity position for a palmar or circumferential burn places the wrist in 30° to 40° of extension and 0° (i.e., neutral) for a dorsal hand burn. For dorsal and volar burns the therapist should flex the metacarpophalangeals (MCPs) to 70° to 90°, fully extend the proximal interphalangeals (PIPs) and distal interphalangeals (DIPs), and palmarly abduct the thumb to the index and middle fingers with the thumb interphalangeal (IP) joint extended (Salisbury, Reeves, & Wright, 1990). A splint applied in the first 72 hours after a burn may not fit the patient 2 hours after application because of significant edema that usually follows a burn injury. The therapist should closely monitor the patient to make necessary adjustments to the splint.

The therapist can position the wrist in 0° to 30° of extension, the MCPs in 60° to 80° of flexion, the PIPs and DIPs in full extension, and the thumb in palmar abduction and extension to splint a crushed hand (Colditz, 1995). Splinting a crushed hand into this position provides rest to the injured tissue and decreases pain, edema, and inflammation (Stanley & Tribuzi, 1992).

Resting hand splints are appropriate "for protecting tendons, joints, capsular and ligamentous structures, and also irritated, surgically released, or transposed nerves" (Leonard, 1990, p. 909). These diagnoses usually require the expertise of experienced therapists and may warrant different splints for day wear and resting hand splints for nighttime. (See Chapter 9 for splint interventions for nerve injuries.)

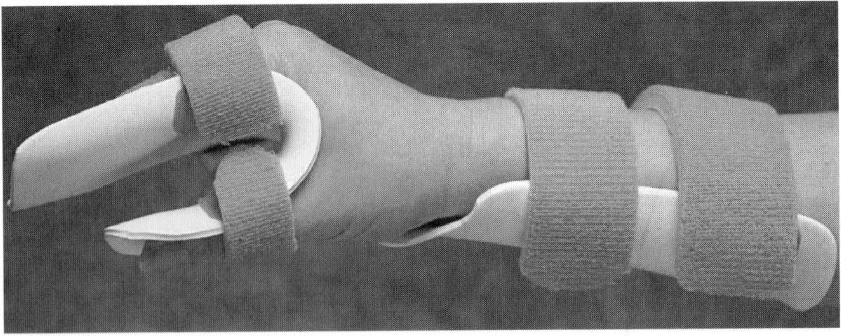

FIGURE 6-2 A resting hand splint with the hand in an antideformity (intrinsic plus) position

Therapists sometimes use resting hand splints to treat stroke patients who are at risk for developing contractures because of increased tone or spasticity (Malick, 1972). (See Chapter 10 for more information on splinting an extremity that has increased tone or spasticity.)

Table 6-1 lists common hand conditions that may require a resting hand splint and includes information regarding suggested hand positioning and wearing schedules. Beginning therapists should remember that these are general guidelines and that physicians and experienced therapists may have their own specific protocols for positioning and wearing.

TABLE 6-1 Conditions That Require a Resting Hand Splint

Hand Condition	Suggested Wearing Schedule	Position
RHEUMATOID ARTHRITIS		
Acute exacerbation*	Fitted to maintain as close to a functional (midjoint) position as possible until exacerbation is over, removed for hygiene and exercise purposes, and worn during the day and at nighttime as necessary.	Wrist—neutral or 20° to 30° extension depending on patient tolerance, 15° to 20° MCP flexion, and 5° to 10° ulnar deviation; thumb—position of comfort in between radial and palmar abduction
TRAUMA		
Crush injuries of the hand*	Fitted after the injury to reduce pain, edema, and swelling and to provide rest to injured tissues; worn at nighttime; and possibly worn as necessary during exacerbation periods	Wrist—extension of 0° to 30°; MCPs—flexion of 60° to 80°; PIP and DIPs—full extension; thumb—palmar abduction and extension
BURNS		
Dorsal or volar hand burns*	Worn after the burn injury; continuously worn until healing begins; and removed for dressing changes, hygiene, and exercises	Wrist—volar or circumferential burn (30° to 40° of extension), dorsal burn (0° = neutral); MCPs—flexion of 70° to 90°; PIP and DIPs—full extension; thumb—palmar abduction and extension

*Diagnosis may require additional types of splinting.

Purpose of the Resting Hand Splint

The resting hand splint has three purposes: to immobilize, to position in functional alignment, and to retard further deformity (Ziegler, 1984; Malick, 1972). When inflammation and pain are present in the hand, the joints and surrounding structures become swollen and result in hand positions not properly aligned.

The resting hand splint may retard further deformity for some patients. The therapist may provide a splint for a patient with arthritis who has early signs of ulnar drift by placing the patient in a comfortable neutral position with the joints in midposition. Rest by means of immobilization reduces symptoms. Joints are then "receptive to proper positioning so that optimal range of motion is maintained" (Ziegler, 1984, p. 34).

Features

The therapist must know the splint's components to make adjustments for a correct fit. The resting hand splint has four main components: the forearm trough, the pan, the thumb trough, and the C bar (Figure 6-3) (Fess & Philips, 1987).

The forearm trough (usually volarly based) is at the base of the splint and supports the weight of the forearm. The therapist should apply biomechanical principles to make the trough about two-thirds the length of the forearm to allow elbow flexion. The width should be one-half the circumference of the forearm. The proximal end of the splint should be flared or rolled to avoid a pressure area.

The pan of the splint supports the fingers and the palm. The therapist must conform the pan to the arches of the hand, thus helping to maintain hand functions such as grasping and cupping motions. The pan should be wide enough to house the width of the index, middle, ring, and little fingers when they are in a slightly abducted position. The sides of the pan should be curved so that they measure approximately ½ inch in height. The curved sides add strength to the pan and ensure that the fingers do not slide off the sides of the pan.

The thumb trough supports the thumb and should extend approximately ½ inch beyond the end of the thumb. This extension allows the entire thumb to rest in the trough. The width and depth of the thumb trough should be one-half the circumference of the thumb, which should be in a palmar abduction position. The therapist should place the carpometacarpal (CMC) joint in 40° to 45° of palmar abduction (Tenney & Lisak, 1986) and extend the thumb's IP and MCP joints.

The C bar keeps the web space of the thumb positioned in palmar abduction. If the web space tightens, it inhibits grasp. From the radial side of the splint the thumb, the web space, and the digits should resemble a C (see Figure 6-3).

Fabrication of a Resting Hand Splint

The first step in the fabrication of a resting hand splint is drawing a pattern similar to the one shown in Figure 6-4. Beginning splintmakers may learn to fabri-

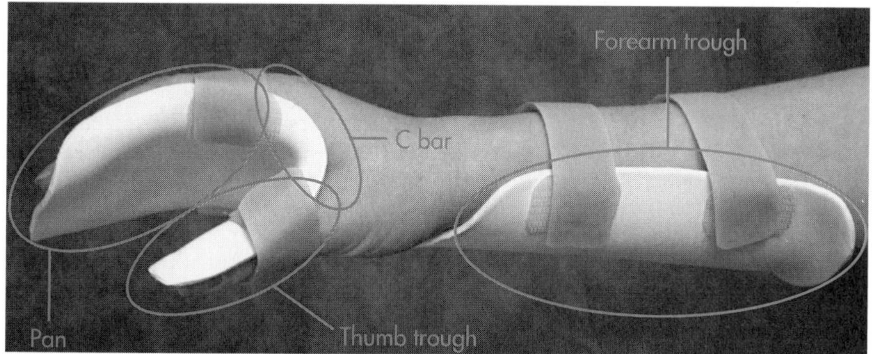

FIGURE 6-3

The components of a resting hand splint are the forearm trough, pan, thumb trough, and C bar.

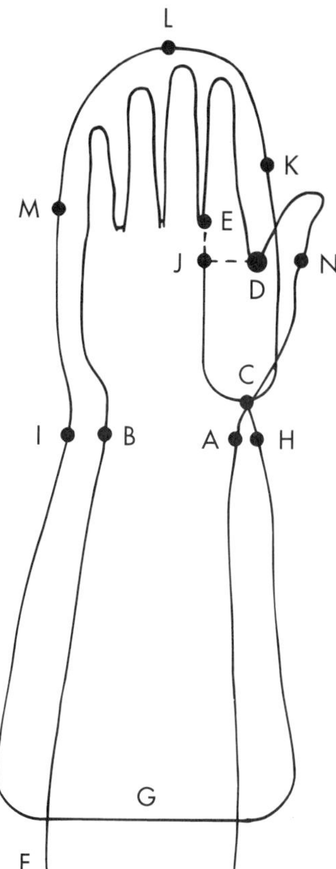

FIGURE 6-4 A detailed resting hand splint pattern

cate splint patterns by following detailed written instructions and by looking at pictures of splint patterns. As therapists gain more experience, they will be able to easily draw splint patterns without having to follow detailed instructions or pictures. The following are the detailed steps for fabricating a resting hand splint:

1. Place the patient's hand flat and palm down with the fingers slightly abducted on a paper towel. Trace the outline of the upper extremity from one side of the elbow to the other.
2. While the patient's hand is yet on the piece of paper, mark the following areas: (1) the radial styloid *A* and the ulnar styloid *B*, (2) the carpometacarpal joint of the thumb *C*, (3) the apex of the thumb web space *D*, (4) the web space between the second and third digits *E*, and (5) the olecranon process of the elbow *F*.
3. Remove the patient's hand from the piece of paper. Draw a line across indicating the two-thirds length of the forearm. Then label this line *G*. After doing this, extend line *G* about 1 to 1½ inches beyond each side of the outline of the arm. Then mark an *H* about 1 inch from the outline to the radial side of *A*. Mark an *I* about 1 inch from the outline to the ulnar side of *B*.
4. Draw a dotted, vertical line from the web space of the second and third digits *(E)* proximally down the palm about 3 inches. Draw a dotted, horizontal line from the bottom of the thumb web space *(D)* toward the ulnar side of the hand until the line intersects the dotted, vertical line. Mark a *J* at the intersection of these two dotted lines. Mark an *N* about 1 inch from the outline to the radial side of *D*.
5. Draw a solid, vertical line from *J* toward the wrist. Then curve this line so that it meets *C* on the pattern (see Figure 6-4). This part of the pattern is known as the thumb trough. After reaching *C*, curve the line upward until it reaches halfway between *N* and *D*.
6. Mark a *K* about 1 inch to the radial side of the index finger's PIP joint. Mark an *L* 1 inch from the top of the outline of the middle finger. Mark an *M* about 1 inch to the ulnar side of the little finger's PIP joint.
7. Draw the line that ends to the side of *N* through *K*, and extend the line upward and around the corner through *L*. From L, round the corner to connect the line with *M* and then pass it through *I*. Continue drawing the line and connect it with the end of *G*. Connect the radial end of *G* to pass through *H*. From *H*, extend the line toward *C*. Curve the line so that it connects to *C* (Figure 6-4).
8. Cut out the pattern. Cut the solid lines of the thumb trough also. Do *not* cut the dotted lines.

Laboratory Exercise 6-1

1. Practice making a resting hand splint pattern on another person. Use the detailed instructions provided to draw the pattern. Cut out the pattern and make necessary adjustments.
2. Use the outline of the hand below to draw the resting hand splint pattern without using the detailed instructions.

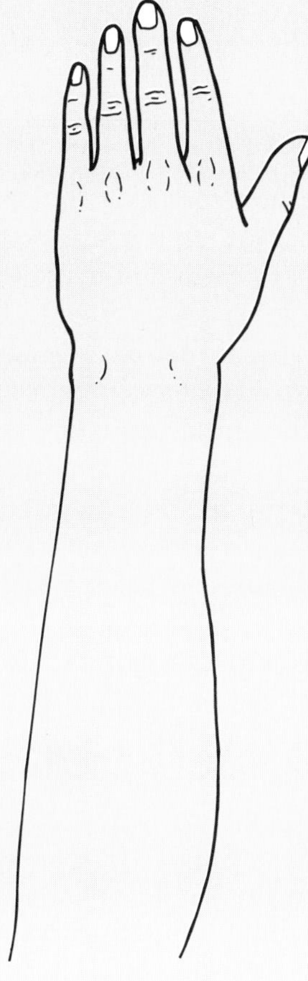

9. Place the pattern on the patient. Moistening the paper towel allows detailed assessment of the pattern fit. Make necessary adjustments (e.g., additions, deletions) on the pattern.
10. With a pencil, trace the splint pattern onto the sheet of thermoplastic material.
11. Heat the thermoplastic material.
12. Cut the pattern out of the thermoplastic material and reheat.
13. Instruct the patient to rest the elbow on the table. The arm should be vertical and the hand relaxed. Although some thermoplastic materials in the vertical position may stretch during the molding process, the vertical position allows the best control of the wrist position. Mold the plastic form onto the patient's hand and make necessary adjustments.
14. Add straps to the pan, the thumb trough, and the forearm trough (Figure 6-5).

Technical Tips for a Proper Fit

1. For patients who have fleshier forearms the splint pattern requires an allowance of more than 1 inch on each side. To be accurate, measure the circumference of the patient's forearm and make the splint pattern one half of this measurement.
2. Choose a thermoplastic material that has strength or rigidity, and avoid materials that have excessive stretch characteristics. The splint material must be strong enough to support the entire hand, wrist, and forearm. A thermoplastic material that the therapist can reheat several times is beneficial if the splint requires adjustment.
3. Make sure that the splint supports the wrist area well. If the thumb trough is cut beyond the thumb carpometacarpal joint, the wrist support is compromised.
4. Measure the patient's joints with a goniometer to ensure a correct therapeutic position before splinting. Be cautious of splinting the wrist in too much ulnar or radial deviation.
5. When applying the straps, be sure to place a strap proximal to the PIPs, proximal to the thumb IP joint, and across the proximal and distal forearm (Figure 6-4).
6. Contour the splint's pan to the hand to preserve the hand's arches. The pan should be wide enough to comfortably support the width of the index, middle, ring, and little fingers.
7. Make sure the C bar conforms to the thumb web space (Figure 6-6).
8. Verify that the thumb trough is long and wide enough. Stretch or trim the thumb trough as necessary.

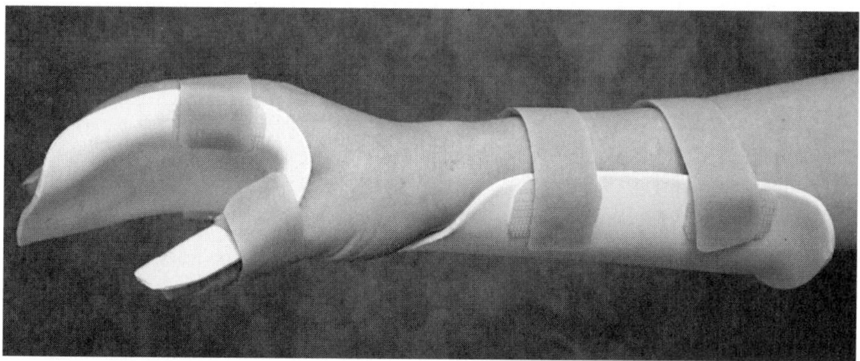

FIGURE 6-5 Strap placement for a resting hand splint.

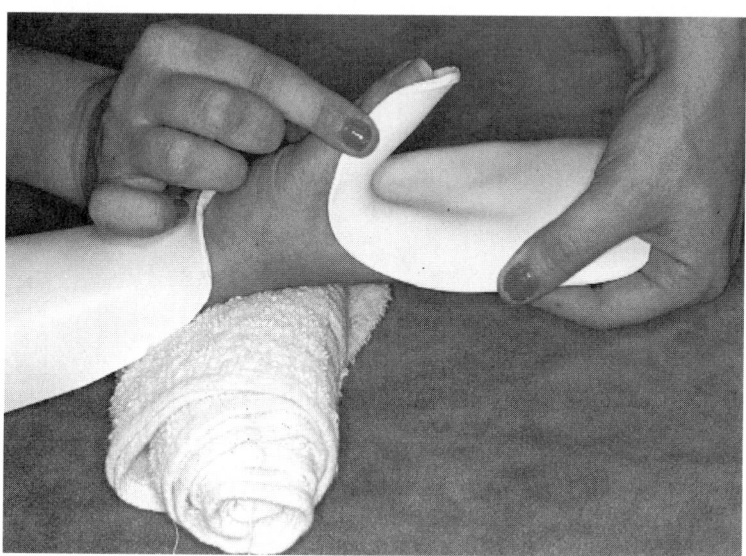

FIGURE 6-6 C-bar conformity to the thumb web space on a resting hand splint

Laboratory Exercise 6-2*

Rita and Jim are 2 patients who sustained burns on their hands Their wounds have healed, and they must wear splints at night to prevent contractures. The therapist fabricated the following splints. Look at each picture and try to identify the problem with each.

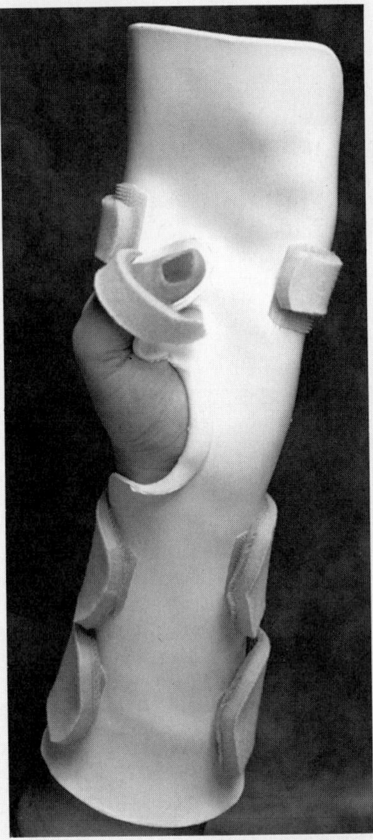

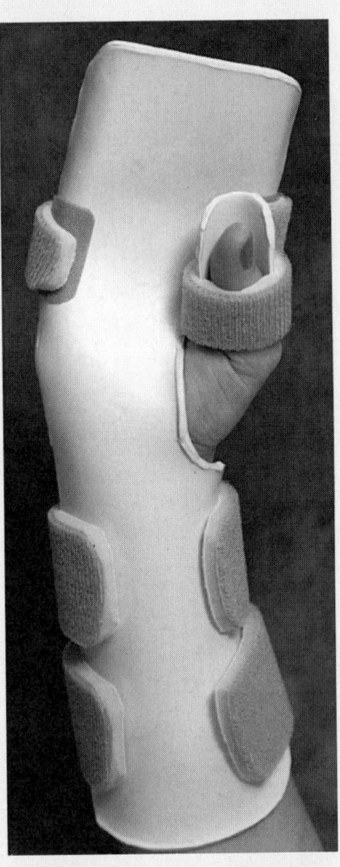

1. What is the problem with this splint?

____

____

____

____

____

2. What is the problem with this splint?

____

____

____

____

____

*See Appendix A for the answer key.

Laboratory Exercise 6-2—cont'd

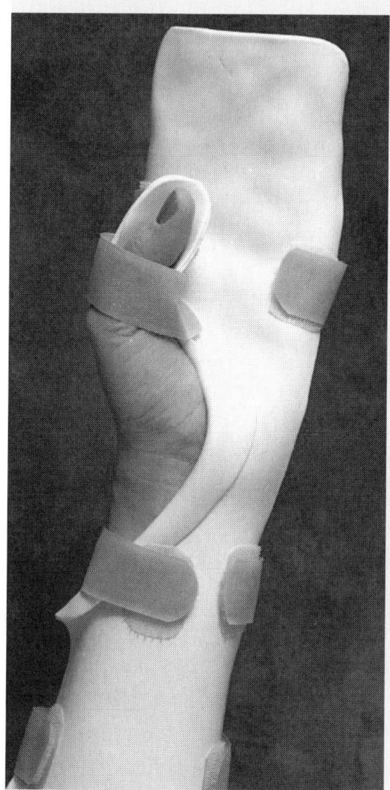

3. What is the problem with this splint?

____

____

____

____

____

Splint-Wearing Schedule

Wearing schedules for resting hand splints vary depending on the diagnostic condition, splint purpose, and physician order (see Table 6-1). Patients suffering from rheumatoid arthritis often wear resting hand splints at night. A patient who has rheumatoid arthritis may also wear a resting hand splint during the day for additional rest, but the patient should remove the splint at least once each day for hygiene and appropriate exercise. A patient who has bilateral hand splints may choose to alternate splints each night.

Patients commonly wear resting hand splints during the healing of burns. After wounds heal, patients may wear day splints with pressure garments or elastomer molds to increase ROM by controlling scarring. In addition to daytime splints, a burn patient may wear a resting hand splint at night to maintain maximum elongation of the healing skin and provide rest and functional alignment.

Precautions for a Resting Hand Splint

The therapist should be aware of precautions when applying a splint to a patient. If the diagnosis permits, the therapist should instruct the patient to remove the splint for a range-of-motion schedule to prevent stiffness and control edema.

1. The therapist should monitor the patient for pressure areas from the splint. With burn injuries and other open wound injuries the therapist should make adjustments frequently as bandage bulk changes.
2. To prevent infection, the therapist must teach the patient or caregiver to clean the splint when open wounds with exudate are present. After removing the splint, the patient or caregiver can clean it using warm, soapy water; hydrogen peroxide; or rubbing alcohol, and dry it with a clean cloth.
3. For a resting hand splint for a patient in an intensive care unit (ICU), supplies and tools should be kept as sterile as possible. Careful planning about supply needs before going into the unit helps prevent repetitious trips. The splint-maker may enlist the help of a second person, aide, or therapist to assist with a burn patient. The therapist working in a sterile environment should follow the facility's protocol on universal precaution procedures.
4. Depending on facility regulations, various actions may be taken to ensure optimal wear and care of a splint. The therapist should consider hanging a wearing schedule above the patient's bed. This precaution is especially helpful if others are involved in applying and removing the splint. A photograph of the patient wearing the splint and posting the picture at the bedside or in the patient's chart may help with correct splint application. The therapist should inform nursing staff members of the wearing schedule and care instruction.
5. When splinting a patient in ICU, the therapist should follow up at least once after the splint's application regarding the fit and the patient's tolerance for the splint. Splints on burn-injured patients require frequent adjustments, and as the patient recovers, the splint design may change several times.
6. A patient who has rheumatoid arthritis may benefit from a splint that is made from thinner thermoplastic (less than ⅛ inch). This type of splint reduces the weight over affected joints (Melvin, 1982).

Laboratory Exercise 6-3

Practice fabricating a resting hand splint on a partner. Before starting, determine the position in which you should place your partner's hand. Use a goniometer to measure the angles of wrist extension, MCP flexion, and thumb palmar abduction to ensure a correct position.

After fitting the splint and making all adjustments, use Form 6-1 as a self-evaluation check-off sheet. Use Grading Sheet 6-1 as a classroom grading sheet.

FORM 6-1* Resting Hand Splint

Name: ______________________________

Date: ______________________________

Position of resting hand splint:

Functional position (midjoint) ❍ Antideformity position (intrinsic plus) ❍

Answer the following questions after the patient wears the splint for 30 minutes. (Mark *NA* for nonapplicable situations.)

Evaluation Areas				Comments
Design				
1. The wrist position is at the correct angle.	Yes ❍	No ❍	NA ❍	
2. The MCPs are at the correct angle.	Yes ❍	No ❍	NA ❍	
3. The thumb is in the correct position.	Yes ❍	No ❍	NA ❍	
4. The wrist has adequate support.	Yes ❍	No ❍	NA ❍	
5. The pan is wide enough for all the fingers.	Yes ❍	No ❍	NA ❍	
6. The length of the pan and thumb trough are adequate.	Yes ❍	No ❍	NA ❍	
7. The splint is two-thirds the length of the forearm.	Yes ❍	No ❍	NA ❍	
8. The splint is one-half the width of the forearm.	Yes ❍	No ❍	NA ❍	
Function				
1. The splint completely immobilizes the wrist, fingers, and thumb.	Yes ❍	No ❍	NA ❍	
2. The splint is easy to apply and remove.	Yes ❍	No ❍	NA ❍	
Straps				
1. The straps avoid bony prominences.	Yes ❍	No ❍	NA ❍	
2. The straps are secure and rounded.	Yes ❍	No ❍	NA ❍	

*See Appendix B for a perforated copy of this form.

Continued.

FORM 6-1 Resting Hand Splint—cont'd

Evaluation Areas				Comments
Comfort				
1. The edges are smooth with rounded corners.	Yes ❍	No ❍	NA ❍	
2. The proximal end is flared.	Yes ❍	No ❍	NA ❍	
3. Impingements or pressure areas are not present.	Yes ❍	No ❍	NA ❍	
Cosmetic Appearance				
1. The splint is free of fingerprints, dirt, and pencil or pen marks.	Yes ❍	No ❍	NA ❍	
2. The splinting material is not buckled.	Yes ❍	No ❍	NA ❍	

Discuss adjustments or changes you would make based on the self-evaluation:

____

____

____

____

____

____

____

GRADING SHEET 6-1*

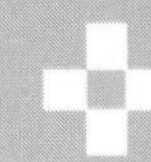

Resting Hand Splint

Name: ______________________________

Date: ______________________________

Position of resting hand splint:

Functional position (mid joint) ❍ Antideformity position (intrinsic plus) ❍

Grade: ______________

1 = beyond improvement, not acceptable
2 = requires maximal improvement
3 = requires moderate improvement
4 = requires minimal improvement
5 = requires no improvement

Evaluation Areas		**Comments**
Design		
1. The wrist position is at the correct angle.	1 2 3 4 5	
2. The MCPs are at the correct angle.	1 2 3 4 5	
3. The thumb is in the correct position.	1 2 3 4 5	
4. The wrist has adequate support.	1 2 3 4 5	
5. The pan is wide enough for all the fingers.	1 2 3 4 5	
6. The length of the pan and thumb trough are adequate.	1 2 3 4 5	
7. The splint is two-thirds the length of the forearm.	1 2 3 4 5	
8. The splint is one-half the width of the forearm.	1 2 3 4 5	

*See Appendix C for a perforated copy of this grading sheet.

Continued.

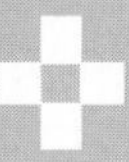

GRADING SHEET 6-1

Resting Hand Splint—cont'd

Evaluation Areas		Comments
Function		
1. The splint completely immobilizes the wrist, fingers, and thumb.	1 2 3 4 5	
2. The splint is easy to apply and remove.	1 2 3 4 5	
Straps		
1. The straps avoid bony prominences.	1 2 3 4 5	
2. The straps are secure and rounded.	1 2 3 4 5	
Comfort		
1. The edges are smooth with rounded corners.	1 2 3 4 5	
2. The proximal end is flared.	1 2 3 4 5	
3. Impingements or pressure areas are not present.	1 2 3 4 5	
Cosmetic Appearance		
1. The splint is free of fingerprints, dirt, and pencil or pen marks.	1 2 3 4 5	
2. The splinting material is not buckled.	1 2 3 4 5	

Case Study*

Read the following scenario and answer the questions based on information in this chapter:

A 39-year-old man suffering from bilateral dorsal hand burns has just been admitted to the ICU. The patient has second- and third-degree hand burns resulting from a torch exploding in his hands. The patient is receiving intravenous pain medication and is not alert. Approximately fourteen hours have passed since his admission, and you have just received orders to fabricate bilateral hand splints.

1. Which type of splint is appropriate for dorsal hand burns?
   a. Bilateral resting hand splints with the hand in a functional (midjoint) position
   b. Bilateral resting hand splints with the hand in an antideformity (intrinsic plus) position
   c. Bilateral wrist cock-up splints
2. What is the appropriate wrist position?
   a. Neutral
   b. 30° of flexion
   c. 30° of extension
3. What is the appropriate MCP position?
   a. 70° to 90° of extension
   b. 70° to 90° of flexion
   c. Full extension
4. What is the appropriate thumb position?
   a. Radial abduction
   b. Palmar abduction
   c. Full flexion
5. Which of the following statements is false regarding the splint process for the scenario above?
   a. The supplies should be sterile.
   b. An extremely stretchable material is necessary to fabricate the splints over the bandages.
   c. The therapist should give a splint-wearing schedule to the ICU nurse for inclusion in the treatment plan.

*See Appendix A for the answer key.

Review Questions

1. What are two common diagnostic conditions in which a therapist can use a resting hand splint?
2. In what position should the therapist place the wrist, MCPs, and thumb for a functional resting hand splint?
3. In what position should the therapist place the wrist, MCPs, and thumb for an antideformity resting hand splint?
4. What are the three purposes for using a resting hand splint?
5. What are the four main components of a resting hand splint?
6. Which equipment must be sterile to make a resting hand splint in a burn unit?

References

American Society of Hand Therapists. (1992). Splint classification system. Garner, NC: American Society of Hand Therapists.

Colditz, J. (February, 1995). Personal communication.

Fess, E.E., & Philips, C.A. (1987). Hand splinting principles and methods (2nd ed.). St. Louis: Mosby.

Geisser, R. W. (1984). Splinting the rheumatoid arthritic hand. In E. M. Ziegler (Ed.), Current concepts in orthotics: A diagnosis-related approach to splinting. Germantown, WI: Rolyan Medical Products.

Leonard, J. (1990). Joint protection for inflammatory disorders. In J. M. Hunter, L. H. Schneider, E. J. Mackin, & A. D. Callahan (Eds.), Rehabilitation of the hand: Surgery and therapy (3rd ed.). St. Louis: Mosby.

Malick, M.H. (1972). Manual on static hand splinting. Pittsburgh: Hamarville Rehabilitation Center.

Marx, H. (1992). Rheumatoid arthritis. In B. G. Stanley, & S. M. Tribuzi (Eds.), Concepts in hand rehabilitation. Philadelphia: F. A. Davis Co.

Melvin, J. L. (1982). Rheumatic disease: Occupational therapy and rehabilitation (2nd ed.). Philadelphia: F. A. Davis Co.

Ouellette, E. A. (1991). The rheumatoid hand: Orthotics as preventative. Seminars in Arthritis and Rheumatism, 21, 65-71.

Salisbury, R. E., Reeves, S. U., & Wright, P. (1990). Acute care and rehabilitation of the burned hand. In J. M. Hunter, L. H. Schneider, E. J. Macklin, & A. D. Callahan (Eds.), Rehabilitation of the hand: Surgery and therapy (3rd ed, pp. 831-840). St. Louis: Mosby.

Stanley, B.G., & Tribuzi, S.M. (1992). Concepts in hand rehabilitation. Philadelphia: F.A. Davis Co.

Tenney, C. G., & Lisak, J. M. (1986). Atlas of hand splinting. Boston: Little, Brown and Company.

Ziegler, E. M. (1984). Current concepts in orthotics: A diagnostic-related approach to splinting. Germantown, WI: Rolyan Medical Products.

CHAPTER SEVEN

Thumb Spica Splints (Thumb Immobilization Splints)

HELENE LOHMAN, MA, OTR/L

Chapter Objectives

1. Discuss the diagnostic indications for a thumb spica splint.
2. List appropriate thumb and wrist positions in a thumb spica splint.
3. Identify the three components of a thumb spica splint.
4. Describe the indications for supporting the joints of the thumb.
5. Discuss the process of pattern making and splint fabrication for a thumb spica splint.
6. Describe elements of a proper fit of a thumb spica splint.
7. List general and specific precautions for a thumb spica splint.
8. Use clinical judgment to evaluate fit problems of a thumb spica splint.
9. Use clinical judgment to evaluate a fabricated thumb spica splint.
10. Apply knowledge about thumb spica splinting to a case study.

A commonly prescribed splint in clinical practice is the thumb spica splint. Other names for this splint are the *thumb immobilization splint* (American Society of Hand Therapists, 1992), the *short or long opponens splint* (Tenney & Lisak, 1986), and the *thumb gauntlet splint.* The purpose of this splint is to immobilize, protect, rest, and position one or all of the thumb joints while allowing the other digits to be free. The application of this splint varies according to diagnostic conditions. For example, this splint provides patients who have tendonitis or rheumatoid arthritis with rest, support, and protection of the thumb. The therapist also uses this splint postoperatively to control motion in patients suffering from rheumatoid arthritis after joint arthrodesis or replacement. In addition, the thumb spica splint can position the thumb before surgery (Geisser, 1984) and provide support and positioning after traumatic thumb injuries such as sprains, joint dislocations, and ligament injuries. One of the most frequent injuries for the application of this splint is *gamekeeper's thumb,* which involves the ulnar collateral ligament of the metacarpophalangeal (MCP) joint.

Diagnostic Indications

Therapists fabricate thumb spica splints in general and specialized hand therapy practices. Specific diagnostic conditions requiring a thumb spica splint include but are not limited to the following: scaphoid fractures, stable fractures of the proximal phalanx of the first metacarpal, tendon transfers, radial or ulnar collateral ligament strains, repair of MCP joint collateral ligaments, wrist arthrodeses, de Quervain's tenosynovitis, median nerve injuries, MCP joint dislocations, and uncomplicated extensor pollicis longus (EPL) repairs. Treatment of many of these diagnoses requires the expertise of experienced hand therapists. In general clinical practice, therapists commonly treat patients suffering from de Quervain's tenosynovitis, rheumatoid arthritis, fractures, and ligament injuries. (Table 7-1 contains guidelines for these hand conditions.) The beginning therapist should keep in mind that physicians and experienced therapists may have their own guidelines for positioning and splint-wearing schedules. The therapist should also be aware that thumb palmar abduction may be uncomfortable for some patients. Therefore the thumb may be positioned midway between radial and palmar abduction.

Splinting for de Quervain's Tenosynovitis

de Quervain's tenosynovitis, which results from repetitive thumb motions and wrist deviation, is a form of tenosynovitis affecting the abductor pollicis longus (APL) and EPL in the first dorsal compartment of the thumb. This condition may be recognized from pain over the radial styloid, edema in the first dorsal compartment, and positive results from the Finkelstein's test.

During the acute phase of this condition, conservative management involves immobilization of the thumb and wrist. This splint may cover the volar or dorsal forearm or radial aspect of the forearm and hand. The therapist can position the wrist in 15° of extension, 40° to 50° palmar abduction of the thumb carpometacarpal (CMC) joint, and 5° to 10° of flexion in the MCP joint (Totten, 1990). Usually the therapist allows the interphalangeal (IP) joint to be free for functional activities and includes the joint in the splint if pain is present with IP flexion and resisted IP extension (Baxter-Petralia & Penney, 1992). This splint is worn continuously with removal for hygiene and exercise (Figure 7-1).

TABLE 7-1 **Conditions That May Require a Thumb Spica Splint**

Hand Condition	Suggested wearing schedule	Type of splint, wrist position
SOFT TISSUE INFLAMMATION		
de Quervain's tenosynovitis	During an acute flare-up, the therapist fabricates a thumb spica splint, which the patient wears continuously with removal for hygiene and exercise. The IP joint is included only if pain is present with IP flexion and resisted IP extension.	Long forearm-based or radial gutter splint—the wrist in 15° of extension, the thumb CMC joint palmarly abducted 40° to 45°, and the thumb MCP joint in 5° to 10° of flexion. To allow slack for inflamed tendons, the thumb CMC joint is sometimes positioned in radial abduction and extension instead of palmar abduction
RHEUMATOID ARTHRITIS		
Periods of pain and inflammation in the thumb joints	The therapist fabricates a thumb spica splint for the patient to wear continuously during periods of pain and inflammation. The patient removes the splint for exercise and hygiene. The therapist adjusts the wearing schedule according to the patient's pain and inflammation levels.	Long forearm-based thumb spica splint—the wrist in 20° to 30° of extension, the thumb CMC joint palmarly abducted 45°, or midway between radial and palmar abduction depending on patient's tolerance; and the MCP joint (if included) in 5° of flexion
TRAUMATIC INJURIES OF THE THUMB		
Gamekeeper's thumb (ulnar collateral ligament)	The patient wears a thumb spica splint continuously for 3 to 4 weeks with removal for hygiene.	Short opponens splint—the MCP joint immobilized and the thumb CMC joint palmarly abducted 25° to 30°

Splinting for Rheumatoid Arthritis

Rheumatoid arthritis often affects the thumb joints, particularly the CMC joint. Splinting for rheumatoid arthritis can reduce pain, slow deformity, and stabilize the thumb joints (Ouellette, 1991). The disease involves three stages, each of which has a different splinting approach even though the therapist may apply the same thumb spica splint (Colditz, 1995).

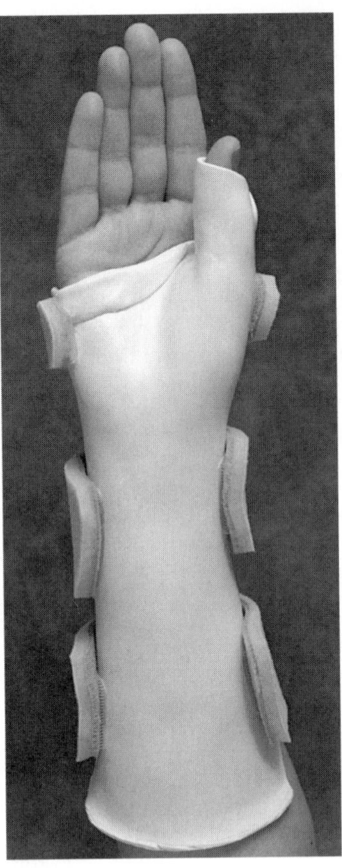

FIGURE 7-1 A long thumb spica splint for de Quervain's Tenosynovitis including the immobilization of the thumb IP joint

The first stage involves an inflammatory process. The goal of splinting in this stage is to rest the joints and reduce inflammation. The patient wears the thumb spica splint continuously during periods of inflammation and periodically thereafter for pain control as necessary. When the disease progresses, the hand requires mechanical support because the joints are less stable and painful with use. The patient wears a thumb spica splint for support while doing daily activities and perhaps at night for pain relief. In the third stage, pain is usually not a factor but joints may be grossly deformed and unstable. In lieu of surgical stabilization a thumb spica splint may provide support to increase function during certain activities. At this stage, splinting is rarely helpful for the patient at night (Colditz, 1995).

One approach to splinting is to immobilize the thumb in a long thumb spica splint with the wrist in 20° to 30° of extension, the CMC joint in 45° of palmar abduction (if tolerated), and the MCP joint in 0° to 5° of flexion (Tenney & Lisak,

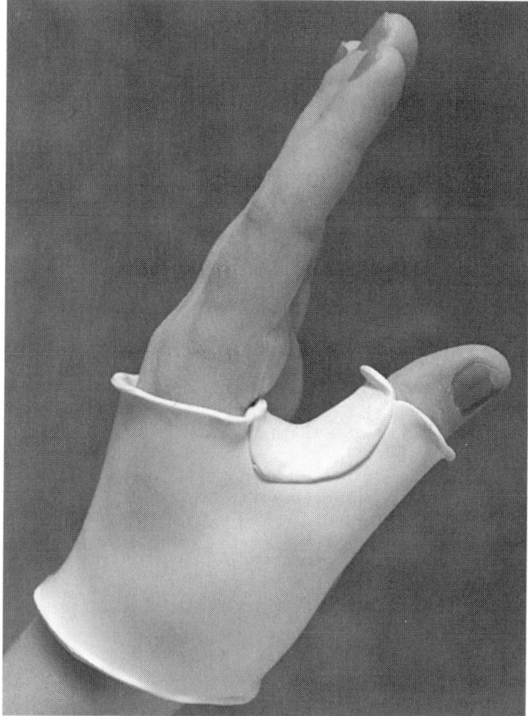

FIGURE 7-2 A hand-based thumb spica splint

1986). Resting the hand in this position is extremely beneficial during periods of inflammation or if the thumb is unstable at the CMC joint (Marx, 1992).

Some patients benefit from splints that position the thumb joints without incorporating the wrist as shown in Figure 7-2 (Colditz, 1990; Melvin, 1989). Positioning the thumb in enough palmar abduction for functional activities is important. The CMC and MCP joints are stabilized in the thumb post because "the structure of the thumb makes it impossible to immobilize the CMC joint and simultaneously allow full MCP joint motion" (Melvin, 1989, p. 413). On the other hand, some therapists stabilize the thumb CMC joint with a short splint that is properly molded and positioned (Colditz, 1995).

With a hand-based thumb spica splint the therapist must incorporate the IP joint into the splint if the joint is painful and inflamed. The patient wears this splint constantly for a minimum of 2 to 3 weeks with removal for hygiene and exercise. The therapist adjusts the wearing schedule according to the patient's pain and inflammation levels.

Often when a physician refers a patient who has rheumatoid arthritis for splinting, deformities have already developed. If the therapist attempts to place the patient's joints in the ideal position, excessive stress on the joints may result. The therapist should always splint an arthritic hand in a position of comfort (Colditz, 1984).

When fabricating a splint on a patient who has rheumatoid arthritis, the therapist should be aware that the patient may have fragile skin. Padding the splint for comfort to prevent skin irritation may be necessary. The selected splinting material should be easily adjustable to accommodate changes in swelling and repositioning as the disease progresses. Asking patients about their swelling patterns is important because splints fabricated during the day should allow enough

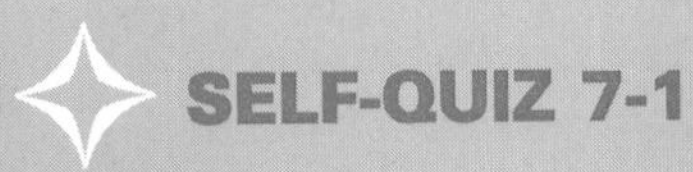

SELF-QUIZ 7-1*

Please circle either true (T) or false (F).

1. T F The main purpose of a thumb spica splint is to protect the thumb.
2. T F A therapist should apply a thumb spica splint only during the chronic phase to a patient suffering from de Quervain's tenosynovitis.
3. T F Fabricating either a long forearm thumb spica splint or a radial gutter thumb spica splint is best for a patient suffering from de Quervain's tenosynovitis.
4. T F Splinting material more than ⅛-inch thick is best for splinting a rheumatoid arthritic hand because this material adds more support.
5. T F If a patient suffering from rheumatoid arthritis has pain in the wrist, the therapist includes the wrist in the thumb spica splint.
6. T F When splinting a patient who has rheumatoid arthritis, the therapist must always place the hand in the ideal position.
7. T F During the acute phase of healing for gamekeeper's thumb, the patient wears the splint continuously for 3 to 4 weeks with removal only for hygiene.

*See Appendix A for the answer key.

room for nocturnal swelling. Thermoplastic material less than ⅛-inch thick is best for small hand splints. Splints fabricated from heavier splinting material have the potential for aggravating other joints (Melvin, 1989). Therapists must carefully evaluate all hand splints for potential stress on other joints and should instruct patients to wear the splints at night, periodically during the day, and during stressful daily activities.

Splinting for Ulnar Collateral Ligament Injury

Injury to the ulnar collateral ligament, a condition also known as *gamekeeper's* thumb or *skier's thumb,* is a common injury that can occur at the MCP joint of the thumb. Gamekeeper's thumb was the original name of the injury because gamekeepers stressed this joint when they killed birds by twisting the necks (Colditz, 1990). The therapist can manage a mild tear of the ligament by splinting the MCP joint in a short opponens with the thumb CMC joint in 25° to 30° of palmar abduction and the MCP joint immobilized in neutral to slight flexion to protect the healing ligament. The patient wears the splint continuously for 3 to 4 weeks with removal for hygiene purposes (Tenney & Lisak, 1986).

Features of the Thumb Spica Splint

The thumb spica splint is a static splint because it has no movable parts (Fess & Philips, 1987). The splint has numerous design variations; it can be a volar (Figure 7-3), dorsal (Figure 7-4), or radial gutter (Figure 7-5). The splint may not include the wrist depending on the patient's diagnosis and the associated pain at the wrist. If the wrist is included, the position will vary according to the diagnosis.

A variance exists in the splinting components fabricated for the final splint product based on the joints included and hand position. The therapist should have a good understanding of the purpose and fabrication process for the different splinting components. Central to any thumb spica splint are the opponens bar, a C bar, and a thumb post (Figure 7-6) (Fess & Philips, 1987). The opponens bar and C bar position the thumb, usually in palmar abduction. The thumb post, which is an extension of the C bar, immobilizes the MCP only or both the MCP and IP joints.

The position of the thumb in a splint varies from palmar abduction to radial abduction depending on the patient's diagnosis. With some conditions such as arthritis the therapist can assist prehension by stabilizing the thumb CMC joint in palmar abduction and opposition. Certain diagnostic protocols (such as those for EPL repairs, tendon transfers for thumb extension, and extensor tenolysis of the thumb) require the thumb to have an extension and a radial abduction position (Cannon, et al., 1985).

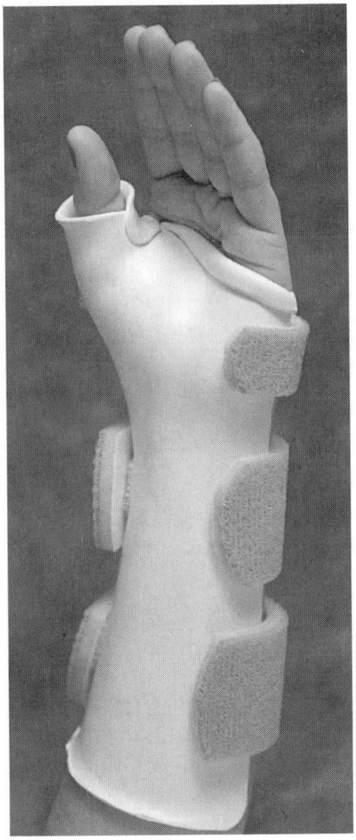

FIGURE 7-3 A volar thumb spica splint

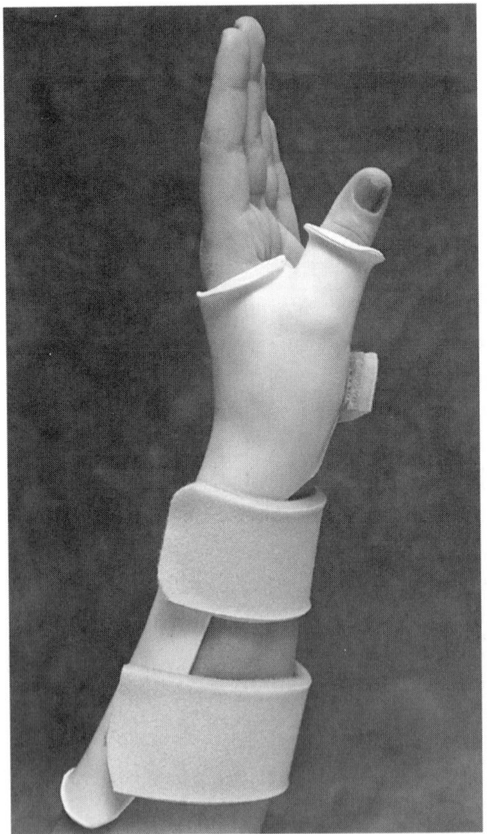

FIGURE 7-4 A dorsal thumb spica splint

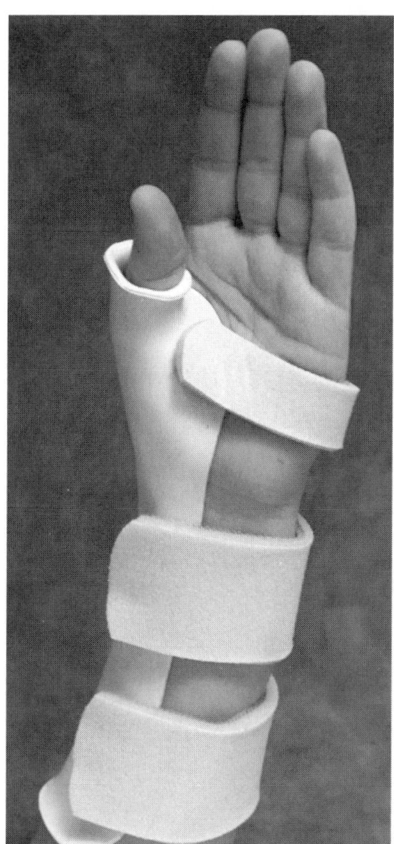

FIGURE 7-5 A radial gutter thumb spica splint

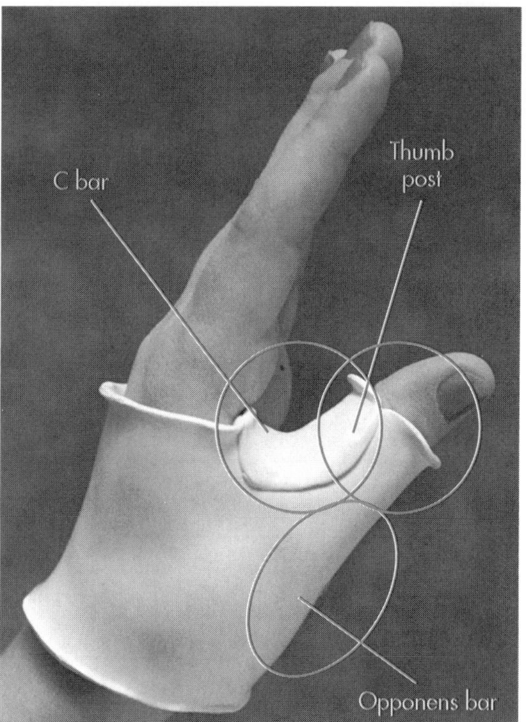

FIGURE 7-6 The opponens bar in conjunction with a C bar and a thumb post

Laboratory Exercise 7-1*

These components are in various types of thumb spica splints. They are also part of other splints such as the wrist cock-up and resting hand splint. Label the splinting components on the following figure.

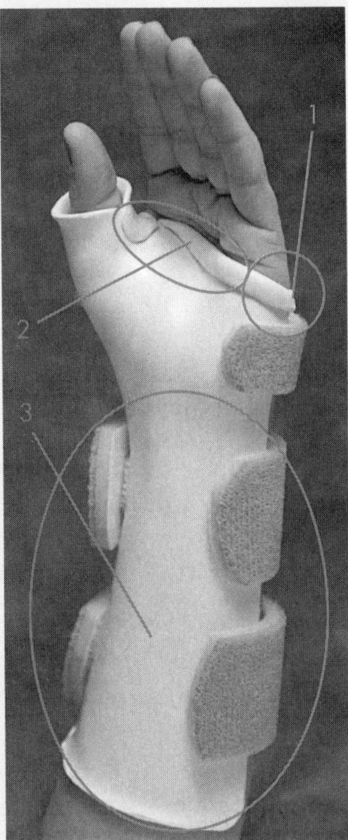

1. ______________________
2. ______________________
3. ______________________

*See Appendix A for the answer key.

The thumb spica splint may do one of the following: (1) stabilize only the CMC joint, (2) include the CMC and MCP joints, or (3) encompass the CMC, MCP, and IP joints. The physician's order may specify which thumb joints to include in the splint. In some situations the therapist may be responsible for determining which joints the splint should stabilize. The therapist uses diagnostic protocols and patient pain to make this decision. Usually the therapist should fabricate a splint that is the most supportive and least restrictive in movement. Certain diagnostic protocols (such as those for severe de Quervain's tenosynovitis, thumb replantations, tendon transfers, and tendon repairs) often require the inclusion of the IP joint in the splint (Tenney & Lisak, 1986). Working with thumb replantations, tendon transfers, and tendon repairs requires more advanced clinical skills.

Fabrication of a Thumb Spica Splint

The thumb spica splint (also known as a *thumb immobilization splint radial design*) (American Society of Hand Therapists, 1992) provides support on the radial side of the hand while stabilizing the thumb. The therapist usually places the thumb in a palmar abducted position so that the thumb opposes the second metacarpal. The therapist leaves the IP joint free for functional movement but can adapt the splint pattern to include the IP joint if more support becomes necessary.

Figure 7-7 represents a detailed radial gutter thumb spica pattern that excludes the interphalangeal joint. (Refer to Figure 7-5 for a picture of the completed splint product.)

1. Position the forearm and hand palm down on a piece of paper. The fingers should be in a natural resting position and slightly abducted. Draw an outline of the hand and forearm to the elbow. As you gain experience with pattern drawing, you will not need to draw the entire hand and forearm outline. The experienced therapist can estimate the placement of key points on the pattern.
2. While the patient's hand is on the paper, mark an *A* at the radial styloid and a *B* at the ulnar styloid. Mark the second and fifth metacarpal heads *C* and *D*, respectively. Mark the IP joint of the thumb *E*, and mark the olecranon process of the elbow *F*. Then remove the patient's hand from the paper pattern.
3. Place an X two-thirds the length of the forearm on each side. Place another X on each side of the pattern approximately 1 to 1½ inches outside and parallel to the two X markings for two-thirds the length of the forearm. Mark these two Xs *H*.

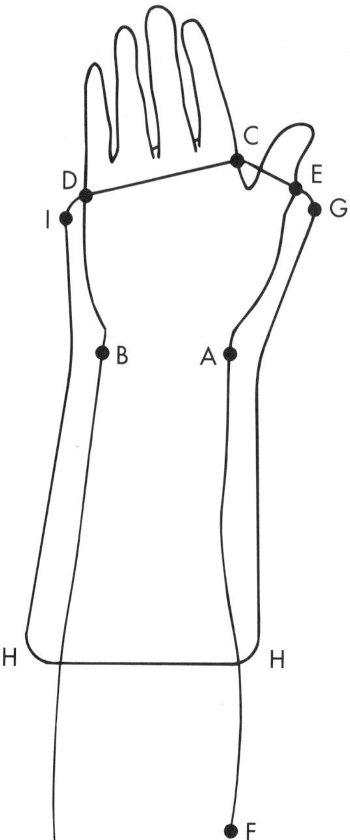

FIGURE 7-7 A detailed pattern for a radial gutter thumb spica splint

4. Draw an angled line connecting the second and fifth metacarpal heads (*C* to *D*). Extend this line approximately 1 to 1½ inches to the ulnar side of the hand and mark it *I*.
5. Connect *C* to *E*. Extend this line approximately 1 to ½ inches. Mark the end of the line *G*.
6. Draw a line from *G* down the radial side of the forearm, and make sure that the line follows the size of the forearm. To ensure that the splint is two-thirds the length of the forearm, end the line at *H*.
7. Begin a line from *I* and extend it down the ulnar side of the forearm, and make certain that the line follows the increasing size of the forearm. End the line at *H*.

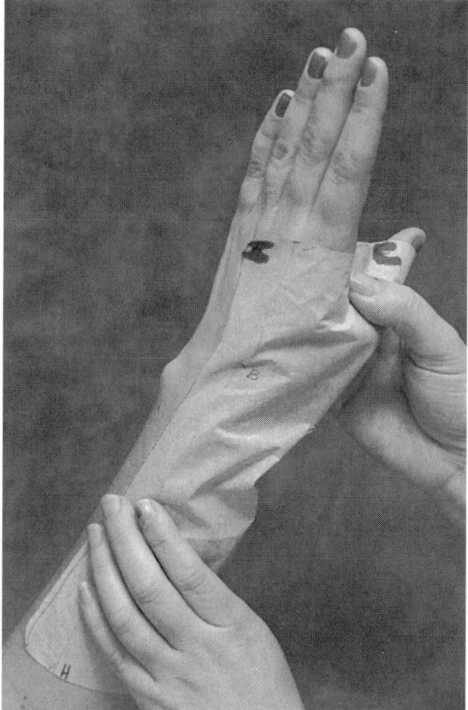

FIGURE 7-8

To ensure a proper fit, place the paper pattern on the patient.

8. For the proximal edge of the splint, draw a straight line that connects both *Hs.*
9. Make sure that the splint pattern lines are rounded at *G, I,* and the two *Hs.*
10. Cut out the pattern.
11. Place the splint pattern on the patient (Figure 7-8). Make certain that the splint's edges end midforearm on the volar and dorsal surface of the patient's hand and forearm. Check that the splint is two-thirds the forearm length and one-half the forearm circumference. Check the thumb position and make any necessary adjustments (e.g., additions, deletions) on the splint pattern.
12. Carefully trace the thumb spica splint pattern on a sheet of thermoplastic material.
13. Heat the thermoplastic material.

Laboratory Exercise 7-2

1. Practice making a pattern for a radial gutter thumb spica splint on another person. Use the detailed instructions on the previous pages to draw the pattern. Make necessary adjustments to the pattern after cutting it out.
2. Practice drawing a pattern for a radial gutter thumb spica splint on the following outline of the hand without using detailed instructions. Label the landmarks.

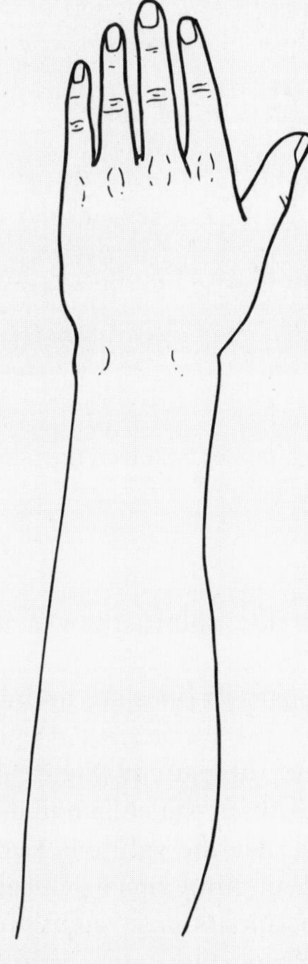

14. Cut the pattern out of the thermoplastic material.
15. Reheat the material, mold the form onto the patient's hand, and make necessary adjustments.
16. Add three straps (two across the forearm and one across the dorsal aspect of the hand, connecting the hypothenar bar to the metacarpal bar).

Technical Tips for Proper Fit

1. Before molding the splint, place the arm on a table top with the elbow in 90° flexion and the forearm in a neutral position. Position the thumb and wrist according to diagnostic indications.
2. Monitor joint positions by measuring during and after splint fabrication. A common mistake when splinting is incorrect placement of the thumb in a midposition between palmar abduction and radial abduction when the diagnostic protocol calls for palmar abduction. Light pressure on the MCP joint when fabricating the splint can help position the thumb correctly in palmar abduction (Figure 7-9).
3. Follow the natural curves of the longitudinal, distal, and proximal arches. Position the splint area that covers the thenar eminence just proximal to the proximal palmar crease. Be especially careful to check that the index finger has full flexion because of its close proximity to the opponens bar, C bar, and thumb post.
4. When molding the piece around the thumb, overlap the extra splinting material into the thumb web space (Figure 7-10). Be certain the thumb IP joint remains in extension during molding to facilitate later splint application and removal. Be extremely careful making adjustments with a heat gun on the thumb post or the result may be an inappropriate fit.
5. For a thumb spica splint that allows IP mobility, make sure the distal end of the thumb post on the volar surface has been rolled to allow full IP flexion (Figure 7-11).

Precautions for a Thumb Spica Splint

The cautious splintmaker should check for areas of skin pressure over the ulnar styloid, the superficial branch of the radial nerve at the radial styloid, and the volar and dorsal surface of the thumb MCP joint. Specific precautions for the molding of the splint include the following:

1. If the thumb post extends too far distally on the volar surface of the IP joint, the result is restriction of the IP joint flexion.
2. Because of its close proximity to the opponens bar, C bar, and thumb post, the radial base of the first metacarpal and first web space has a potential for skin irritation.

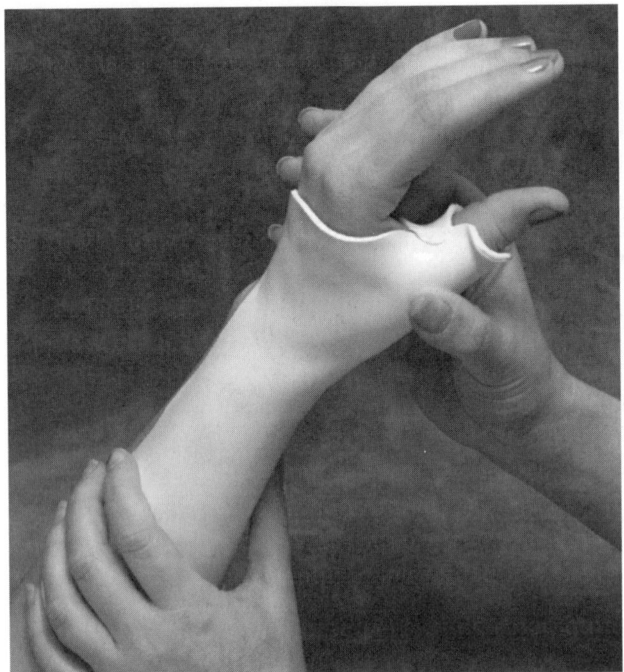

FIGURE 7-9

Provide light pressure on the thumb MCP joint to position the thumb correctly in palmar abduction.

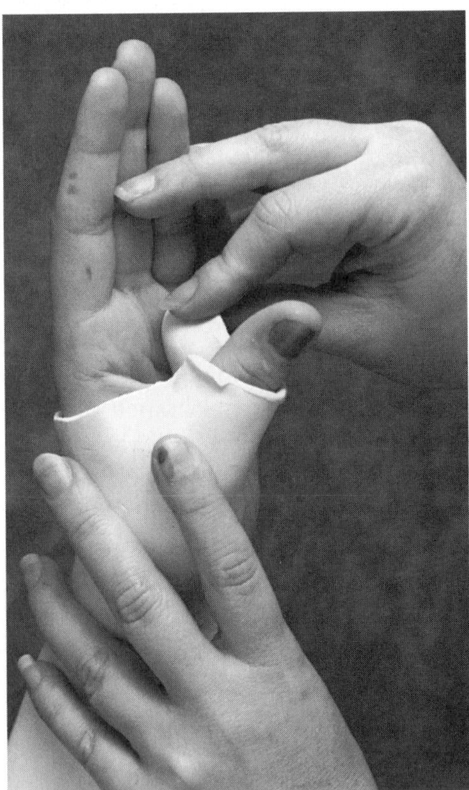

FIGURE 7-10

Overlap the extra splinting material into the thumb web space.

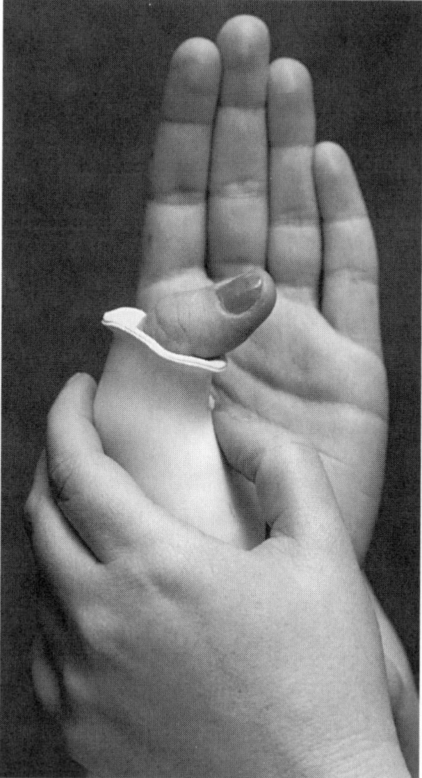

FIGURE 7-11
Roll the distal end of the thumb post to allow full IP flexion.

3. With a radial gutter splint, monitor the splint for a pressure area at the midline of the forearm on the volar and dorsal surface.
4. Be careful to fabricate a thumb splint that is supportive and not too constrictive. Constriction results in decreased circulation and possible skin breakdown. Make allowances for edema when fabricating the thumb post.
5. Make sure to position the thumb in the correct degree of palmar abduction. If the protocol calls for 45° of palmar abduction, positioning in more palmar abduction can cause excessive stress on the ulnar collateral ligament of the thumb MCP joint (Cannon, et al., 1985).
6. If using a thermoplastic material that has memory properties, be aware that the material shrinks when cooling. Therefore the thumb post opening must remain large enough for comfortable application and removal of the splint.

Laboratory Exercise 7-3* Splint Evaluation

The illustration below shows a thumb spica splint for a 35-year-old woman working as a secretary. She has a long history of rheumatoid arthritis. Her physician ordered a thumb spica splint after the patient complained of pain and inflammation in the thumb MCP joint. Keeping in mind the diagnostic protocols for thumb spica splinting, identify two problems with the illustrated splint.

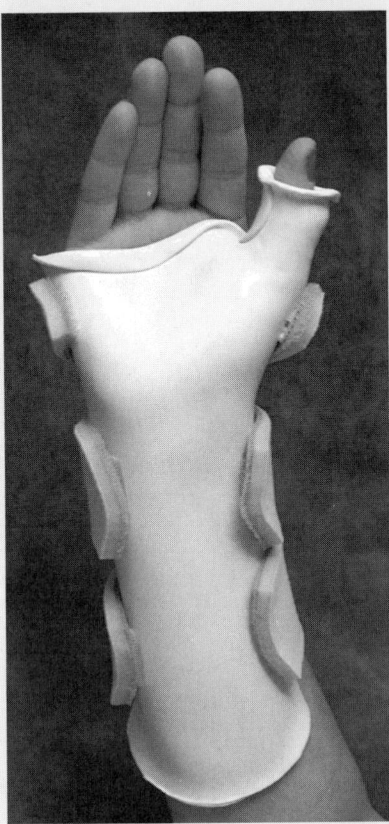

1. List two problems with this splint.

   a. ______________________________

   b. ______________________________

2. Which problems might arise from continual splint wear?

   ____

   ____

*See Appendix A for the answer key.

Laboratory Exercise 7-4*

On a partner, practice fabricating a radial gutter thumb spica splint that does not immobilize the thumb IP joint. Before starting, use a goniometer to ensure that the wrist is in 15° of extension, the CMC joint of the thumb in 45° of palmar abduction, and the MCP joint of the thumb in 5° to 10° of flexion. Check the finished product to ensure that full finger flexion and thumb IP flexion are possible after you fit the splint and make all adjustments. Use Form 7-1 as a check-off sheet for a self-evaluation of the thumb spica splint. Use Grading Sheet 7-1 as a classroom grading sheet.

FORM 7-1* Thumb Spica Splint

Name: ____________________

Date: ____________________

Type of thumb spica splint:

Volar Dorsal Radial gutter Hand based

Thumb joint positions: ____________________

Answer the following questions after the splint is worn for 30 minutes. (Mark *NA* for non-applicable situations.)

Evaluation Areas				**Comments**
Design				
1. The wrist position is at the correct angle.	Yes ❍	No ❍	NA ❍	
2. The thumb position is at the correct angle.	Yes ❍	No ❍	NA ❍	
3. The thenar eminence is not restricted or flattened.	Yes ❍	No ❍	NA ❍	
4. The thumb post is adequately supported and is not constricted.	Yes ❍	No ❍	NA ❍	
5. The splint is two-thirds the length of the forearm.	Yes ❍	No ❍	NA ❍	
6. The splint is one-half the width of the forearm.	Yes ❍	No ❍	NA ❍	
Function				
1 The splint allows thumb IP flexion.	Yes ❍	No ❍	NA ❍	
2. The splint allows full MCP flexion of the fingers.	Yes ❍	No ❍	NA ❍	
3. The splint provides thumb support that allows functional activities.	Yes ❍	No ❍	NA ❍	

*See Appendix B for a perforated copy of this form.

FORM 7-1 Thumb Spica Splint—cont'd

Evaluation Areas		Comments
Straps		
1. The straps avoid bony prominences.	Yes ❍ No ❍ NA ❍	
2. The straps are secure and ends are rounded.	Yes ❍ No ❍ NA ❍	
Comfort		
1. The edges are smooth with rounded corners.	Yes ❍ No ❍ NA ❍	
2. The proximal end is flared.	Yes ❍ No ❍ NA ❍	
3. Impingements or pressure areas are not present.	Yes ❍ No ❍ NA ❍	
Cosmetic Appearance		
1. The splint is free of fingerprints, dirt, and pencil or pen marks.	Yes ❍ No ❍ NA ❍	
2. The splinting material is not buckled.	Yes ❍ No ❍ NA ❍	

Discuss adjustments or changes you would make based on the self-evaluation:

____

____

____

____

____

____

____

____

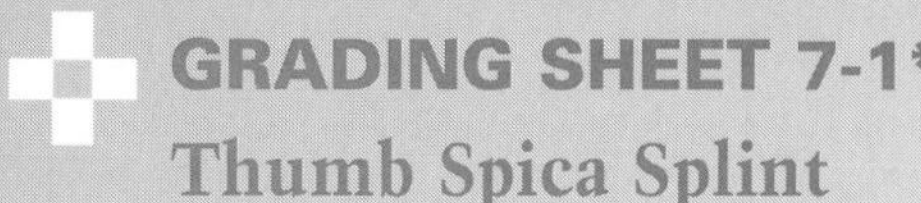

GRADING SHEET 7-1*
Thumb Spica Splint

Name: ______________________

Date: ______________________

Type of thumb spica splint:

Volar Dorsal Radial gutter Hand based

Thumb joint positions: ____________

Grade: ____________

1 = beyond improvement, not acceptable
2 = requires maximal improvement
3 = requires moderate improvement
4 = requires minimal improvement
5 = requires no improvement

Evaluation Areas		Comments
Design		
1. The wrist position is at the correct angle.	1 2 3 4 5	
2. The thumb position is at the correct angle.	1 2 3 4 5	
3. The thenar eminence is not restricted or flattened.	1 2 3 4 5	
4. The thumb is adequately supported and is not constricted.	1 2 3 4 5	
5. The splint is two-thirds the length of the forearm.	1 2 3 4 5	
6. The splint is one-half the width of the forearm.	1 2 3 4 5	
Function		
1. The splint allows thumb IP flexion.	1 2 3 4 5	
2. The splint allows full MCP flexion of the fingers.	1 2 3 4 5	
3. The splint provides thumb support that allows functional activities.	1 2 3 4 5	

*See Appendix C for a perforated copy of this grading sheet.

GRADING SHEET 7-1

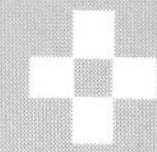

Thumb Spica Splint—cont'd

Evaluation Areas						Comments
Straps						
1. The straps avoid bony prominences.	1	2	3	4	5	
2. The straps are secure and rounded.	1	2	3	4	5	
Comfort						
1. The edges are smooth with rounded corners.	1	2	3	4	5	
2. The proximal end is flared.	1	2	3	4	5	
3. Impingements or pressure areas are not present.	1	2	3	4	5	
Cosmetic Appearance						
1. The splint is free of fingerprints, dirt, and pencil or pen marks.	1	2	3	4	5	
2. The splinting material is not buckled.	1	2	3	4	5	

Comments:

Case Study*

Read the following scenario and answer the questions based on information in this chapter:

Mrs. S is a 46-year-old, right-hand dominant woman working as a housekeeper. Much of her work involves dusting, mopping floors, and washing dishes. Mrs. S complained that the base of her thumb was swollen and painful with motion. Clinical examination revealed pain over the radial styloid and swelling of the first dorsal compartment. The physician diagnosed the condition as de Quervain's tenosynovitis.

1. With which of the following splints should you fit the patient?
   a. A forearm-based or radial gutter thumb spica splint
   b. A short opponens splint
   c. A wrist cock-up splint
2. What is the function of Mrs. S's splint?
   a. To position the thumb correctly during the healing phase
   b. To protect the tendons during the chronic phase of the tenosynovitis
   c. To provide rest, support, and protection for the inflamed tendons
3. For this splint, how should you position the wrist?
   a. 20° to 30° of extension
   b. 10° to 15° of extension
4. For this splint, how should you position the thumb?
   a. 40° to 45° of palmar abduction
   b. Midpoint between palmar abduction and radial abduction
   c. 20° to 30° of palmar abduction
5. Which joints should you immobilize in a splint if the patient experiences pain with IP active flexion?
   a. CMC and MCP
   b. CMC, MCP, and IP
6. Which of the following is the correct wearing schedule?
   a. 3 times daily and all night
   b. Only when the thumb is painful
   c. Continuously with removal for hygiene and exercise

*See Appendix A for the answer key.

Review Questions

1. What are the general reasons for provision of a thumb spica splint?
2. What are some of the clinical indications for including the IP joint of the thumb in a thumb spica splint?
3. What is a proper wearing schedule for a patient suffering from rheumatoid arthritis who wears a thumb spica splint?
4. Which type of thumb spica splint should a therapist fabricate for a patient suffering from de Quervain's tenosynovitis? When should the therapist include the IP joint in the splint?
5. Which type of thumb spica splint should a therapist fabricate for an injury of the thumb ulnar collateral ligament?
6. What are three specific precautions for a thumb spica splint?

References

American Society of Hand Therapists. (1992). Splint classification system. Garner, NC: American Society of Hand Therapists.

Baxter-Petralia, P. & Penney, V. (1992). Cumulative trauma. In B. G. Stanley & S. M. Tribuzi (Eds.), Concepts in hand rehabilitation (pp. 419-443). Philadelphia: F. A. Davis Co.

Cannon, N. M., Foltz, R. W., Koepfer, J. M., Lauck, M. R., Simpson, D. M., & Bromley R. S. (1985). Manual of hand splinting. New York: Churchill Livingstone Inc.

Colditz, J. C. (1984). Arthritis. In M. H. Malick & M. C. Kasch (Eds.), Manual on management of specific hand problems (pp. 112-136). Pittsburgh: AREN Publications.

Colditz, J. C. (1990). Anatomic considerations for splinting the thumb. In J. M. Hunter, L. H. Schneider, E. J. Mackin, & A. D. Callahan (Eds.), Rehabilitation of the hand (pp. 353-363). St. Louis: Mosby.

Colditz, J. C. (April, 1995). Personal communication.

Fess, E. E., & Philips, C. A. (1987). Hand splinting principles and methods (2nd ed.). St. Louis: Mosby.

Geisser, R. W. (1984). Splinting the rheumatoid arthritic hand. In E. M. Ziegler (Ed.), Current concepts in orthosis (pp. 29-49). Germantown, WI: Rolyan Medical Products.

Marx, H. (1992). Rheumatoid arthritis. In B. G. Stanley & S. M. Tribuzi (Eds.), Concepts in hand rehabilitation (pp. 395-418). Philadelphia: F. A. Davis Co.

Melvin, J. L. (1989). Rheumatic disease in the adult and child (3rd ed.). Philadelphia: F. A. Davis Co.

Ouellette, E. (1991). The rheumatoid hand: orthotics as preventive. Seminars in Arthritis and Rheumatism 21,(2) 65-72.

Tenney, C. G., & Lisak, J. M. (1986). Atlas of hand splinting. Boston/Toronto: Little, Brown & Co Inc.

Totten, P. L. (1990). Therapist's management of de Quervain's disease. In J. M. Hunter, L. H. Schneider, E. J. Mackin, & A. D. Callahan (Eds.), Rehabilitation of the hand (pp. 308-317). St. Louis: Mosby.

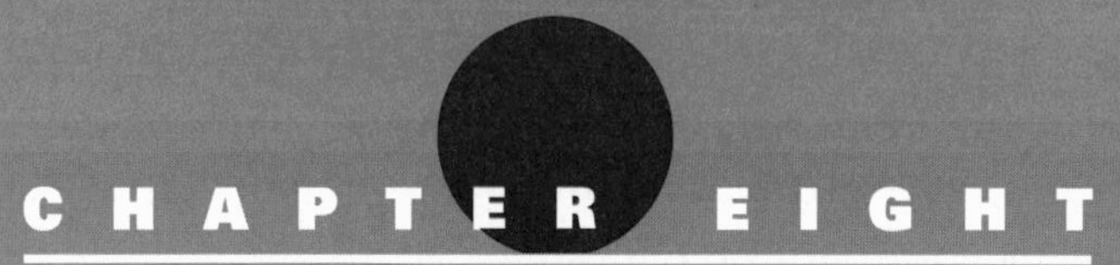

CHAPTER EIGHT

Dynamic Splinting

JEAN WILWERDING-PECK, OTR/L, CHT

Chapter Objectives

1. Understand the biomechanics of dynamic splinting.
2. Identify effects of force on soft tissue.
3. Understand the way to apply appropriate tension.
4. Identify common uses of dynamic splinting.
5. List the goals of dynamic splinting.
6. List the materials necessary for fabrication of a dynamic splint.
7. Explain the risks of applying dynamic force.
8. Understand the fabrication steps of three dynamic splints.
9. Identify instances in which dynamic splinting is appropriate.
10. Explain sources of force in dynamic splinting.

Dynamic splints or mobilizing splints (American Society of Hand Therapists, 1992) have movable parts and are most often designed to apply force across joints (Brand, 1990). Forces use constant or adjustable tension, or both, to achieve one of the following (Fess, 1990):

1. Substitute for loss of muscle function
2. Correct a deformity caused by muscle-tendon tightness or joint contracture
3. Maintain active or passive range of motion
4. Provide controlled motion after tendon repair or joint arthroplasty
5. Aid in fracture alignment and wound healing

This chapter provides basic information on the principles of dynamic splinting. Specifically, this chapter reviews the construction process of dynamic splints for a flexor tendon repair, radial nerve injury, and proximal interphalangeal (PIP) flexion contracture. Early attempts at dynamic splint construction may seem tedious and frustrating, but the process becomes easier with practice and experience.

BIOMECHANICS OF DYNAMIC SPLINTING

Anatomical Considerations

To fabricate a dynamic splint accurately, a therapist must know principles of hand biomechanics and the way the application of external force affects normal hand biomechanics (Fess, 1990). Knowledge of complex mathematical calculations is not required for a therapist to have a basic understanding of biomechanics to avoid harm and provide the best results.

The goal of splinting is to restore a joint so that it glides through the normal full range and has minimal inflammation and scar tissue. Application of an external force to a healing joint raises questions such as the following: At what stage of the healing process should the therapist apply force? How much force should the therapist apply? Where should the therapist apply force? The therapist should never apply force to an injured joint until the inflammation and pain are under control (Fess & Philips, 1987). Mild inflammation is acceptable, but edema should not fluctuate. A dynamic splint applied too early after injury may result in increased inflammation and decreased motion.

Soft tissue structures respond to prolonged stress by changing or re-forming. This activity is called *creep* and involves the adaptation of soft tissue from the application of prolonged force (Brand & Hollister, 1993). Soft tissue responds to excessive force with a reintroduction of the inflammatory process. By applying controlled stress to the tissue over a prolonged period, the therapist can create tension gentle enough to allow creep without tissue injury. If it remains within the elastic limits, the stress from a dynamic splint can positively effect the gradual realignment of collagen fibers and result in increased tensile strength of the tissue. The opportunity to affect collagen formation is greatest during the proliferative stage of wound healing but continues to a lesser degree for several months while the scar matures (Colditz, 1990).

Torque and Mechanical Advantage

To offer the patient the greatest benefit from a dynamic splint, the therapist must understand relevant theories of physics. *Torque* is defined as the effect of force on the rotational movement of a point (Fess & Philips, 1987). Torque amount is calculated by multiplying the force by the length of the moment arm. The greater the length of the lever arm, the greater the mechanical advantage of the applied

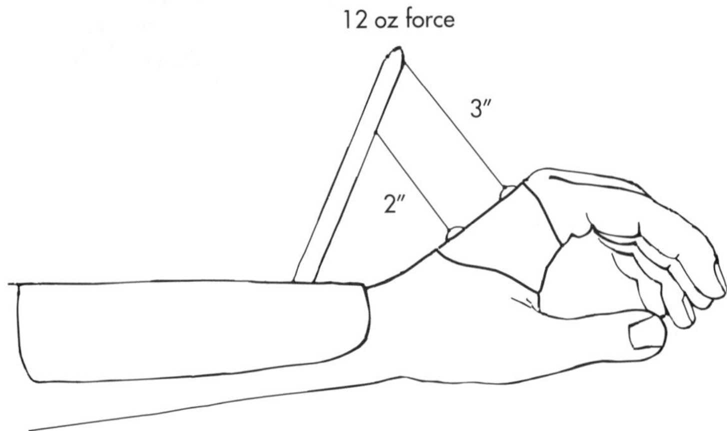

FIGURE 8-1
The 2-inch moment arm produces 24 inch ounces of torque. The 3-inch moment arm produces 36 inch ounces of torque.

force (Figure 8-1). A correlation exists between the distance from a pivot point and the amount of force required. A force applied close to the pivot point (i.e., short moment arm) must be greater than the force applied on a longer moment arm. This force is called *torque* because it acts on the rotational movement of a joint. In practical terms the therapist should place the force as far as possible from the mobilized joint without affecting other joints (Brand & Hollister, 1993).

Application of Force

In dynamic splinting the therapist applies force to a joint or finger through the application of nail hooks or finger loops. When applying force to increase passive joint range of motion, the therapist must keep the direction of pull at a 90° angle to the axis of the joint (Cannon et al., 1985). As range of motion improves, the therapist must adjust the outrigger to maintain the 90° angle (Figure 8-2) (Fess & Philips, 1987). The outrigger should not pull toward ulnar or radial deviation.

When excessive force is applied to the skin for a prolonged period, tissue damage can result. The amount of pressure the skin can tolerate dictates the maximum tolerable force. As a general rule, the amount of acceptable pressure or force per unit area is 50 g/cm^2 (Brand & Hollister, 1993). As the area over which force is applied, becomes larger, the pressure per unit area becomes less. A leather sling with a skin contact area on a finger of approximately 4 cm^2 should provide a maximum pressure of 200 g (Fess & Philips, 1987). A smaller sling with less skin contact area concentrates pressure and is less tolerable.

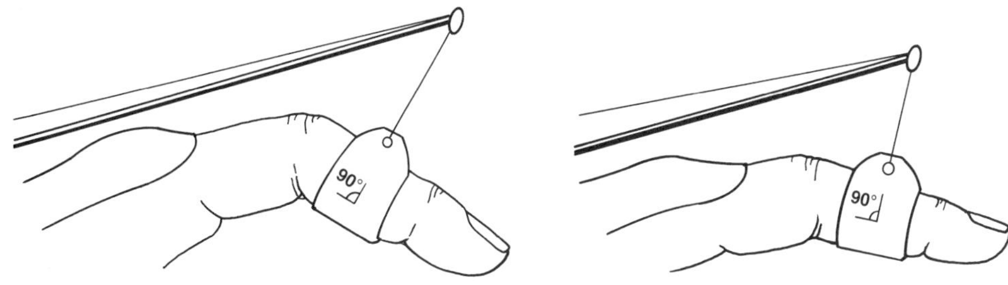

FIGURE 8-2

The line of tension must be maintained at 90° from the long axis of the bone.

Skin grafts, immature scar tissue, and fragile skin of older patients have less tolerance for sling pressure. The patient's tolerance ultimately determines the amount of force. The patient should report the sensation of a gentle stretch, not pain (Fess, 1990). To avoid harm to the patient, the therapist should monitor the splint for the first 30 minutes of wear and at every treatment session thereafter.

Diagnostic Implications

The uses for dynamic splints become more familiar with clinical experience and exposure to various hand injuries. To fit a dynamic splint, the therapist must understand the patient's injury, surgical procedures, and the physician's protocol for treatment. When in doubt, the therapist should always seek clarification.

Substitution for Loss of Motor Function

Whether the patient suffers from a peripheral nerve injury, spinal cord injury, or other debilitating diseases, a splint can increase the functional use of a hand. The goals of splinting for loss of muscle function are to substitute for loss of function, prevent overstretching of nonfunctioning muscles, and prevent joint contractures. Dynamic and static splints can accomplish these goals (Fess & Philips, 1987).

A common peripheral nerve injury is radial nerve palsy. Because of the inability to extend the wrist and metacarpophalangeal (MCP) joints and because of the lack of palmar abduction and extension of the thumb, a hand with radial nerve damage has limited functional use. A splint suspends the hand by means of fingerloops, thus allowing the patient to perform composite extension and flexion of the hand.

A patient who has a C7 spinal cord injury may also use a movable splint. The patient's active wrist extension is the force that transmits motion to the finger flexion in this tenodesis splint.

Patients who have debilitating diseases such as amyotrophic lateral sclerosis,

Guillain-Barré syndrome, or other neurological disorders may also benefit from specialized dynamic splints. Traditionally, patients who suffered from spasticity were not candidates for dynamic splinting (see Chapter 10).

Correction of a Joint Deformity

Joint range of motion that is limited and passive may be the result of multiple factors, including prolonged immobilization, trauma, and significant scar formation. Any patient who has limited passive joint motion may be a candidate for a dynamic splint. However, if a large discrepancy exists between active and passive joint motion, the goal of treatment should focus on active range of motion and strengthening (Colditz, 1990). The best results from dynamic splinting are attained when the therapist initiates treatment soon after edema and pain are under control. As previously mentioned, the best way to lengthen tissue is to provide a tolerable force over a long period. Research indicates a correlation between the amount of time a stiff joint is held at its end range and the resulting gain in passive joint motion (Flowers & LaStayo, 1994). The focus of dynamic splinting should be on increasing the amount of time the splint is worn rather than increasing the force. A general goal for a dynamic splint is to increase passive range of joint motion by 10° per week (Brand, 1990).

Provision of Controlled Motion

A therapist uses a dynamic splint to control motion after the completion of joint implant arthroplasty and flexor tendon repair. Because of the altered joint mechanics of a patient who has arthritis and undergoes joint replacement surgery, the dynamic splint has multiple functions. First, the dynamic splint provides controlled motion and precise alignment while remediating soft tissue deformity. After joint replacement, the splint may provide force on one finger, in extension and radial deviation (Figure 8-3). Second, the splint provides stability for the healing structures while allowing the patient to strengthen previously weakened structures (Fess & Philips, 1987).

After the repair of a flexor tendon, the therapist uses a dynamic splint to provide controlled motion to the healing structures. The reasons for controlled motion are threefold. First, moving the tendons that force the nutrient-rich synovial fluid into the tendon enhances healing. Second, tendons allowed early mobilization display increased tensile strength compared with immobile tendons. Third, by allowing 3 to 5 mm of tendon excursion, the therapist reduces adhesion formation between tendons and surrounding structures (van Strien, 1990).

Aid in Fracture Alignment and Wound Healing

The therapist uses dynamic splinting for the treatment of selected intraarticular fractures of the finger (Schenck, 1994). By providing constant traction at various

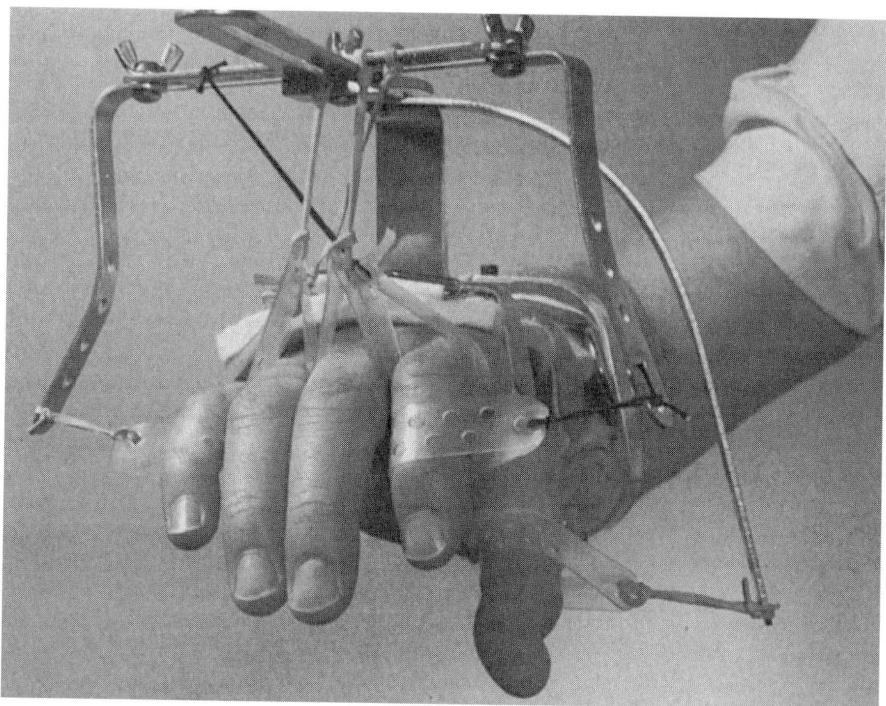

FIGURE 8-3
After implant arthroplasty, tension to one finger may be in two separate directions. (From Hunter, J. M., Schneider, L. H., Mackin, E. J., & Callahan. [1990]. Rehabilitation of the hand: Surgery and therapy [3rd ed., p. 921]. St. Louis: Mosby.)

joint angles, the therapist allows the fracture to heal while it maintains glide of surrounding soft tissues. The therapist may also use dynamic splints to assist in the healing of wounds such as severe burns to affect collagen alignment and scar formation.

Features of a Dynamic Splint

Two features unique to dynamic splinting are the use of an outrigger and the application of force. The outrigger is a projection from the splint base that the therapist uses to position a mobilizing force. The outrigger material depends on the amount and position of necessary force. If the outrigger and attachment to the base are not secure, the mobilizing force becomes altered (Colditz, 1983).

An outrigger can be high or low profile (Figure 8-4). Each type has advantages and disadvantages. A high-profile outrigger requires adjustment less frequently to maintain the 90° angle of pull on the joint. However, a high-profile outrigger is

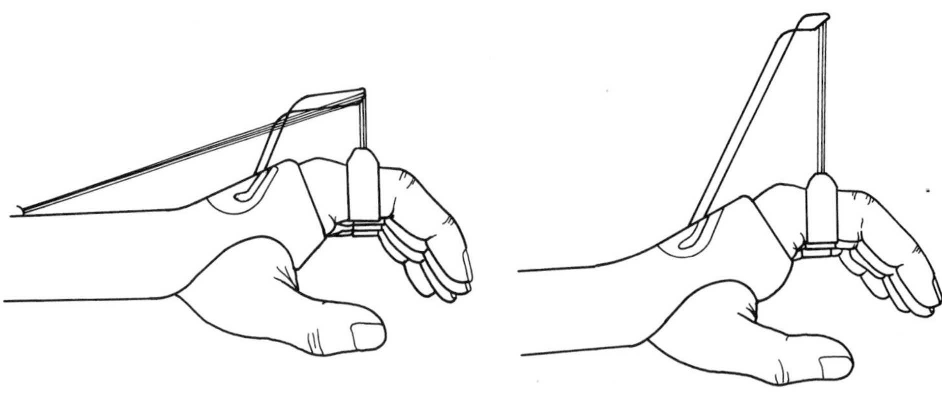

FIGURE 8-4 A low-profile outrigger (*left*) versus a high-profile outrigger (*right*)

bulky and may decrease the patient's compliance with wearing the splint. A low-profile outrigger requires adjustments more frequently but is more aesthetically pleasing and less cumbersome (Fess, 1990).

Various materials are appropriate for outriggers. The therapist may roll a thermoplastic material that has a high level of self-adherence to form a thick, tubular outrigger. This material offers easy adjustment by reheating the plastic. With this material the splint is usually more cumbersome and a strong bond between the outrigger and the base is often difficult. A therapist can also form an outrigger from ⅛-inch wire rod. This diameter is thick enough to provide stability yet pliable enough to manipulate with pliers. Construction of an outrigger using a wire rod requires precise shaping, a skill that necessitates practice. Adjustable wire outrigger kits are available commercially. Although using the kit may increase the splint cost, the application is usually easier because of adjustability of the components.

The therapist can use various methods for applying force to a finger or hand. Finger loops from strong pliable material are usually best because of the increased conformability to the shape of the finger and the decreased chance for tissue maceration (Fess & Philips, 1987). The therapist can supply force by using rubber bands, springs, or elastic thread. Whereas rubber bands are more readily available and easy to adjust, springs offer more consistent tension throughout the range. Elastic thread is the easiest to apply and adjust. A long rubber band stretched over the maximum length of the splint provides more constant tension than a short rubber band (Brand & Hollister, 1993). A nonstretchable string or outrigger line is necessary to connect the finger loop to the source of the force (Figure 8-5). The choice is usually based on clinical experience and preference.

Although dynamic splints have movable parts, a trend toward using static pro-

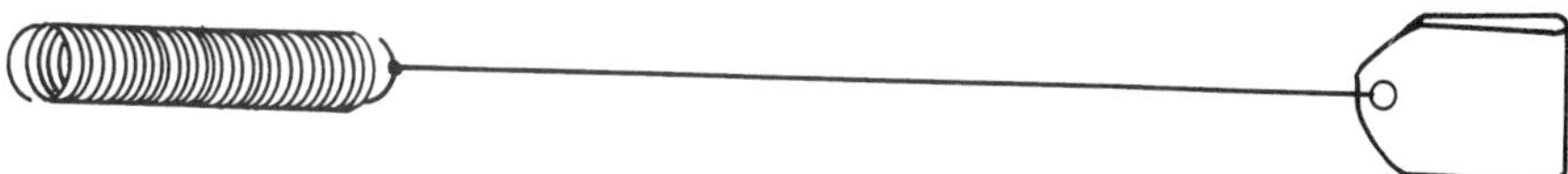

FIGURE 8-5
The therapist uses nonstretchable nylon string to attach finger loops to the source of tension.

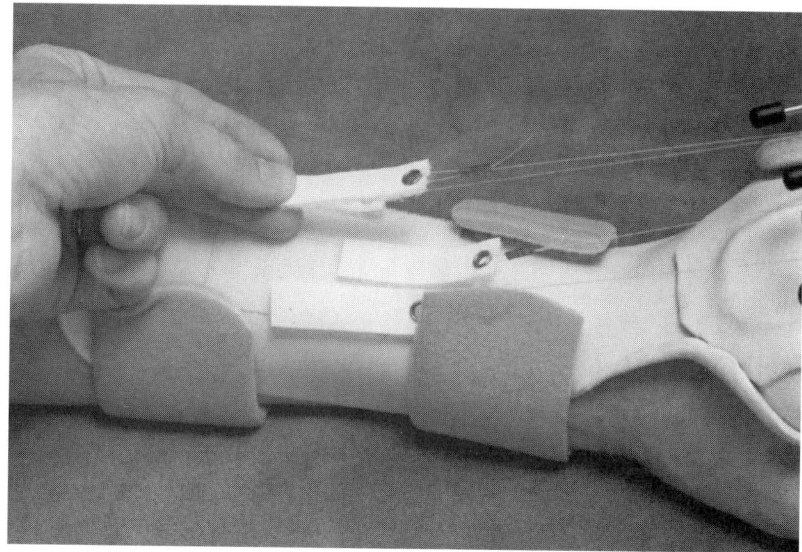

FIGURE 8-6
The patient may adjust velcro tabs used for static progressive tension.

gressive force with resistive contractures is emerging. The therapist uses a tab of velcro loop in place of the rubber band or spring and places a velcro hook on the base of the splint. The patient increases the tension by gradually moving the velcro tab more proximally on the splint base. The force is static rather than dynamic but is readily adjustable by the patient throughout the wearing time (Figure 8-6).

Technical Tips for Dynamic Splinting

When applying an outrigger to the base, the therapist must make sure that both surfaces to be bonded are clean. If a plastic has a glossy finish, the two surfaces may require light scratching to increase the self-adherence. The therapist then heats both surfaces and applies the bonding agent. After placing the outrigger appropriately on the base, the therapist holds the surfaces firmly together and smooths the edges until the plastic cools.

The therapist should use caution when spot heating near an outrigger wire. The wire is better than the plastic at conducting heat, so the wire may push through the thermoplastic. When splinting over bandages or a dressing, the therapist may place a damp paper towel over the area to prevent the thermoplastic from adhering to the dressing. Finally, the therapist should check the line of pull so that it is a 90° angle on the finger loops from front and side views.

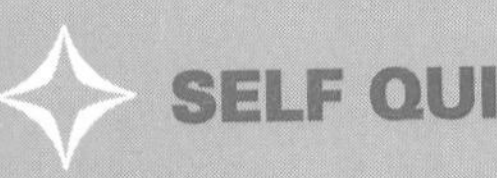

SELF QUIZ 8-1*

Please circle either true (T) or false (F).

1. T F A therapist should apply a dynamic splint to an extremity only when pain and inflammation are well controlled.
2. T F Creep occurs when soft tissue adapts through application of a prolonged force.
3. T F Patients who have new tissue or skin grafts have a high tolerance for pressure to those areas.
4. T F The focus of dynamic splinting should be on increasing the tension rather than on the amount of time the splint is worn.
5. T F A general goal for a dynamic splint is to increase passive range of motion by 10° per week.

*See Appendix A for the answer key.

Materials and Equipment for a Dynamic Splint

In addition to the equipment necessary to fabricate a static splint, a variety of items are required to fabricate a dynamic splint. The following is a list of materials and equipment therapists use for dynamic splinting, though all items are not necessary for every splint.

1. Thermoplastic with a high level of self-adhesion
2. Finger loops
3. Nail hooks, an emery board, and super glue
4. Solvent

5. Nonstretchable nylon string (outrigger line)
6. An outrigger kit
7. A wire rod (⅛ inch) with tools to bend
8. Rubber bands, springs, elastic string, or velcro tabs
9. Safety pins or other material to make a hook

Fabrication of a Flexor Tendon Splint

A therapist commonly uses a dynamic splint for a patient who has an injury to one or more finger flexor tendons. The goal of the splint is to maintain the hand in a protected position while allowing controlled motion of the fingers (May, Silfverskiöld, & Sollerman, November, 1992). This dynamic splint is one of the least complicated to fabricate because an outrigger is not required. The therapist should check the physician's preference because various protocols exist for tendon repairs.

1. Apply the nail hooks to the patient's fingernails so that the super glue thoroughly dries before application of the force. Explain to the patient the reason for the application of the hooks, and assure the patient that removal of the hooks is possible. To increase the adherence of the hook, roughen the fingernail with an emery board and then clean the fingernail with an alcohol wipe. The hook may require an adjustment with two pairs of pliers to fit the contour of the nail. When applying the hook, do not use an excessive amount of glue. Glue that comes in a gel form may be easier to manage. Give the patient extra hooks and application instructions because a hook may come off.
2. Form the splint base over the dorsal surface of the forearm, wrist, and hand. The ideal hand position is 30° to 45° of wrist flexion, 50° to 70° of MCP flexion, and the interphalangeals (IPs) in full extension (May et al., September, 1992). If the hand has just been removed from the cast, the patient may not tolerate the ideal position. If this occurs, splint as close as possible to the ideal position and adjust the splint when tolerable.
3. Using the heat gun, create a bubble over the radial and ulnar styloids to avoid pressure.
4. Apply hook and loop velcro for straps across the palm, wrist, and forearm.
5. Attach a safety pin to the strap that is approximately 3 inches proximal to the wrist crease (Figure 8-7).
6. Apply traction to the nail hooks and attach it to the safety pin. Use elastic thread because of its amount of elasticity. Apply the force to hold the fingers in flexion, but allow the patient to achieve full active extension of the IP joints against the force of the elastic. Attaining full PIP extension is essential to avoid a PIP flexion contracture. As the extensors regain strength, increase the tension to maximum comfortable flexion and yet allow full extension.

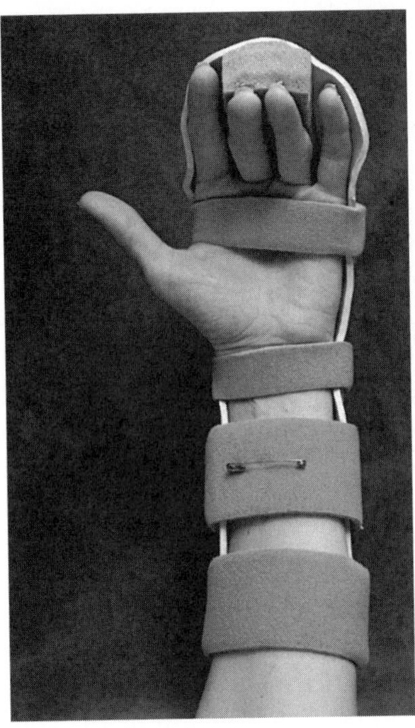

FIGURE 8-7
The safety pin is fixed to the strap 3 inches proximal to the wrist crease.

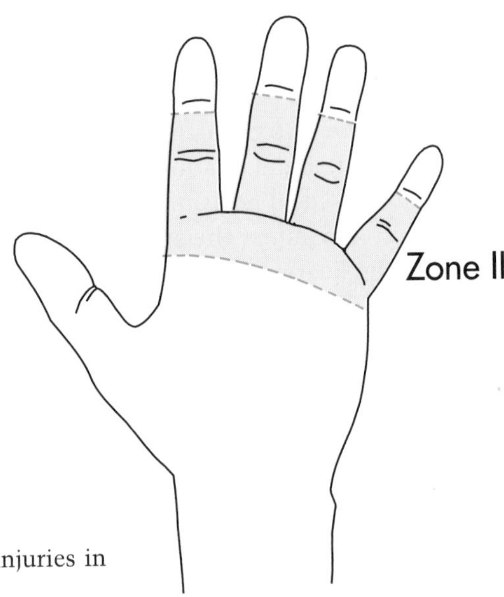

FIGURE 8-8
A palmar pulley may be best for tendon injuries in zone II.

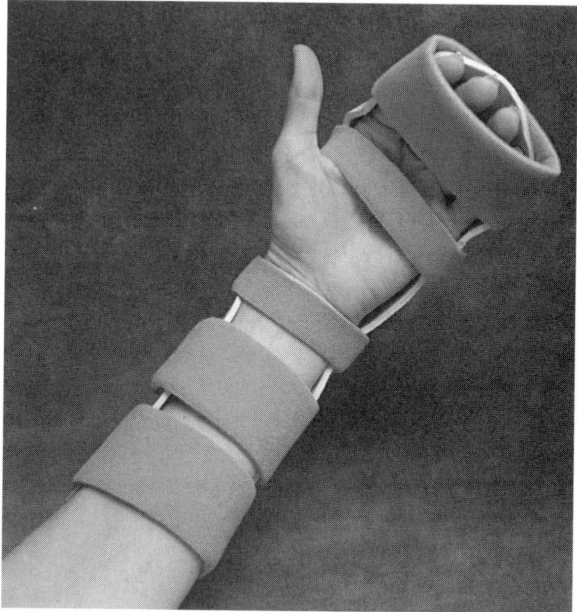

FIGURE 8-9
The patient may use a strap to secure fingers in extension for night wear.

Flexor tendon injuries in zone II are most susceptible to adhesions (Figure 8-8) (Duran, Coleman, Nappi, & Klerekoper, 1990). A palmar pulley may help provide greater excursion of the tendon for these lesions. A therapist can create this pulley by attaching a safety pin to the palmar strap. The elastic thread runs through the palmar pulley as the patient actively exercises approximately 10 minutes every hour. The treatment rationale is to increase excursion of the tendon, limit scar formation, and increase tensile strength of the repair (May, et al., November, 1992).

Because the patient may not feel comfortable sleeping with the fingers in traction, the therapist may apply a strap to the distal aspect of the fingers in order to maintain full interphalangeal extension (Figure 8-9). This application may also reduce extension deficits of the interphalangeal joints (May et al., November, 1992). However, the therapist should caution the patient that the strap is only intended for night wear and that maintaining traction is necessary during the day. The therapist should issue the patient a written home program consisting of a splint-wearing schedule, instructions regarding splint care, and home exercises.

Fabrication of a Dynamic PIP Extension Splint

A dynamic PIP extension splint helps a patient who has decreased passive extension of the PIP joints. Because the PIP joints are not limited at the same joint angles, the therapist may use an outrigger kit that has separate extender rods for each finger. The commercial outrigger usually contains a wire outrigger, extender rods, an Allen wrench, rubber caps for the rods, and adjustment wheels to secure the rods on the outrigger. Instead of rubber bands or springs, the therapist uses velcro tabs to provide static progressive force.

1. Fabricate a dorsal splint from the proximal forearm to the PIP joints, and make certain that the splint conforms to the palmar arches. (See Chapter 5 for a pattern. Note that this splint pattern must be adjusted to extend proximal to the PIP joints.)
2. Use a palmar bar to assist in stabilizing the MCP joints. Because the goal of this splint is to increase composite extension, place the wrist in 30° of extension with the MCPs in the maximum extension tolerable (Figure 8-10).
3. Be sure the distal aspect of the dorsal splint conforms to the shape of the fingers to reduce pressure points.
4. Add adhesive padding between the splint material and dorsum of the fingers for increased comfort.
5. Add straps at the level of the palmar bar, wrist, and forearm.
6. Bend the ends of the outrigger wire that are to be attached to the splint base to increase the stability of the outrigger. The wire may require adjustments to conform to the splint base.

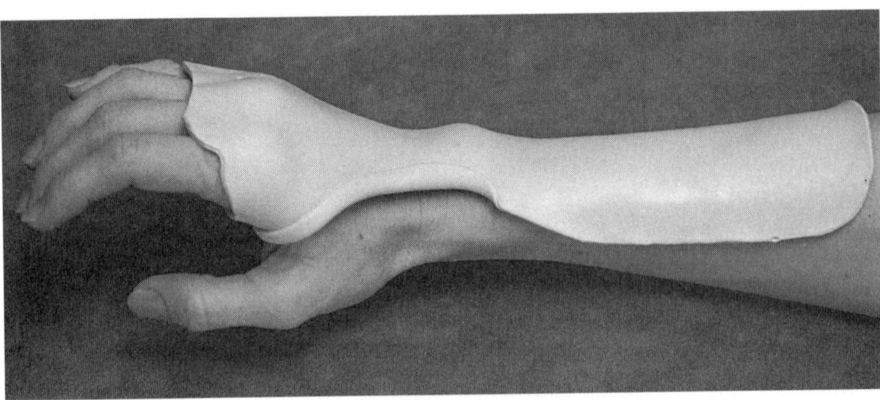

FIGURE 8-10

The wrist is maintained in a functional position with the MCPs in maximum extension.

7. Attach extender rods loosely to the wire outrigger to approximate proper positioning of the outrigger. Place each extender rod parallel to the long axis of the finger, and be sure that the finger loop and cord approach the digit to provide a 90° angle of pull.
8. With the outrigger in place, mark the splint where the ends of the wire are to be attached to the base (Figure 8-11).
9. Remove the splint from the patient. If the extender rods are in the way, remove them before attaching the outrigger to the base.
10. Cut a piece of thermoplastic material large enough to extend beyond the outrigger base by at least ½ inch.
11. Heat the outrigger wire over a heat gun, and slightly embed the wire into the splint base.
12. Apply solvent to the warm piece of thermoplastic material to increase the bonding.

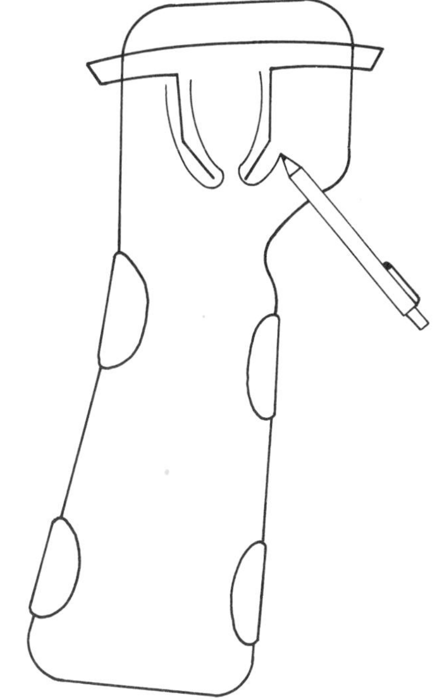

FIGURE 8-11

The outrigger is outlined on the base before attachment to the splint.

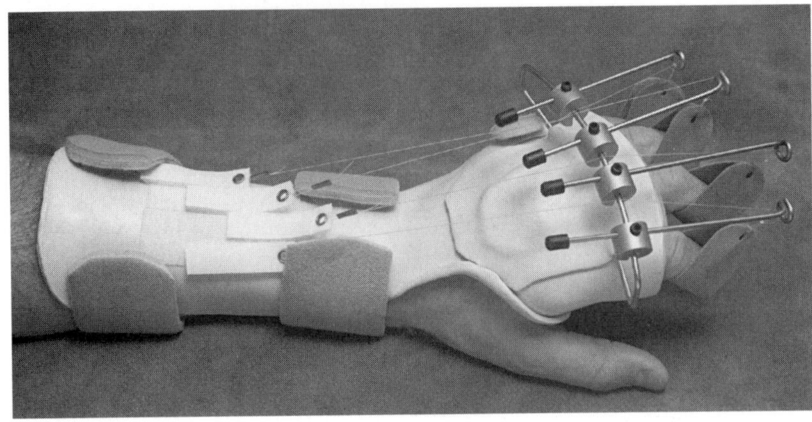

FIGURE 8-12
The therapist places velcro tabs to provide gentle tension.

13. Place the warm thermoplastic material over the outrigger base, and secure the material to the splint base.
14. Add straps to the splint at the palm, wrist, and forearm to prevent shifting of the splint while other adjustments are made.
15. Apply a velcro hook to the dorsal aspect of the forearm part of the splint (from the mid area to the proximal area) for attachment of the tabs.
16. Loosely reattach the extender rods to the outrigger.
17. Apply the splint to the patient's hand.
18. With the loops in place on the fingers and nylon string through the rods, position the extender rod parallel to the finger to ensure a 90° angle of pull. Gently tighten the rods in place by using the Allen wrench.
19. Secure velcro tabs in place so that the tension provides a gentle force (Figure 8-12).
20. Remove the splint from the patient and finish securing the extender rods. If the rods extend more than ½ inch proximal to the adjustment wheels, cut the rods by using heavy-duty wire cutters.
21. Place rubber protective caps on the end of each rod.

Fabrication of a Radial Palsy Splint

The radial nerve palsy splint does not involve the application of force to mobilize a joint, a process that typically defines dynamic splinting (Colditz, 1995). Instead of a mobilizing force, the splint uses a static line to support the fingers. The splint does, however, use an outrigger, which makes the construction similar to that of a dynamic splint.

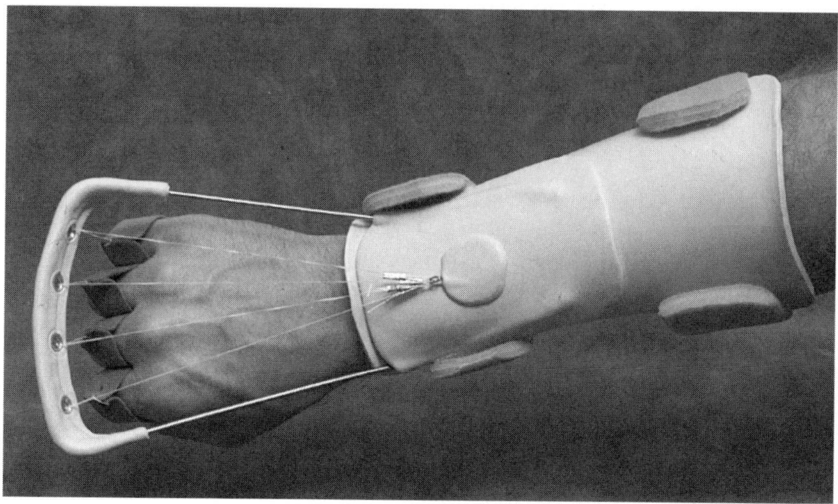

FIGURE 8-13

The therapist must form the outrigger wider than the hand at the level of the MCPs.

A lesion to the radial nerve results in loss of active wrist, thumb, and finger MCP extension. The inability to actively extend and stabilize the wrist limits the functional use of the hand. The goal of this splint is to create a limited tenodesis action to allow functional grip (Colditz, 1987). The splint includes a dorsal base with a low-profile outrigger that spans from the wrist to each proximal phalanx.

1. Fabricate the dorsal forearm base of the radial nerve splint from a thermoplastic material that has self-adherence properties. Rest the splint on the dorsal aspect of the forearm, and extend the splint from the proximal aspect of the forearm to just proximal to the distal radiocarpal joint. The base must be at least one-half the circumference of the forearm to prevent distal migration of the splint. The base must be at least half the circumference of the forearm to prevent distal migration of the splint (Figure 8-13).
2. Apply straps to stabilize the splint base during formation of the outrigger.
3. Make the outrigger from ⅛-inch wire rod. The outrigger must be wider than the hand at the level of the MCPs by approximately ½ inch (Figure 8-13).
4. To form the outrigger properly, draw an outline of the hand marking MCP and PIP joints. Draw a curved line halfway between the joints and extend it ½ inch beyond the hand on each side. Form the distal aspect of the outrigger along this curved line.

5. After forming the outrigger, secure it to the base by using a piece of thermoplastic material prepared with solvent.
6. Drape an additional piece of thermoplastic material over the distal aspect of the outrigger (over the phalanges). Punch holes directly above each finger.
7. To decrease wear on the cord, place metal eyelet reinforcements in each hole.
8. Form a hook from a paper clip and place it in the middle of the dorsal forearm splint (Figure 8-14).
9. Place the splint on the patient to secure the finger loops and cord. The length of the cord should allow full finger extension when the wrist drops to neutral (Figure 8-15). During active finger flexion, the wrist extends slightly.

Laboratory Exercise 8-1

Practice fabricating a radial nerve splint on a partner. After fitting the splint and making all adjustments, use Form 8-1. This check-off sheet is a self-evaluation of the radial nerve splint. Use Grading Sheet 8-1 as a classroom grading sheet.

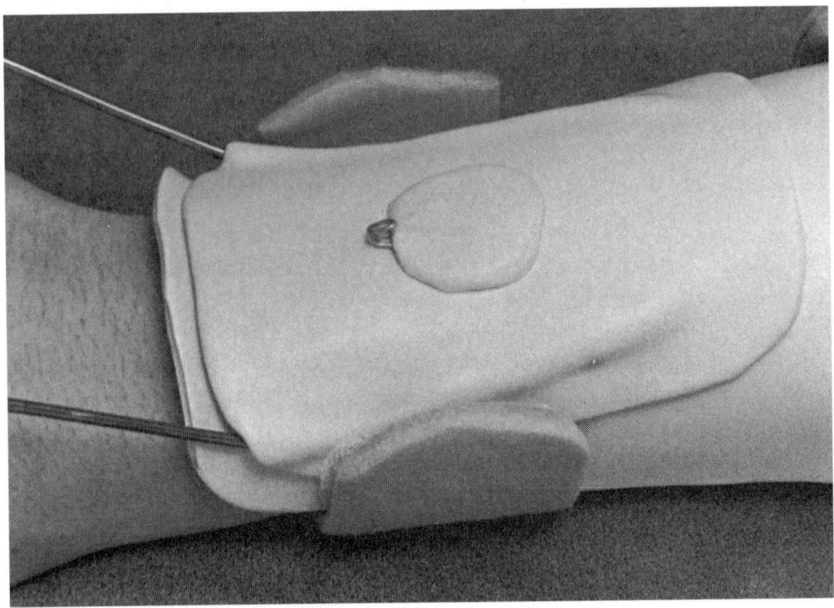

FIGURE 8-14 An anchor hook formed from a paper clip

A

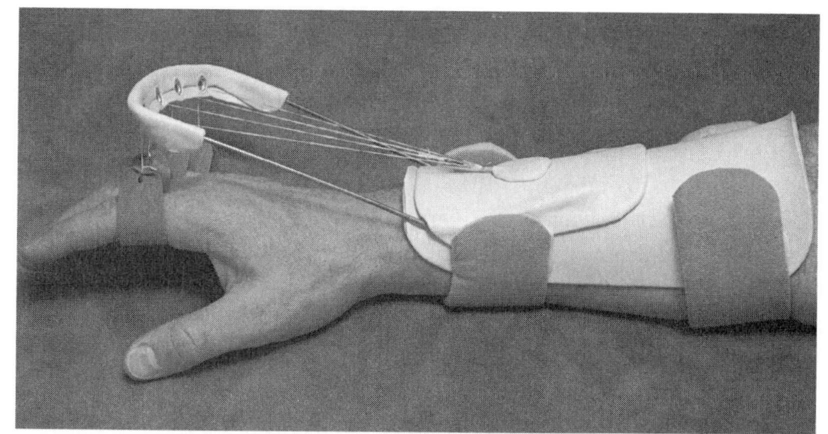

B

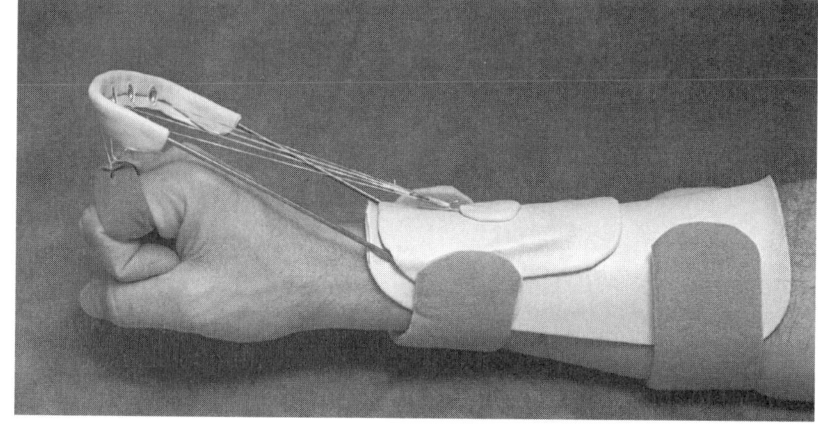

FIGURE 8-15

Neither the outrigger (**A**) nor the line (**B**) must impede composite flexion.

PRECAUTIONS FOR DYNAMIC SPLINTING

In addition to the guidelines just mentioned, therapists should consider other specific precautions during application of dynamic splints. The first rule of dynamic splinting and of all treatment is to do no harm. Therapists can follow this rule by paying strict attention to a few basic guidelines (Fess, 1990), including the following:

1. Be aware that the patient must be responsible enough to care for the splint and follow a wearing schedule. Use extreme caution when applying a dynamic splint to a child who cannot follow instructions (see Chapter 12).
2. Keep in mind normal functional anatomy and biomechanics of the extremity.
3. Apply minimum force. The amount of force should provide a low-grade stretch tolerable to the patient over a long period (Colditz, 1990). A patient probably will not wear a splint that causes discomfort.
4. Keep in mind the risks of wearing an ill-fitting splint (e.g., pressure points, skin breakdown, prolonged immobilization of noninvolved structures).
5. Remember aesthetics. A patient is more likely to wear a splint that has a finished, professional appearance.
6. Monitor and adjust the splint frequently for accurate fit.
7. Listen to the patient. The splint must fit well, have a tolerable amount of tension, and cause minimal interference with daily activities. Complaints by the patient require reevaluation of the splint's fit.
8. Use extreme caution when applying an external force to a hand that has decreased sensation. An increased risk of skin breakdown exists if a therapist applies an excessive amount of force in the absence of sensory feedback.
9. The altered joint mechanics of a patient who has rheumatoid arthritis make static splinting more appropriate than dynamic splinting. A therapist may complete dynamic splinting of a patient who has rheumatoid arthritis only with rare, specific indications (Cailliet, 1994).

FORM 8-1* Radial Nerve Splint

Name: ______________________________

Date: ______________________________

Answer the following questions after the splint has been worn for 30 minutes. (Mark *NA* for nonapplicable situations.)

Evaluation Areas		Comments
Design		
1. The forearm trough is the proper length and width.	Yes ❍ No ❍ NA ❍	
2. The outrigger wire is at the appropriate angles and ½ inch wider than the MCPs at the level of the hand.	Yes ❍ No ❍ NA ❍	
3. The thermoplastic material on the MCP aspect of the outrigger is secure.	Yes ❍ No ❍ NA ❍	
4. The line to the outrigger is at a 90° angle from the long axis of the bone when the hand is at rest.	Yes ❍ No ❍ NA ❍	
5. The anchor hook is secure.	Yes ❍ No ❍ NA ❍	
6. The thermoplastic patch adequately secures the outrigger.	Yes ❍ No ❍ NA ❍	
Function		
1. The wrist is maintained in neutral when the fingers are in extension.	Yes ❍ No ❍ NA ❍	
2. The outrigger or lines do not impede composite flexion of the fingers.	Yes ❍ No ❍ NA ❍	
3. The fit of the trough and straps prevents distal migration of the splint.	Yes ❍ No ❍ NA ❍	
4. The slings do not migrate distally with finger flexion and extension.	Yes ❍ No ❍ NA ❍	

*See Appendix B for a perforated copy of this form.

Continued.

FORM 8-1 Radial Nerve Splint—cont'd

Evaluation Areas		Comments
Comfort		
1. Excessive pressure is not present on the radial or ulnar styloids.	Yes ❍ No ❍ NA ❍	
2. The edges are smooth with rounded corners.	Yes ❍ No ❍ NA ❍	
3. The proximal and distal ends are flared.	Yes ❍ No ❍ NA ❍	
4. Impingements or pressure areas are not present.	Yes ❍ No ❍ NA ❍	

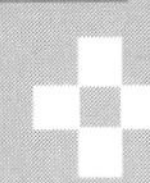

GRADING SHEET 8-1*
Radial Nerve Splint

Name: ______________________

Date: ______________________

Wrist position at rest:

Grade: ________

1 = beyond improvement, not acceptable
2 = requires maximal improvement
3 = requires moderate improvement
4 = requires minimal improvement
5 = requires no improvement

Evaluation Areas		**Comments**
Design		
1. The forearm trough is the proper length and width.	1 2 3 4 5	
2. The outrigger wire is at the appropriate angles and ½ inch wider than the MCPs at the hand level.	1 2 3 4 5	
3. The thermoplastic on the distal aspect of the outrigger is secure.	1 2 3 4 5	
4. The line to the outrigger is at a 90° angle from the long axis of the bone when the hand is at rest.	1 2 3 4 5	
5. The anchor hook is secure.	1 2 3 4 5	
6. The thermoplastic material patch adequately secures the outrigger.	1 2 3 4 5	
Function		
1. The wrist is maintained in neutral when the fingers are in extension.	1 2 3 4 5	
2. The outrigger or lines do not impede composite flexion of the fingers.	1 2 3 4 5	
3. The fit of the trough and straps prevents distal migration of the splint.	1 2 3 4 5	
4. The slings do not migrate distally with active finger flexion and extension.	1 2 3 4 5	

*See Appendix C for a perforated copy of this grading sheet.

Continued.

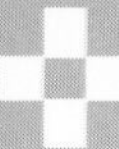

GRADING SHEET 8-1
Radial Nerve Splint—cont'd

Evaluation Areas						Comments
Comfort						
1. Excessive pressure is not present on the radial or ulnar styloids.	1	2	3	4	5	
2. The edges are smooth with rounded corners.	1	2	3	4	5	
3. The proximal and distal ends are flared.	1	2	3	4	5	
4. Impingements or pressure areas are not present.	1	2	3	4	5	

Comments:

Case Study*

Read the following scenario and answer the questions based on information in this chapter:

Michael is a 12-year old, right-handed boy who is out of school for the summer. After a rough landing from his bike ramp, he was unable to move his right elbow without significant pain. At the hospital the physician determined that Michael had a comminuted fracture of the right humerus. In addition, Michael was unable to actively extend his thumb, wrist, and MCPs, and he was unable to abduct his thumb. An electromyogram revealed damage to the radial nerve. The physician has ordered occupational therapy for fabrication of a splint.

1. Which clinical evaluation is required before fabrication of the splint?
   a. Evaluate ability to actively extend wrist, MCPs, and thumb
   b. Evaluate sensory deficits
   c. Evaluate functional use of injured hand
   d. All of the above

2. What is the primary goal for this splint?
   a. Prevent further injury
   b. Protect damaged nerve by immobilizing wrist
   c. Increase functional use of hand
   d. Limit composite flexion of fingers

3. Which outrigger is most appropriate for this splint?
   a. High profile
   b. Low profile

4. What is the most desirable source of finger and wrist support for this splint?
   a. Static tension
   b. Rubber band tension
   c. Spring tension
   d. Elastic string tension

5. What is the position of the wrist during composite flexion of the fingers?
   a. Flexion of 30°
   b. Neutral
   c. Extension of 45°

*See Appendix A for the answer key.

Review Questions

1. What are four possible goals of dynamic splinting?
2. What are the complications associated with application of too much force?
3. What is the angle of pull between the long axis of the bone and the outrigger line that the therapist must maintain?
4. What is the acceptable force per unit area for sling pressure?
5. What patient information should the therapist gather before considering a patient for a dynamic splint?
6. What is the difference between a high-profile and low-profile outrigger? What are the advantages and disadvantages of each?
7. What are three methods for the application of force?
8. What are the steps for attaching an outrigger wire to a splint base?
9. What are three precautions with dynamic splinting?

References

American Society of Hand Therapists. (1992). Splint classification system. Garner, NC: American Society of Hand Therapists.

Brand, P., & Hollister, A. (1993). Terminology, mechanical resistance, and external stress: Effect at the surface. In J. D. Ryan (Ed.), Clinical mechanics of the hand (pp. 5, 99, & 140). St. Louis: Mosby.

Brand, P. W. (1990). The forces of dynamic splinting: Ten questions before applying a dynamic splint to the hand. In J. M. Hunter, L. H. Schneider, E. J. Mackin, & A. D. Callahan (Eds.), Rehabilitation of the hand. St. Louis: Mosby.

Cailliet, R. (1994). Functional anatomy and joints: Injuries and disease. In Hand pain and impairment (pp. 23 & 244). Philadelphia: F. A. Davis Co.

Cannon, N., Foltz, R., Koepfer, J., Lauck, M., Simpson, D., & Bromley, R. (1985). Mechanical principles. In Manual of hand splinting (pp. 6-7). New York: Churchill Livingstone.

Colditz, J. (1983). Low profile dynamic splinting of the injured hand. Am J Occup Ther, 37, 182-188.

Colditz, J. (1987). Splinting for radial nerve palsy. J Hand Ther, 1, 18-23.

Colditz, J. C. (1990). Dynamic splinting of the stiff hand. In J. M. Hunter, L. H. Schneider, E. J. Mackin, & A. D. Callahan (Eds.), Rehabiltation of the hand. St. Louis: Mosby.

Colditz, J. C. (May, 1995). Personal communication.

Duran, R. J., Coleman, C. R., Nappi, J. F., & Klerekoper, L. A. (1990). In J. M. Hunter, L. H. Schneider, E. J. Mackin, & A. D. Callahan (Eds.), Rehabilitation of the hand. St. Louis: Mosby.

Fess, E. E. (1990). Principles and methods of splinting for mobilization of joints. In J. M. Hunter, L. H. Schneider, E. J. Mackin, & A. D. Callahan (Eds.), Rehabilitation of the hand. St. Louis: Mosby.

Fess, E. E., & Philips, C. A. (1987). Hand splinting principles and methods (2nd ed.). St. Louis: Mosby.

Flowers, K., & LaStayo, P. (1994). Effect of total end range time on improving passive range of motion. J Hand Ther, 7, 150-157.

May, E., Silfverskiöld, K., & Sollerman, C. (Sept., 1992). Controlled mobilization after flexor tendon repair in zone II: A prospective comparison of three methods. J Hand Surg, 17A, 942-952.

May, E., Silfverskiöld, K., & Sollerman, C. (Nov., 1992). The correlation between controlled range of motion with dynamic traction and results after flexor tendon repair in zone II. J Hand Surg, 17, 1133-1139.

Schenck, R. (1994). The dynamic traction method. Hand Clin, 10, 187-197.

van Strien, G. (1990). Postoperative management of flexor tendon injuries. In J. M. Hunter, L. H. Schneider, E. J. Mackin, & A. D. Callahan (Eds.), Rehabilitation of the hand. St. Louis: Mosby.

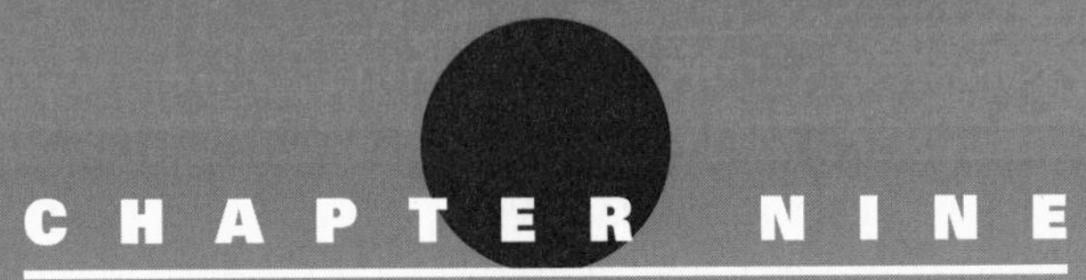

CHAPTER NINE

Splinting for Nerve Injuries

HELENE LOHMAN, MA, OTR/L
BRENDA M. COPPARD, MS, OTR/L

Chapter Objectives

1. List the three purposes for splinting nerve palsies.
2. Define the terms *neurapraxia, axonotmesis,* and *neurotmesis.*
3. Identify low and high nerve lesions.
4. Explain causes of radial, ulnar, and median nerve lesions.
5. Review the sensory and motor distributions of the radial, median, and ulnar nerves.
6. Explain the functional effects of radial, ulnar, and median nerve lesions.
7. Identify the splinting approaches and rationale for radial, ulnar, and median nerve palsies.
8. Identify the advantages and disadvantages of different splint application positions for carpal tunnel syndrome.
9. Use clinical judgment to evaluate a problematic splint for a nerve lesion.
10. Use clinical judgment to evaluate a fabricated, hand-based ulnar nerve splint.
11. Apply documentation skills to a case study.

Splint interventions for nerve lesions require thorough knowledge of static and dynamic splinting principles and sound critical-thinking skills. Kinesiology and anatomy comprehension are paramount to understanding the motor, sensory, and vasomotor implications of a nerve injury. Good manual muscle-testing skills are also necessary to evaluate the muscles as the nerve returns (Colditz, 1990).

Nerves are at risk for injury when laceration, avulsion, stretch, crush, compression, or contusion occurs (Callahan, 1984). Often bone, tendon, ligamentous, vessel, and soft-tissue injuries accompany nerve injuries.

Peripheral nerve lesions usually occur to the median, radial, and ulnar nerves. The location of the lesion determines the impairment of vasomotor, muscular, sensory, and functional involvement (Boscheinen-Morrin, Davey, & Conolly, 1987). This chapter discusses splinting for radial, median, and ulnar nerve injuries and compressions.

Purposes for Splinting Nerve Palsies

The three purposes for splinting an extremity that has a nerve palsy are protection, prevention, and assistance with function (Arsham, 1984). If a nerve has undergone surgical repair, the physician may initially order application of a cast or splint to place the hand, wrist, and/or elbow in a protective position, thus reducing the amount of tension on the repaired nerve.

Prevention of contractures is important because nerve lesions result in various degrees of muscle denervation. For example, with a median nerve injury a short opponens splint prevents a contracture of the thumb web space (Fess & Philips, 1987).

Sometimes a patient does not seek immediate medical attention after the occurence of a nerve injury and after the development of a contracture that requires splint intervention. For example, if a person suffers from a clawhand deformity as a result of an ulnar nerve injury, the therapist can fabricate a dynamic ulnar gutter splint to stretch the soft tissues and mobilize the ring and little finger proximal interphalangeal (PIP) joints into extension (Callahan, 1984). The therapist should keep in mind that once metacarpophalangeal (MCP) and PIP stiffness have occurred, treatment should focus on regaining maximum passive range of motion. Splinting interventions for the muscle imbalance may then be an option (Fess, 1986).

Nerve Compression Classification

Nerve compressions are categorized by the extent of damage to the axon and sheath (Skirven, 1992). Nerve compression lesions often contribute to peripheral neuropathies. When a specific portion of a peripheral nerve is compressed, the peripheral axons that are within the nerve sustain the greatest injury. As the compression worsens, the motor, proprioceptive, light touch, and vibratory sensory axons become more vulnerable (Spinner, 1990). All the fibers may be paralyzed after they endure severe and prolonged compression. As shown in Figure 9-1, the three classifications of nerve compressions are (1) neurapraxia, (2) axonotmesis, and (3) neurotmesis (Spinner, 1990; Pec'ina, Krmpotic'-Nemanic', & Markiewitz, 1991).

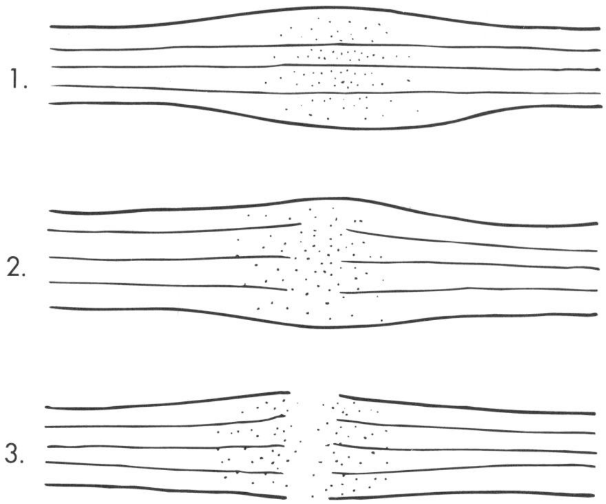

1.

2.

3.

FIGURE 9-1

The three classifications of nerve injuries are (1) neurapraxia, (2) axonotmesis, and (3) neurotmesis.

Neurapraxia

Neurapraxia has been defined as a "nerve concussion with a transient physiological block" (Boscheinen-Morrin, et al., p. 54, 1987). The prognosis for persons with neurapraxia is extremely good; recovery is usually spontaneous. "Most neurapractic lesions respond to conservative treatment within three months" (Spinner, p. 523, 1990).

Axonotmesis

When axonotmesis occurs, the axon is severed and the sheath remains intact. In addition, wallerian degeneration exists distal to the level of the compression (Spinner, 1990). Wallerian degeneration occurs when the axons degenerate but the connective tissue remains open and unblocked. Regenerating fibers reaching the proximal end usually form a neuroma that requires surgical removal before repair (Boscheinen-Morrin, et al., 1987).

Neurotmesis

Neurotmesis results in partial or complete severance of the axon and the sheath, and surgical intervention is required to excise any neuromas. Occasionally grafting is necessary if the gap is too large for approximation of the two nerve ends (Spinner, 1990).

Locations of Nerve Lesions

The location of a nerve lesion's damage affects the result. Lesions are referred to as *low* or *high*. Low lesions occur distal to the elbow, and high lesions occur proximal to the elbow (Barr & Swan, 1988). High lesions affect more muscles and may affect a larger sensory distribution than low lesions. Therefore knowledge of relevant anatomy is important.

Substitutions or Trick Motions

When a nerve lesion occurs, "there is no opposing balancing force to the intact active muscle group" (Colditz, p. 647, 1990). If a nerve lesion remains unsplinted, the intact musculature will overpower the denervated muscles and the person will learn to adapt to the imbalance (Colditz, 1990). An example of a substitution or trick movement is the pinch that occurs after a median nerve injury. With the help of the adductor pollicis the flexor pollicis longus pinches objects against the radial side of the index finger. A therapist may think that motor return has occurred for the abductor pollicis brevis, flexor pollicis brevis, opponens pollicis, and first and second lumbricals. However, the movement observed is actually a substitution.

Prognosis

Many factors affect the prognosis of recovery from a nerve injury. These factors include the following: the extent of the injury, the cleanliness of the wound, the method of repair, and the patient's age (Skirven, 1992). Correct alignment of axons and avoidance of tension on the damaged nerve improves the prognosis. A clean wound has a better prognosis than a dirty wound (Boscheinen-Morrin, et al., 1987). A nerve injury that an experienced microsurgeon repairs and is "timed appropriately according to the nature and extent of the injury is essential for a favorable outcome" (Skirven, 1992, p. 324).

Age is also a factor in the speed of recovery. A child's potential for regeneration is greater than an adult's (Skirven, 1992). Full sensory and motor return is visible in a child but rarely in an adult. Because nerve regeneration is slow, the therapist should complete periodic monitoring. In addition, the therapist should document results of the evaluation and any changes to the splinting or exercise program.

Radial Nerve Injuries

Of the three basic upper extremity nerve lesions, radial nerve palsies are the most common and typically occur from midhumeral fractures or compressions (Colditz, 1987; Arsham, 1984). Other causes of superficial radial nerve palsies at the wrist include the following: pressure, edema, and trauma on the nerve from

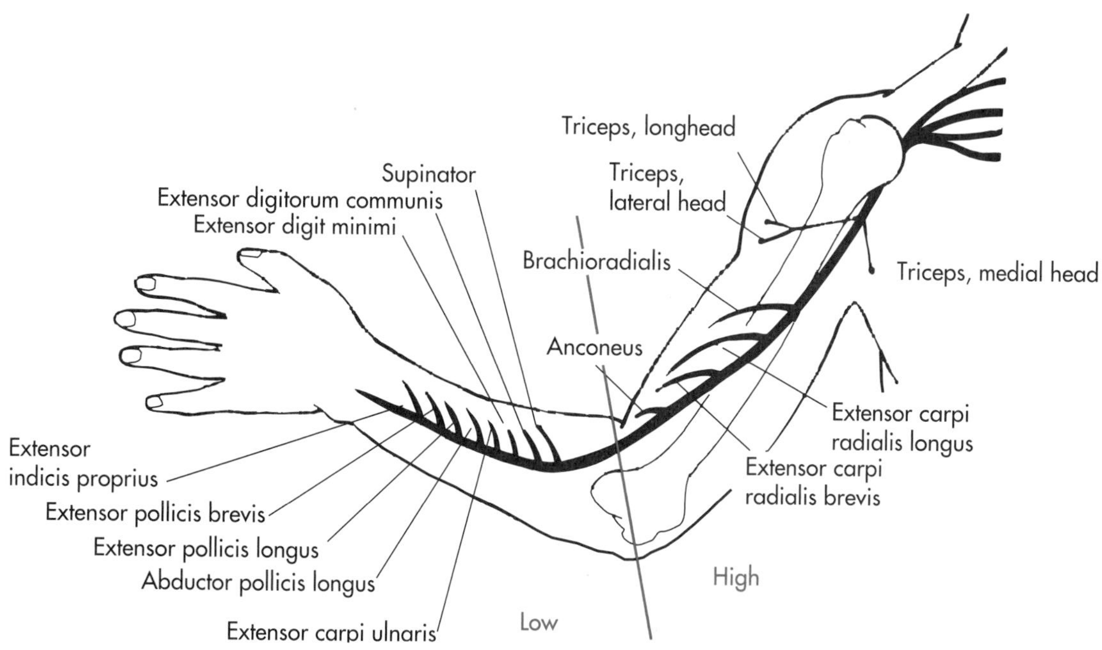

FIGURE 9-2 Radial nerve motor innervation

crush injuries; de Quervain's tendonitis; handcuffs; and a tight or heavy wristwatch (Eaton & Lister, 1992). The location of the radial nerve injury determines which muscles are affected (Figure 9-2).

Three lesions are visible when the radial nerve is injured (Colditz, 1990). The first type of lesion involves a high injury at the level of the humerus that results in wristdrop and lack of finger MCP extension (Figure 9-3). With this type of lesion the triceps are rarely affected unless the injury is extremely high. After spiraling around the humerus and crossing the elbow, the radial nerve divides into a motor and sensory branch (Eaton & Lister, 1992). The motor branch is the posterior interosseous nerve, and the sensory branch is the superficial branch of the radial nerve.

The second type of lesion involves the posterior interosseous nerve. Compression usually causes this palsy, but lacerations or stab wounds can also be sources of lesions.

The third type of lesion that is visible when the radial nerve is injured involves the sensory branch. This last type of lesion does not result in a functional loss because the sensory innervation occurs to the dorsoradial surface of the hand.

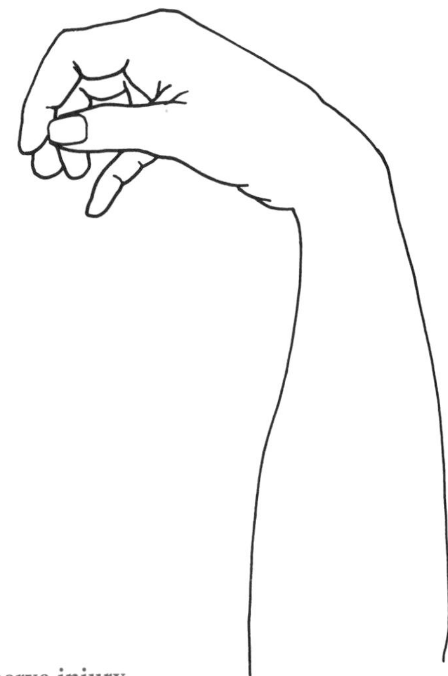

FIGURE 9-3 Wrist drop deformity from a radial nerve injury

Functional Involvement from Radial Nerve Lesions

Table 9-1 shows the muscles and motions that are affected and the lesion locations.

After crossing the elbow and dropping below the supinator, the radial nerve divides and forms the posterior interosseous nerve (Colditz, 1990). Lesions and compressions of the posterior interosseous nerve at the forearm level can affect the following muscles:

1. Extensor digitorum communis
2. Extensor carpi ulnaris
3. Abductor pollicis longus
4. Extensor pollicis longus
5. Extensor pollicis brevis
6. Extensor indicis proprius
7. Extensor digiti minimi

Loss of these muscles results in a loss of MCP extension of all the digits, loss of thumb radial abduction, and loss of thumb extension. With attempts at wrist ex-

TABLE 9-1

Radial Nerve Lesions

Affected muscles	Weak and lost motions
FOREARM LEVEL (POSTERIOR INTEROSSEOUS NERVE)	
Extensor digitorum communis	Lost MCP extension of all digits
Extensor carpi ulnaris	
Extensor indicis proprius	
Extensor digiti minimi	
Abductor pollicis longus	Lost thumb radial abduction
Extensor pollicis longus	Lost thumb extension
Extensor pollicis brevis	
ELBOW LEVEL	
Extensor carpi radialis longus	Lost radial wrist extension
Extensor carpi radialis brevis	
Supinator	Weak supination
Extensor digitorum communis	Lost MCP extension
Extensor carpi ulnaris	
Extensor indicis proprius	
Extensor digiti minimi	
Abductor pollicis longus	Lost thumb abduction
Extensor pollicis longus	Lost thumb extension
Extensor pollicis brevis	
AXILLA LEVEL	
Brachioradialis	Weak elbow flexion
Triceps	Lost elbow extension
Extensor carpi radialis longus	Lost radial wrist extension
Extensor carpi radialis brevis	
Supinator	Weak supination
Extensor digitorum communis	Lost MCP extension
Extensor carpi ulnaris	
Extensor indicis proprius	
Extensor digiti minimi	
Abductor pollicis longus	Lost thumb abduction
Extensor pollicis longus	Lost thumb extension
Extensor pollicis brevis	

tension, strong wrist radial deviation is present. With finger extension attempts the MCPs flex and the PIPs extend because the extensor digitorum muscle is affected.

In addition to the muscles just indicated, a radial nerve injury at the elbow level can affect the following muscles:

1. Extensor carpi radialis longus
2. Extensor carpi radialis brevis
3. Supinator

In addition to the motions lost at the forearm level, an injury at the elbow level involves a loss of radial wrist extension, MCP joint extension, thumb extension, thumb radial abduction, and weakened forearm supination.

When a high-level lesion or compression occurs in the upper arm (i.e., axilla level), the injury can affect the triceps and brachioradialis muscles. Loss of these muscles results in lost elbow extension, weak supination, absent wrist and finger extensors, and lost thumb extension and abduction.

The functional results of an axilla-level lesion are a loss of wrist stabilization in an extended position, loss of finger and thumb extension, and loss of thumb abduction. A patient who suffers from a high radial nerve lesion has poor grip and

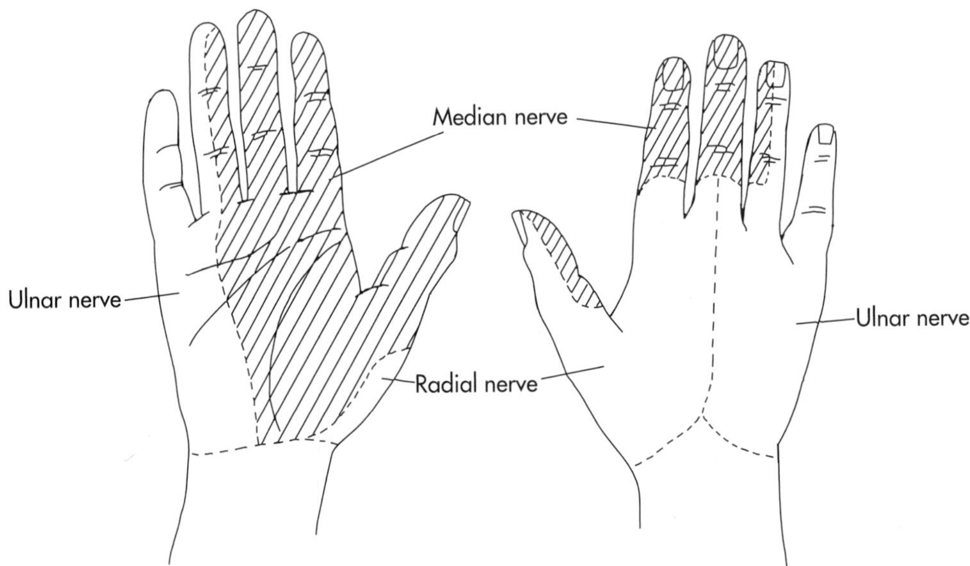

FIGURE 9-4 Radial, median, and ulnar nerve sensory distribution

coordination because of the lack of wrist extensor opposition to the flexors (Bosheinen-Morrin, et al., 1987; Fess, 1986).

Significant loss of sensation is not present with radial nerve injuries. The superficial sensory branch of the radial nerve supplies sensation to the dorsum of the index and middle fingers and half of the ring finger to the PIP joint level. Figure 9-4 shows a representation of sensory distribution from the radial nerve.

Radial Nerve Injury Splint Intervention

The patient benefits from a splint intervention in addition to a therapeutic program. Several splint options exist for radial nerve injuries.

Wrist Cock-Up Splint

The therapist can use a wrist cock-up splint to place the wrist in a functional position of 30° extension (Cannon, et al., 1985). A patient can usually extend the fingers to release an object by using the intrinsic hand muscles (Boscheinen-Morrin, et al., 1987). The therapist should keep in mind the advantages, disadvantages, and patterns of volar and dorsal wrist cock-up splints (see Chapter 5).

Dynamic Extension Splints

Dynamic splinting for a radial nerve injury usually promotes functional hand use (Borucki & Schmidt, 1992). The therapist can fabricate a dorsal wrist cock-up splint as the base for a dynamic extension splint (Arsham, 1984). The dynamic component for this splint should keep the MCPs in extension. However, Colditz (1990) remarks that "one should be cautioned against designs for dynamic wrist and finger extension, because the powerful unopposed flexors often overcome the force of the dynamic splint during finger flexion" (p. 656).

A dynamic MCP extension splint for a radial nerve injury substitutes for the absent muscle power of the MCP extensors. This splint is usually worn throughout the day until the impaired musculature reaches a manual muscle test grade of fair (Callahan, 1984). A patient who does not show clinical improvement in 3 months should return to a physician for possible surgical intervention (Eaton & Lister, 1992).

Because wrist control usually returns first, the therapist can use a hand-based dynamic splint after the forearm-based dynamic splint has been worn (Arsham, 1984; Ziegler, 1984). If only one finger is lagging in extension, the therapist should dynamically incorporate that finger into the splint (Ziegler, 1984). The therapist may use a thumb extension outrigger in the splint design to prevent a contracture.

Another type of dynamic splint that the therapist can use for radial nerve injuries is a splint that was designed at the Hand Rehabilitation Center in Chapel Hill, North Carolina, in 1978 (Colditz, 1990). (See Chapter 8 for fabrication

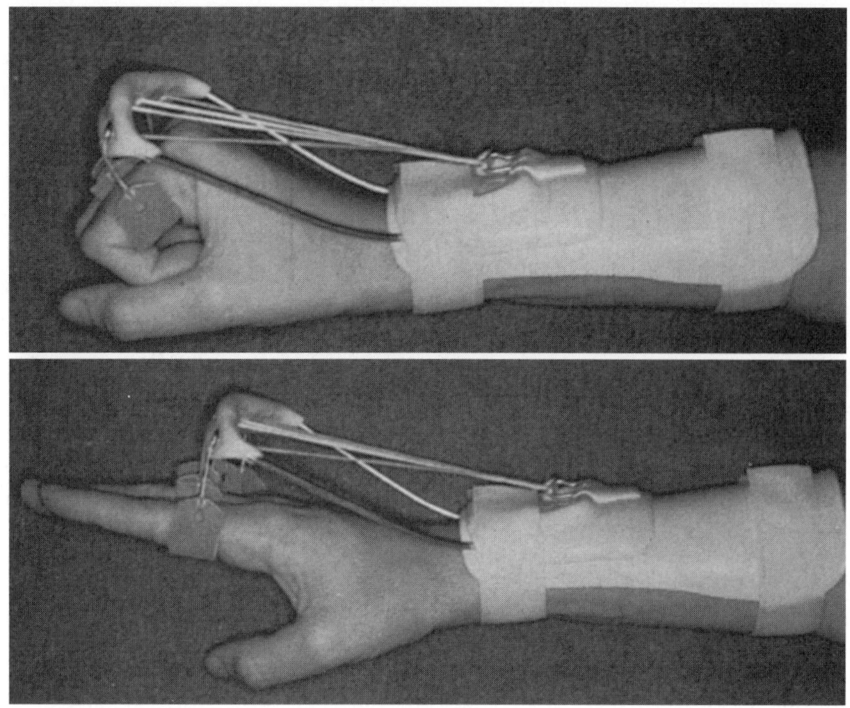

FIGURE 9-5 **A splint for a radial nerve palsy**
(From Hunter, J. M., Schneider, L. H., Mackin, E. J., & Callahan, A. D. [1990]. Rehabilitation of the hand: Surgery and therapy [3rd ed., p. 655]. St. Louis: Mosby.)

instructions.) This dynamic splint reestablishes the tenodesis pattern of the hand (Colditz, 1987) and includes a dorsal base splint with a low-profile outrigger that spans from the wrist to each proximal phalanx. Finger loops are worn on each proximal phalanx, and a nylon cord attached from the finger loops is stretched to a point on the dorsal base. The tenodesis pattern occurs when the patient flexes the wrist and the fingers extend and when the patient extends the wrist and the fingers flex (Figure 9-5).

This splint design has many advantages. First, the design allows the palmar surface of the hand to be relatively free for sensory input. The wrist is not immobilized; it only moves with the natural tenodesis effect (Colditz, 1987). As wrist movement returns, the patient can continue to wear the splint because it does not immobilize the wrist. Therefore a hand-based splint is not required. The low-profile splint also enhances the performance of functional tasks.

Laboratory Exercise 9-1*

Ricardo is a 36-year-old, right-handed man who sustained a left forearm–level posterior interosseous nerve lesion. The physician referred Ricardo to a therapist for splint fabrication and a home program. The therapist wrote the following S.O.A.P. note:

S—"I've been working on my home program every day."

O—Pt. presented with a left forearm level radial nerve injury. Manual muscle testing (MMT) results for the extensor digitorum communis, extensor digiti minimi, extensor indicis, abductor pollicis longus, and extensor carpi ulnaris all scored zero. Semmes-Weinstein Monofilament sensation testing revealed absent sensation on the dorsum of the index and middle fingers and one half of the ring finger to the PIP joint level. Pt. reports no pain in the LUE. A left dorsal-based dynamic MCP extension splint was fabricated and fitted for the pt. Pt. was instructed on donning and doffing the splint and how to grasp and release objects. Pt. was also instructed verbally and given written information on the wearing schedule, splint care, and precautions. Pt. was given a home program to be completed 5x/day. Pt. was taught one-handed ADL techniques.

A—Pt. was receptive to splint and home program. Pt. was able to independently grasp objects while wearing the splint. Anticipate compliance with wearing schedule and home program.

P—Will monitor needs for modifications of the splint and home program.

Several appointments later, the patient regained wrist movements with an MMT score of fair (3). The therapist fabricated a left dynamic MCP extension hand-based splint. The therapist encouraged the patient to continue with ADL and the home program. The therapist also modified the patient's wearing schedule and home program and told the patient to complete the program 5x/day. The patient had no complaints. The patient was able to independently grasp light objects while wearing the splint. Semmes-Weinstein Monofilaments sensation testing revealed impaired sensation on the dorsum of the index and middle fingers and one half of the ring finger to the PIP joint level.

Write the next progress note below:

____

____

____

____

____

____

____

____

____

____

*See Appendix A for the answer key.

Ulnar Nerve Injuries

Lesions to the ulnar nerve can occur from a fracture of the medial epicondyle of the humerus, a fracture of the olecranon process of the ulna, and/or a laceration of the wrist. A compression of the ulnar nerve can occur at the elbow level in the cubital tunnel or at the wrist level within the Guyon's canal (Skirven, 1992). Ulnar compression syndromes are the second most common compression neuropathies in the upper extremity (Norkus & Meyers, 1994). An ulnar nerve lesion can also occur with a median nerve lesion (Enna, 1988).

Regardless of the etiology or location of an ulnar lesion, if a deformity results, it is called a *clawhand.* Anatomically, this deformity occurs because the MCP joints of the ring and little fingers are positioned in hyperextension and incapable of fully extending the PIP and distal interphalangeal (DIP) joints because of the unopposed action of the extensor digitorum communis and the extensor digiti minimi (Figure 9-6). In addition, the lumbricals are not functional (Boscheinen-Morrin et al., 1987).

Functional Nerve Involvement with Ulnar Nerve Injuries

Table 9-2 identifies the muscles the ulnar nerve innervates in a low-level or wrist lesion and a high-level lesion that occurs at or above the elbow. If an ulnar nerve lesion occurs just distal to the elbow, the extrinsic muscles of the hand are lost because they are innervated distal to the elbow. The functional result from a high- or low-level ulnar nerve lesion is loss of pinch and power grip strength (Fess, 1986; Skirven, 1992). The patient is not able to grasp an object fully because of the denervation of the finger abductors, atrophy of the hypothenar emi-

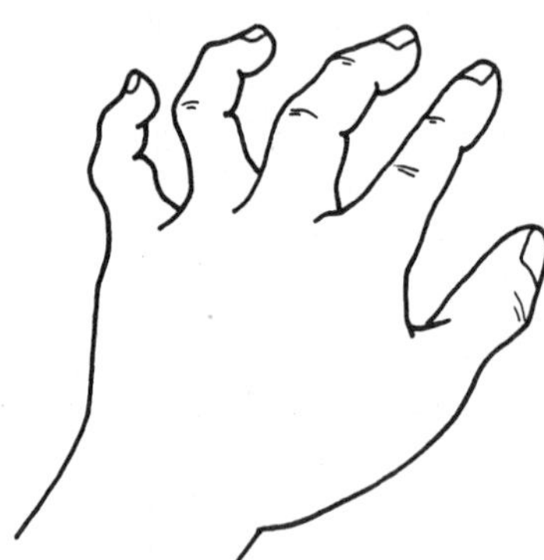

FIGURE 9-6 A clawhand deformity caused by an ulnar nerve injury

nence, inability to elevate the little finger metacarpal to oppose the thumb, and ineffective pinch of the thumb (Boscheinen-Morrin et al., 1987; Salter, 1987). The loss of the first dorsal interosseous muscle and the abductor pollicis leads to unstable pinching of the thumb and index finger (Boscheinen-Morrin et al., 1987). Loss of lateral finger movements and diminished sensory feedback can affect functional occupational activities such as typing on a computer (Salter, 1987).

TABLE 9-2

Ulnar Nerve Lesions

Affected muscles	Weak and lost motions
LOW LEVEL (WRIST LEVEL)	
Abductor digiti minimi	Lost little finger abduction and weak opposition
Flexor digiti minimi	Lost MCP flexion of the little finger and weak opposition
Opponens digiti minimi	Lost little finger opposition
Lumbricals to the fourth and fifth digit	Lost MCP finger flexion and interphalangeal (IP) extension
Dorsal interossei	Lost abduction of the thumb, index, ring, and little fingers
Palmar interossei	Lost adduction of the thumb, index, ring, and little fingers
Flexor pollicis brevis (deep head)	Lost MP and carpometacarpal (CMC) flexion of the thumb and weak opposition
Adductor pollicis	Lost adduction of the CMC joint and weakness in MP joint flexion
HIGH LEVEL (AT OR ABOVE THE ELBOW LEVEL)	
Flexor carpi ulnaris	Weak wrist flexion and adduction
Flexor digitorum profundus to the ring and small fingers	Lost flexion of the distal interphalangeal (DIP) joint of the ring and small fingers
Abductor digiti minimi	
Flexor digiti minimi	
Opponens digiti minimi	
Lumbricals to the fourth and fifth digit	
Dorsal interossei	
Palmar interossei	
Flexor pollicis brevis (deep head)	
Adductor pollicis	

With a high lesion the loss of the flexor digitorum profundus of the ring and small fingers further compromises hand grasp (Skirven, 1992). In addition, the therapist should note weakened wrist ulnar deviation.

Another characteristic of ulnar nerve injuries is a posture called *Froment's sign*, which functionally results in flexion of the thumb IP joint during pinching activities (Cailliet, 1994). Froment's sign occurs because the adductor pollicis brevis, the deep head of the flexor pollicis brevis, and first dorsal interosseous

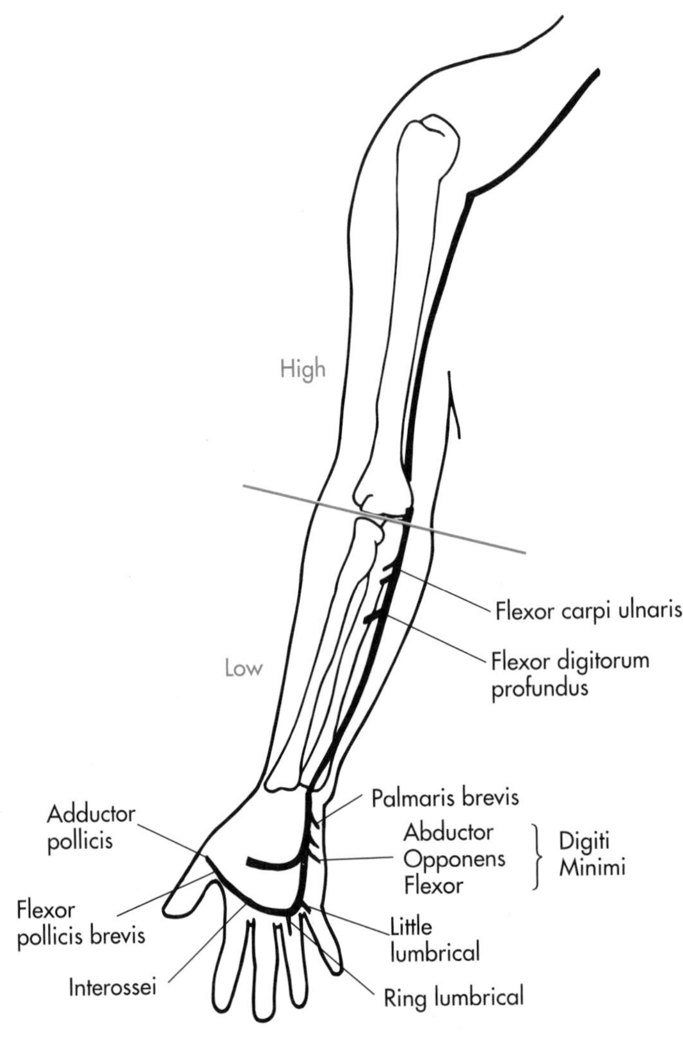

FIGURE 9-7 Ulnar nerve motor innervation

muscle are not working. Because of these losses, performance of the fine dexterity tasks of daily living is remarkably affected.

The sensory distribution of the ulnar nerve innervates the little finger and ulnar half of the ring finger on the volar and dorsal surfaces of the hand (see Figure 9-4). Patients who have ulnar nerve compression can experience numbness, tingling, and paresthesia in this nerve distribution and equal sensory loss in high and low lesions. When splinting for ulnar nerve lesions, the therapist must monitor the areas of decreased sensation for pressure sores. Figure 9-7 illustrates the muscles that an ulnar nerve lesion affects.

Ulnar Nerve Injury Splint Interventions

Splints for ulnar nerve compression or injury at the elbow and wrist levels require patient training to modify activities that contribute to the development of the problem.

Splinting for Ulnar Nerve Compression at the Elbow

In literature, no specified course of conservative management exists for ulnar nerve compression at the elbow (Harper, 1990). However, a commonly discussed treatment for compression at the cubital tunnel is an elbow splint with the elbow flexed 30° to 45° (Harper, 1990; Aiello, 1993). If included, the wrist is positioned in neutral to 20° extension. The patient should wear this splint for 3 months at night (Aiello, 1993).

The elbow splint helps to prevent repetitive or prolonged elbow flexion, especially beyond 60° to 90°. Prolonged elbow flexion is a problem that can stress the ulnar nerve (Harper, 1990; Seror, 1993) and commonly occurs during sleep or with computer usage (Seror, 1993; Cailliet, 1994). If demonstrating dysesthesia and decreased sensibility, the patient should wear the elbow splint during the day (Cannon, et al., 1991).

To fabricate an elbow splint, the therapist chooses a thermoplastic material that has some of the following properties: (1) rigidity so that the thermoplastic material is strong enough to support the weight of the elbow, (2) self-bonding to help with formulation of the crease at the elbow, and (3) conformability and drapability to mold the material over the bony olecranon process (see Chapter 1). When fabricating the splint, the therapist should have an assistant help stabilize the arm or use an ace wrap bandage. The fold of the splinting material should be close to the elbow joint (Figure 9-8).

Hand-Based Ulnar Nerve Splint Intervention

As shown in Figure 9-9, the position for an ulnar nerve lesion involves splinting the ring and little fingers in 30° to 45° of MCP flexion (Callahan, 1984; Cannon, et al., 1985). This position prevents overlengthening of the denervated intrinsic muscles of the ring and little fingers (Colditz, 1990). In addition, this position corrects the clawhand posture of MCP hyperextension and PIP flexion as the long extensors act on the PIP joint in the absence of the intrinsic muscles. Ultimately, this splint will help to facilitate the functional grasp of the patient (Skirven, 1992).

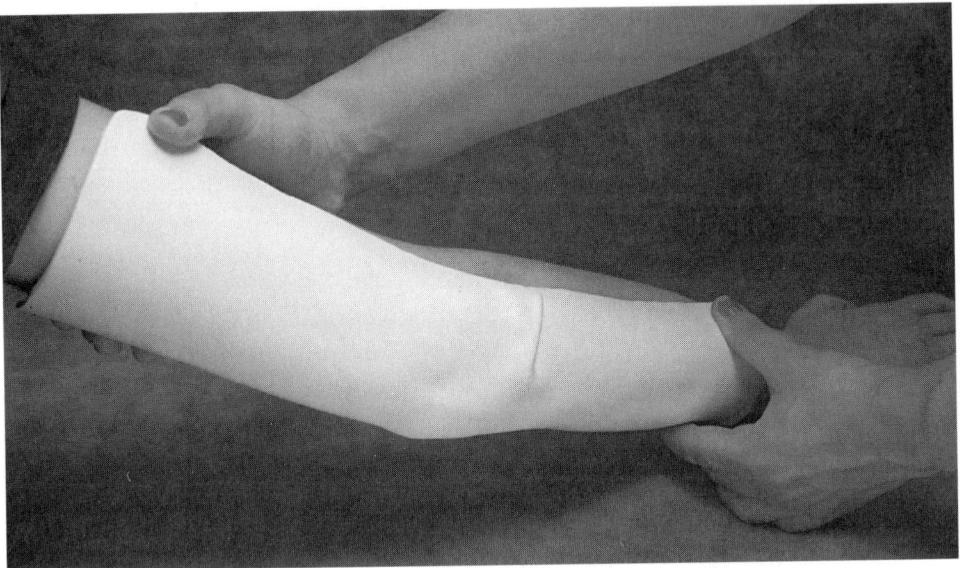

FIGURE 9-8 The arm and elbow position during molding of an elbow splint

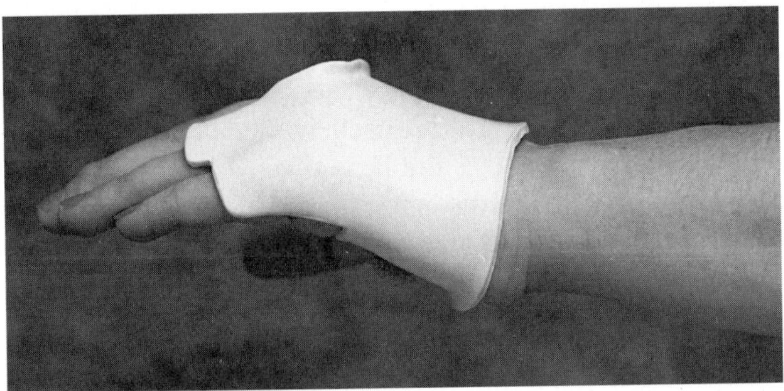

FIGURE 9-9 The hand position for splinting an ulnar nerve injury

The therapist splints the hand in this position by using a dynamic or static splint. A patient usually wears a static splint continuously with removal only for hygiene and exercise. Colditz (1990) suggests the fabrication of a less bulky splint in order to keep from impeding the palmar sensation and function of the hand. One such splint is the figure-of-eight splint design that Kiyoshi Yasaki developed at the Hand Rehabilitation Center in Philadelphia, Pennsylvania (Callahan, 1984).

Dynamic Splinting for Ulnar Nerve Injuries

The therapist can use a dynamic splint that includes finger loops attached to the ring and little finger's proximal phalanx (Figure 9-10). The rubber band traction pulls the two fingers into MCP flexion and is connected to a soft wrist cuff. The patient wears the splint throughout the day with removal for hygiene and exercise. Physicians usually prescribe this type of splint when a need exists for additional force to prevent hyperextension contractures at the MCP joints. In order to supplement this type of splint, a static nighttime splint may be necessary. A static hand-based pattern for an ulnar nerve injury (Figure 9-11) is useful for providing a strong counterforce to prevent a clawhand deformity (Callahan, 1984).

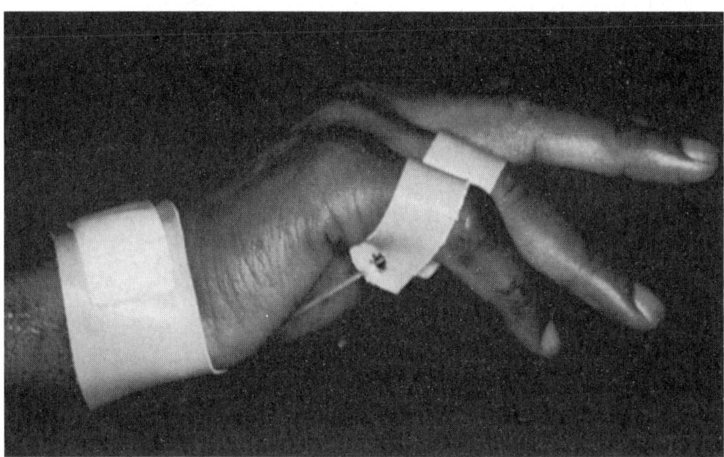

FIGURE 9-10 A dynamic extension splint for an ulnar nerve injury (From Hunter, J. M., Schneider, L. H., Mackin, E. J., & Callahan, A. D. (1990). Rehabilitation of the hand: Surgery and therapy (3rd ed., p. 650). St. Louis: Mosby.)

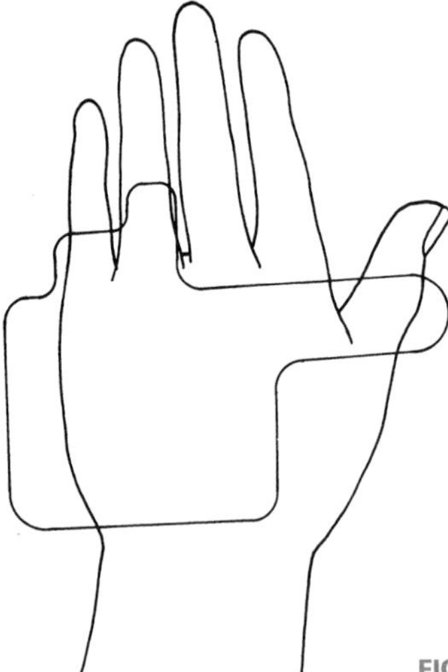

FIGURE 9-11 A hand-based pattern for an ulnar nerve splint

Laboratory Exercise 9-2

On a partner, practice fabricating a hand-based splint in the anticlaw position for a patient who has an ulnar nerve lesion. Before starting, determine the position in which to place the person's hand. Remember to position the MCP joints of the ring and little fingers in approximately 30° to 45° of flexion.

After fitting the splint and making all adjustments, use Form 9-1 at the end of the chapter. This check-off sheet is a self-evaluation of the splint. Use Grading Sheet 9-1 at the end of the chapter as a classroom grading sheet.

Median Nerve Lesions

Median nerve lesions can occur from humeral fractures, elbow dislocations, distal radius fractures, dislocations of the lunate into the carpal canal, and lacerations of the volar wrist (Skirven, 1992). The classic deformity is called an *ape* or *simian hand* because the thenar eminence is flattened and a loss of thumb opposition occurs (Figure 9-12). The thumb is positioned in extension and adduction next to the index finger because of the unopposed action of the extensor pollicis longus and the adductor pollicis (Boscheinen-Morrin et al., 1987). The thumb web space may atrophy and the fingers may show trophic changes. In addition, a slight claw deformity of the index and middle fingers may occur because of the involvement of the lumbricals (Salter, 1987).

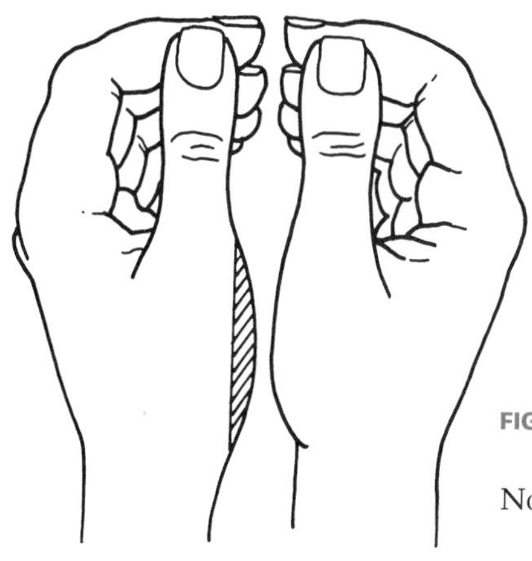

FIGURE 9-12 The classic median nerve deformity called an *ape* or *simian hand*
Note the thenar muscle atrophy of the left hand.

Functional Involvement from a Median Nerve Injury

The median nerve in a low or wrist lesion and a high lesion involving the elbow or neck area innervates certain muscles (Figure 9-13). The functional result from a median nerve lesion is clumsiness with pinch and a decrease in power grip (Boscheinen-Morrin, et al., 1987). The sensory loss in a median nerve injury is equal whether it is a low or high injury. With lack of sensation in the fingers, skilled functions are difficult to perform with the hand. Power grip is affected because the thumb is no longer a stabilizing force as a result of loss of the abductor pollicis brevis, flexor pollicis brevis, and the opponens pollicis. Weakness in the lumbricals of the index and middle fingers further affects skilled movements of the hand (Borucki & Schmidt, 1992). The sensory areas innervated by the median nerve are used for identifying objects, temperature, and texture (Arsham, 1984).

Higher lesions can weaken or impair forearm pronation, wrist flexion, thumb IP flexion, and flexion of the proximal and distal IP joints of the index and middle fingers. Compression syndromes that can occur from higher median nerve injuries are the following: pronator syndrome, anterior interosseous syndrome, and the ligament of Struthers syndrome. Frequently these syndromes require surgical procedures to decompress the nerve (Borucki & Schmidt, 1992). On occasions a physician may request a splint for conservative management of mild cases of pronator teres syndrome. For example, for a mild case of pronator teres syndrome the physician may prescribe a forearm splint in a neutral position between pronation and supination (Table 9-3) (Cailliet, 1994).

Course and sensory distribution of the median nerve occurs to the volar surface of the thumb, index, middle, and radial half of the ring fingers and to the dor-

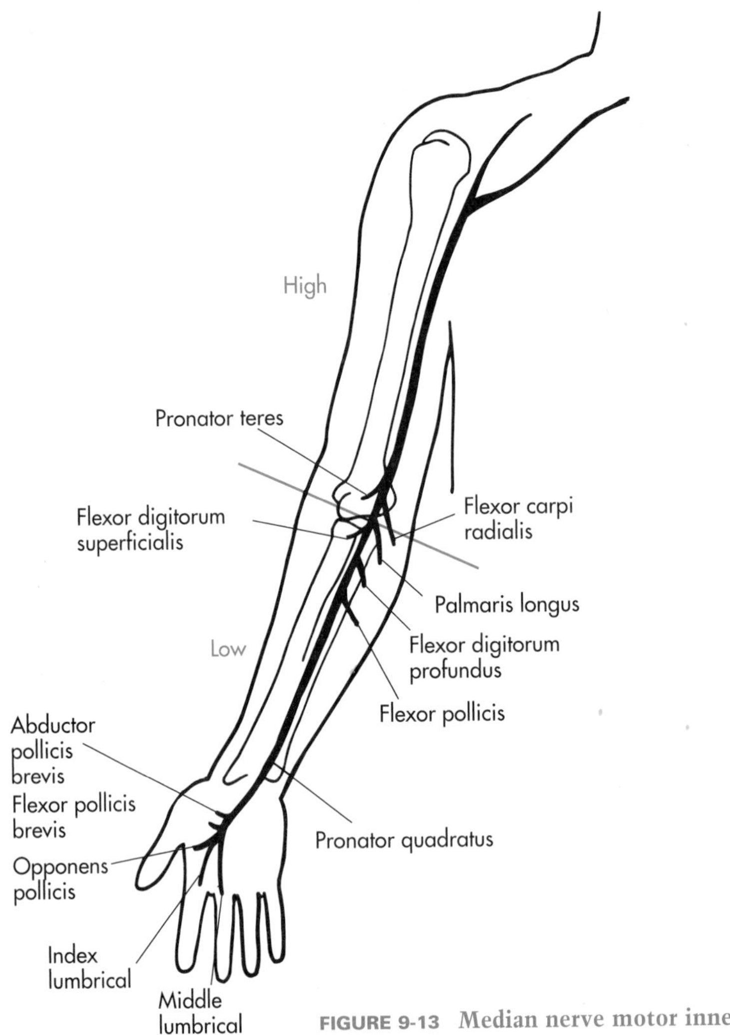

FIGURE 9-13 Median nerve motor innervation

sal surface of the distal phalanxes of the thumb, index, middle and radial half of the ring finger (see Figure 9-4). Patients who have median nerve compression can experience numbness, tingling, and paresthesia in this nerve distribution. Because the area of sensory distribution is so large, the therapist must monitor and educate patients and/or caregivers about skin breakdown.

Splinting Interventions for Median Nerve Injuries

An understanding of the functional effect of the muscular loss from median nerve injury or compression influences splint provision. Usually with a median

TABLE 9-3

Median Nerve Lesions

Affected muscles	Weak and lost motions
LOW LEVEL (WRIST LEVEL)	
Abductor pollicis brevis	Lost abduction of the CMC and MP joints of the thumb, weak extension of the IP joint, and weak opposition
Flexor pollicis brevis (superficial head)	Lost flexion of the MP and CMC joints and weak opposition
Opponens pollicis	Lost thumb opposition
First and second lumbricals	Lost IP extension and MCP flexion of the index and middle fingers
HIGH LEVEL (ELBOW OR NECK LEVEL)	
Flexor pollicis longus	Lost IP thumb flexion and weakness with flexion of the MP and CMC joints
Lateral half of the flexor digitorum profundus to the index and middle fingers	Lost DIP flexion of the index and middle fingers
Pronator quadratus	Lost forearm pronation and elbow flexion
Pronator teres	Lost forearm pronation and elbow flexion
Flexor carpi radialis	Weak flexion and abduction of the wrist
Palmaris longus	Weak wrist flexion
Flexor digitorum superficialis	Lost flexion of the PIP joints index through little fingers and weak flexion of the MCP joints and wrist flexion
Abductor pollicis brevis	
Flexor pollicis brevis (superficial head)	
Opponens pollicis	
First and second lumbricals	

nerve lesion, if the therapist is able to maintain good passive mobility of the joints, extensive splinting may not be necessary and occasional night splinting may be sufficient (Fess, 1986).

Splinting for Carpal Tunnel Syndrome

The most common type of nerve compression is carpal tunnel syndrome (CTS), which compresses the median nerve at the wrist. When manifestations are primarily sensory and occur from overuse or occupational causes, splinting of the wrist can help reduce pain and symptoms (Borucki & Schmidt, 1992). One study (N = 105 adults) about carpal tunnel syndrome indicates a more favorable response to neutral wrist splinting when the patient wears the splint within the first 3 months of symptom onset and when no structural damage is present (Kruger, Kraft, Deitz, Ameis, & Polissar, 1991).

Usually any splint for carpal tunnel syndrome positions the wrist as close to neutral as possible, thus helping maximize available carpal tunnel space, minimize nerve compression, and provide pain relief (Kruger, et al., 1991). Some patients and therapists often prefer volar wrist cock-up splints, which provide good support. Some therapists working on wound control after carpal tunnel release surgery prefer this splinting approach combined with Otoform-K or elastomer putty. A disadvantage of a volar wrist splint for CTS is that the splint may interfere with palmar sensation (Borucki & Schmidt, 1992). A volar wrist cock-up splint designed with poor biomechanics could compress the carpal tunnel area of the wrist.

Other splinting approaches include fabrication of dorsal or ulnar gutter wrist cock-up splints. The dorsal wrist cock-up splint has an advantage because it does not compress the carpal tunnel area. However, a disadvantage of the dorsal wrist cock-up splint is that it does not maintain as much support as the volar wrist cock-up splint. An ulnar gutter wrist cock-up splint may also position the wrist in neutral and is less likely to compress the carpal tunnel (see Chapter 5).

For occupational use the patient may be more comfortable with a soft prefabricated wrist splint, which the therapist should check carefully for a correct fit. In particular, the therapist should note whether the splint supports the wrist at neutral, the arches of the hand have adequate support, and the patient has functional finger flexion and thumb movements. With any splint provision for carpal tunnel syndrome the therapist must educate the patient about the causes and prevention of the syndrome and about an appropriate exercise program.

Splinting Median Nerve Palsies That Have Thumb Symptoms

For a patient who has a median nerve injury or compression involving the thumb the therapist must address loss of thumb opposition for functional grasp and pinch. The therapist splints the thumb in an opposition and palmar abduction position, which assists the thumb for tip prehension. The C bar between the thumb and index finger helps maintain the thumb web space, which is a common site for muscular atrophy to occur from median nerve damage. The splint design can be static or dynamic. A typical static splint for a median nerve injury is a hand-based thumb spica splint (see Chapter 7).

The therapist may choose to fabricate a web spacer for a low-level median nerve lesion (Figure 9-14). This type of splint will allow free wrist mobility, which helps the patient to perform functional activities because of the tenodesis effect of wrist extensors on finger flexors (Borucki & Schmidt, 1992). After the fabrication of a dynamic thumb splint, the therapist may incorporate into the splint-wearing program a static thumb spica splint that the patient wears at night.

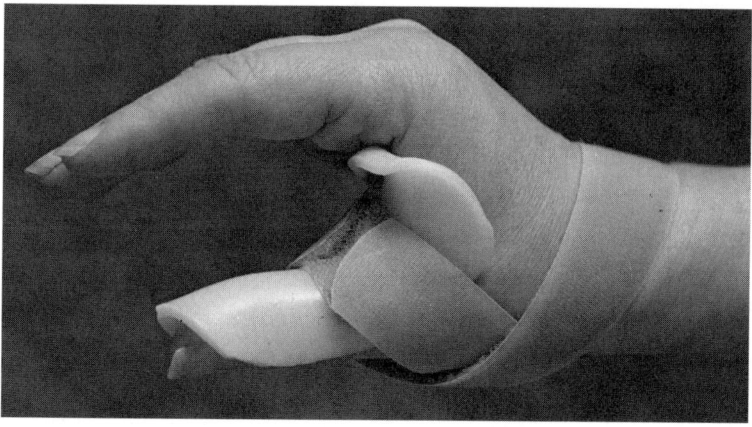

FIGURE 9-14 A thumb web spacer splint for a median nerve injury

TABLE 9-4

Splint Interventions for Peripheral Nerve Lesions

Splint	Position
RADIAL	
Wrist cock-up splint	Wrist in 30° extension
Dynamic dorsal-based MCP extension splint	Wrist in 30° extension MCPs in dynamic extension
Tenodesis splint (described by Colditz)	Dorsal base using the tenodesis effect with MCPs in dynamic extension
ULNAR	
Elbow splint	Elbow in 30° to 45° flexion
Hand-based static anticlaw splint	MCPs of ring and little fingers in 30° to 45° dynamic flexion
Hand-based dynamic anticlaw splint	MCPs of ring and little fingers in 30° to 45° dynamic flexion
MEDIAN	
Dorsal- or volar-based wrist cock-up splint	Wrist in neutral
Ulnar gutter wrist cock-up splint	Wrist in neutral
Thumb web splint or C-bar splint	Thumb in 40° to 45° of palmar abduction

Splinting for nerve injuries involves a comprehensive knowledge of the muscular, sensory, and functional problems. The therapist can use various splinting interventions for nerve injuries (Table 9-4) but should keep in mind that these are general guidelines and that physicians and experienced therapists may have other specific protocols for positioning.

SELF QUIZ 9-1*

Please circle either true (T) or false (F).

1. T F With neurapraxia the prognosis is extremely good because recovery is usually spontaneous.
2. T F Functionally, a patient suffering from a radial nerve injury has a poor grip.
3. T F The main purpose of splinting a nerve injury is to immobilize the extremity.
4. T F The clawhand deformity occurs only with a low-level ulnar nerve injury.
5. T F The therapist should position an elbow splint in 90° flexion for a patient who has an ulnar nerve compression at the elbow level.
6. T F For an ulnar nerve splint the therapist should position the ring and little fingers in approximately 30° to 45° MCP flexion.
7. T F The proper splint for a radial nerve injury is a wrist cock-up or dynamic wrist and MCP extension splint.
8. T F The therapist should immobilize radial, ulnar, and median nerve injuries only in static splints.
9. T F Froment' sign is an identifying posture of a median nerve injury.
10. T F Functionally, a patient suffering from an ulnar nerve injury has loss of pinch strength and power grip.
11. T F The therapist may use a thumb web spacer splint for a median nerve injury.
12. T F Low-level nerve injuries occur only distal to the wrist.

*See Appendix A for the answer key.

FORM 9-1* Anticlaw Splint

Name: ______________________

Date: ______________________

Answer the following questions after the splint has been worn for 30 minutes. (Mark *NA* for nonapplicable situations.)

Evaluation Areas		**Comments**
Design		
1. The splint prevents hyperextension of the MCP joints of the ring and little fingers.	Yes ❍ No ❍ NA ❍	
Function		
1. The splint allows full wrist motions.	Yes ❍ No ❍ NA ❍	
2. The splint allows full function of the middle and index fingers.	Yes ❍ No ❍ NA ❍	
Straps		
1. The straps avoid bony prominences.	Yes ❍ No ❍ NA ❍	
2. Straps are secure and rounded.	Yes ❍ No ❍ NA ❍	
Comfort		
1. The edges are smooth with rounded corners.	Yes ❍ No ❍ NA ❍	
2. The proximal end is flared.	Yes ❍ No ❍ NA ❍	
3. Impingements or pressure areas are not present.	Yes ❍ No ❍ NA ❍	
Cosmetic Appearance		
1. The splint is free of fingerprints, dirt, and pencil or pen marks.	Yes ❍ No ❍ NA ❍	
2. The splinting material is not buckled.	Yes ❍ No ❍ NA ❍	

Discuss possible adjustments or changes you would make based on the self-evaluation:

____

____

____

____

____

____

*See Appendix B for a perforated copy of this form.

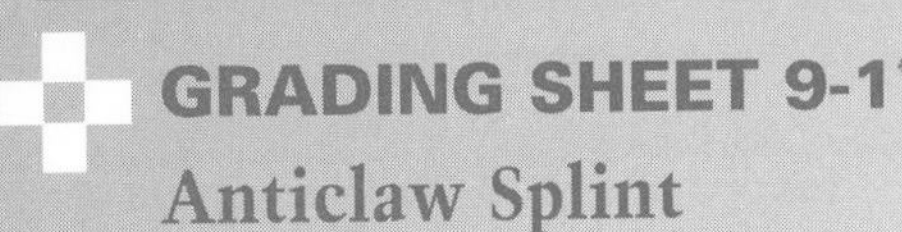

GRADING SHEET 9-1*

Anticlaw Splint

Name: ______________________

Date: ______________________

Grade: __________

1 = beyond improvement, not acceptable

2 = requires maximal improvement

3 = requires moderate improvement

4 = requires minimal improvement

5 = requires no improvement

Evaluation Areas		Comments
Design		
1. The splint prevents hyperextension of the MCP joints of the ring and little fingers.	1 2 3 4 5	
Function		
1. The splint allows full wrist motions.	1 2 3 4 5	
2. The splint allows full function of the middle and index fingers.	1 2 3 4 5	
Straps		
1. The straps avoid bony prominences.	1 2 3 4 5	
2. The straps are secure and rounded.	1 2 3 4 5	
Comfort		
1. The edges are smooth with rounded corners.	1 2 3 4 5	
2. The proximal end is flared.	1 2 3 4 5	
3. Impingements or pressure areas are not present.	1 2 3 4 5	
Cosmetic Appearance		
1. The splint is free of fingerprints, dirt, and pencil or pen marks.	1 2 3 4 5	
2. The splinting material is not buckled.	1 2 3 4 5	

Comments:

*See Appendix C for a perforated copy of this grading sheet.

Case Study*

Read the following scenario and answer the questions based on information in this chapter:

Reggie is a 41-year-old woman working as a carpenter who sustained a median nerve injury from falling off a ladder and fracturing her humerus.

1. Which of the following muscles would a median nerve injury affect based on the location of the lesion?
   a. Flexor pollicis longus
   b. Adductor pollicis
   c. Lateral half of the flexor digitorum profundus to the index and middle fingers
   d. Pronator teres
   e. Opponens pollicis
   f. Extensor pollicis brevis
2. Functionally, which of the following symptoms could occur from a high median nerve lesion?
   a. Loss or weakness in wrist extension
   b. Loss or weakness in thumb adduction
   c. Loss of IP thumb flexion and weakness with flexion of the MP and CMC joints
3. Which of the following is the correct positioning for a hand-based splint with thumb involvement?
   a. A thumb spica splint with the thumb in palmar abduction
   b. A volar wrist cock-up splint
   c. A resting hand splint with the thumb in palmar abduction

*See Appendix A for the answer key.

Review Questions

1. Which factors are important in the prognosis of a peripheral nerve lesion?
2. What are the deformities resulting from radial, ulnar, and median nerve lesions?
3. What are the functional results of radial, ulnar, and median nerve lesions?
4. What are the splinting options for radial nerve palsies? In which position should the therapist splint the hand?
5. What is the proper type, position, and thermoplastic material needed for fabrication of a splint for ulnar nerve compression at the elbow?
6. What is the proper splinting position for a clawhand deformity? Why is this a good position?
7. What are the advantages and disadvantages of the different approaches to wrist splinting for carpal tunnel syndrome?
8. What is the appropriate position in which to splint a median nerve lesion that includes thumb symptoms?

References

Aiello, B. (1993). Ulnar nerve compression in cubital tunnel. In G. L. Clark, E. F. Shaw Wilgis, B. Aiello, D. Eckhaus, & L. V. Eddington (Eds.), Hand rehabilitation: A practical guide. New York: Churchill Livingstone Inc.

Arsham, N. Z. (1984). Nerve injury. In E. M. Ziegler (ed.), Current concepts in orthotics: A diagnosis-related approach to splinting. Germantown, WI: Rolyan Medical Products.

Barr, N. R., & Swan, D. (1988). The hand: Principles and techniques of splintmaking. Boston: Butterworth Publishers.

Borucki, S., & Schmidt, J. (1992). Peripheral neuropathies. In M. L. Aisen (Ed.), Orthotics in neurologic rehabilitation. New York: Demos Publications.

Boscheinen-Morrin, J., Davey, V., & Conolly, W. B. (1987). Peripheral nerve injuries (including tendon transfers). In J. Boscheinen-Morrin, V. Davey, & W. B. Conolly (Eds.), The hand: Fundamentals of therapy. Boston: Butterworth Publishers.

Cailliet, R. (1994). Hand pain and impairment. Philadelphia: F. A. Davis Co.

Callahan, A. (1984). Nerve injuries. In M. H. Makick & M. C. Kasch (Eds.), Manual on management of specific hand problems. Pittsburg: American Rehabilitation Educational Network.

Cannon, N. M. (Ed.). (1991). Diagnosis and treatment manual for physicians and therapists (3rd. ed.). Indianapolis: The Hand Rehabilitation Center of Indiana, P. C.

Cannon, N. M., Foltz, R. W., Koepfer, J. M., Lauck, M. F., Simpson, D. M., & Bromley, R. S. (1985). Manual of hand splinting. New York: Churchill Livingstone Inc.

Colditz, J. C. (1987). Splinting for radial nerve palsy. J Hand Ther, 1, 18-23.

Colditz, J. C. (1990). Splinting peripheral nerve injuries. In J. M. Schneider, E. J. Mackin, & A. D. Callahan (Eds.), Rehabilitation of the hand: Surgery and therapy (3rd ed., pp. 647-657). St. Louis: Mosby.

Eaton, C. J., & Lister, G. D. (1992). Radial nerve compression. Hand clin, 8(2), 345-357.

Enna, C. D. (1988). Peripheral denervation of the hand. New York: Alan R. Liss Inc.

Fess, E. E. (1986). Rehabilitation of the patient with peripheral nerve injury. Hand Clin, 2(1), 207-215.

Fess, E. E., & Philips, C. A. (1987). Hand splinting principles and methods. St. Louis: Mosby.

Harper, B. D. (1990). The drop-out splint: An alternative to the conservative management of ulnar nerve entrapment at the elbow. J Hand Ther, 3, 199-210.

Kruger, V. L., Kraft, G. H., Deitz, J. C., Ameis, A., & Polissar, L. (1991). Carpal tunnel syndrome: Objective measures and splint use. Arch Phys Med Rehabil, 72, 517-520.

Norkus, S. A., & Meyers, M. C. (1994). Ulnar neuropathy of the elbow. Sports Med, 17(2), 189-199.

Pećina, M. M., Krmpotić-Nemanić, J., & Markiewitz, A. D. (1991). Tunnel Syndromes. Ann Arbor, MI: CRC Press Inc.

Salter, M. I. (1987). Hand injuries: A therapeutic approach. Edingburgh, London: Churchill Livingstone Inc.

Seror, P. (1993). Treatment of ulnar nerve palsy at the elbow with a night splint. J Bone Joint Surg Br, 75(2), 322-327.

Skirven, T. (1992). Nerve injuries. In B. G. Stanley & S. M. Tribuzi (Eds.), Concepts in hand rehabilitation (pp. 322-338). Philadelphia: F. A. Davis Co.

Spinner, M. (1990). Nerve lesions in continuity. In J. M. Schneider, E. J. Mackin, & A. D. Callahan (Eds.), Rehabilitation of the hand: Surgery and therapy (3rd ed., pp. 523-529). St. Louis: Mosby.

Ziegler, E. M. (1984). Current concepts in orthotics: A diagnosis-related approach to splinting. Germantown, WI: Rolyan Medical Products.

CHAPTER TEN

Antispasticity Splinting

MICHAEL LOHMAN, MEd, CO, OTR/L

CHAPTER OBJECTIVES

1. Identify and describe the two historic trends in upper-extremity tone-reduction splinting (orthotics).*
2. Compare the strengths and weaknesses of dorsal and volar forearm platforms (troughs).†
3. Discuss the neurophysiologic rationale supporting the use of the finger spreader and hard cone.
4. Discriminate between the passive and dynamic components of spasticity.
5. Describe the difference between submaximum and maximum ranges as they relate to tone-reduction splints.
6. Identify and describe the two major components of orthokinetic splints.
7. Describe one unique characteristic for each of the following materials:
   - Plaster bandage
   - Fiberglass bandage
   - Inflatable splints
   - Cylindrical foam
   - Neoprene
8. Successfully fabricate and clinically evaluate the proper fit of a thermoplastic hard cone.
9. Use clinical judgment to correctly analyze the two case study questions.

*The author uses the terms *splint* and *orthosis* interchangably in this chapter.
†The author uses the terms *platform* and *trough* interchangably in this chapter.

The status of tone-reduction wrist-hand orthotics is like an amorphous quicksand waiting to engulf the unwary therapist. Rehabilitation literature reflects the universal lack of consensus, which Fess and Philips (1987, p. 357) summarize with the following statement:

> Some physicians and therapists feel strongly that the hypertonic extremity should not be splinted, whereas others are equally adamant that splinting has beneficial results. Even among proponents of splinting, numerous disagreements exist concerning splint design, surface of splint application, wearing times and schedules, joints to be splinted, and specific construction materials for splints and splint components.

Current professional standards of practice dictate that significant cumulative data and consistent scientific analysis provide the foundation for objective evaluations and treatment protocols. Literature in tone-reduction splinting does not reflect the development of this core body of knowledge. The paucity of data on the effectiveness of tone-reduction splinting has fostered confusion and contradiction. In the absence of a well-established practice protocol, this chapter is restricted to a discussion of current theoretical and experimental rationales and splint designs. Each practitioner is ultimately responsible for justifying the effectiveness of these techniques in patient treatment.

Basmajian et al (1982, p. 1382) define *spasticity* as "a state of increased muscular tone with exaggeration of the tendon reflexes." Patients who have upper motor neuron (UMN) lesions such as cerebrovascular accidents (CVAs), closed-head injuries, spinal cord injuries, and cerebral palsy often exhibit spasticity (Bishop, 1977). Spasticity can cause deformity (Bloch & Evans, 1977) and limit functional movement (Doubilet & Polkow, 1977). Hand splinting is one treatment technique used to prevent joint deformity and influence muscle tone (Mills, 1984).

Historically experts have documented two major trends in hemiplegic hand splinting. Until the 1950s the direct application of mechanical force to correct or prevent joint contractures (i.e., biomechanical approach) was the preferred practice in dealing with the effects of spasticity. During the 1950s, emphasis shifted to the underlying causes of spasticity. This viewpoint focuses on the effects of sensory feedback provided by the splints in altering muscle tone and promoting normal movement patterns (i.e., neurophysiological approach) (Neuhaus et al., 1981). As differing neurophysiologic theories emerged in the 1950s, therapists advocated divergent treatment and splint management principles. At present, several prevalent neurophysiologic rationales recommend a variety of designs composed of a variety of elements related to design position and material options, including the following: (1) platform design, (2) finger and thumb position, (3) static and dynamic prolonged stretch, and (4) material properties.

Some authors have limited their splint designs to one elemental concern, whereas other authors have combined several design elements to support specific treatment rationales.

Several commercially available, antispasticity hand splints incorporate a variety of design elements. Though this chapter reviews each design element separately, therapists must remember that neurophysiologic splint-design concepts are interrelated and many splints encompass combinations of design elements.

Forearm-Platform Position

A forearm platform is a design element that provides a base of support to control wrist position. Many frequently used tone-reduction splint designs do not affect wrist control but attempt only to influence the digits (Dayhoff, 1975; Bloch & Evans, 1977; Jamison & Dayhoff, 1980; Langlois, Pederson, & MacKinnon, 1991). Other designs attempt to influence wrist position but do not address digit position (Switzer, 1980; MacKinnon, Sanderson, & Buchanan, 1975). Isolated joint control constitutes a fundamental design flaw that can produce a predictable outcome because the tendons of the extrinsic flexors cross the wrist, fingers, and thumb. If the digits are positioned in extension, the unsplinted wrist assumes a greater attitude of flexion (Fess & Philips, 1987). This compensatory sequence can lead to decreased passive motion and contracture development.

Rehabilitation science literature contains adherents for volar-based forearm platforms (Brennan, 1959; Zislis, 1964; Peterson, 1980) and dorsal-based forearm platforms (Kaplan, 1962; Charait, 1968; Snook, 1979). Other authors report that the two positions are equally effective in tone reduction (McPherson, Kreimer, Aalderks, & Gallager, 1982; Rose & Shah, 1987). National distributors market ulnar-based platform splints designed to reduce spasticity (Smith & Nephew Rolyan, 1993; Sammons-Bisell Health Care Corporation, 1995), although literature does not appear to mention ulnar-based forearm platforms (Figure 10-1). A therapist can secure all orthotic forearm platforms to the forearm by using straps, resulting in skin contact with volar and dorsal surfaces simultaneously (Rose & Shah, 1987; Langlois, MacKinnon, & Pederson, 1989). The corresponding cutaneous stimulation provided to flexors or extensors by the forearm platform and straps may be facilitatory or inhibitory. The literature has not yet described research that examines the exact relationship between these variables (Langlois et al., 1991). These variables are, however, discussed later in this chapter.

Research does not indicate which if any of these forearm-platform designs provide the best results to reduce spasticity. However, each forearm-platform design possesses individual qualities that may be relevant in a clinical decision regarding forearm-platform design. A volar forearm platform that extends into the hand provides greater support for the transverse metacarpal arch. Volar designs do not extend thermoplastic material over the ulnar styloid, thus avoiding the possibility of pressure over this key bony prominence. A dorsal forearm platform frees the palmar area and enhances sensory feedback. This style is easier to apply and remove if wrist flexion tightness is present. Pressure is also more evenly distributed over the larger thermoplastic surface of the dorsal forearm platform as

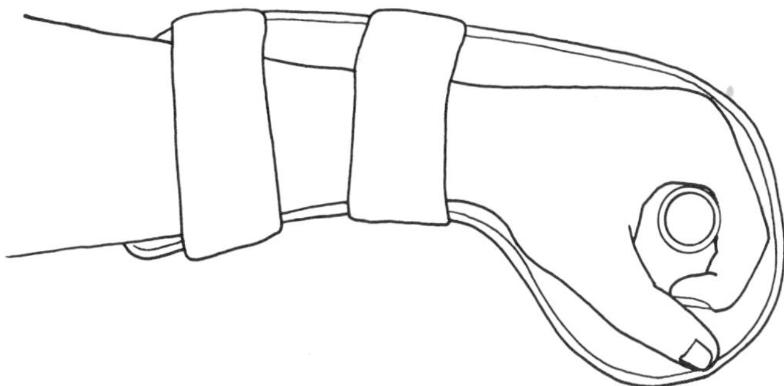

FIGURE 10-1 **A hard cone attached to an ulnar platform**: spasticity cone splint (Sammons, 1995)

opposed to the smaller strap surface that the volar style provides. An ulnar forearm platform provides a more even distribution of pressure for a patient who exhibits a strong component of wrist ulnar deviation with wrist flexion spasticity (Figure 10-1).

Finger and Thumb Position

The finger spreader and hard cone are examples of splint designs based on divergent neurophysiologic treatment theories. Both positioning devices are designed to be adjuncts to specific treatment techniques that promote voluntary hand motion (Bobath, 1978; Farber, 1982; Davies, 1985).

The neurodevelopmental treatment (NDT) theory advocates the use of reflex-inhibiting patterns (RIP) to inhibit abnormal spasticity. Finger and thumb abduction is a key point of control that facilitates extensor muscle tone and inhibits flexor muscle tone (Bobath, 1978; Davies, 1985). The finger-spreader design assists in maintaining the reflex-inhibiting pattern.

Therapists have constructed recent adaptations of the finger-spreader design from rigid thermoplastic material (Doubilet & Polkow, 1977; Langlois et al., 1991). Bobath's (1970) original soft-foam material possesses dynamic qualities that are sacrificed when the therapist substitutes rigid, more durable, and cosmetically appealing materials (Langlois et al., 1989) (Figure 10-2). Doubilet and Polkow (1977) state that positioning the thumb in palmar abduction with the metacarpophalangeal (MCP) and proximal interphalangeal (PIP) joints extended is preferable to radial abduction of the thumb because palmar abduction provides greater fitting security, positions the thumb more comfortably, and produces similar results in spasticity reduction.

In addition to deciding the thumb position, the therapist must consider wrist and interphalangeal joint control. Although some researchers have not extended their RIP designs to include the wrist or interphalangeal joints (Doubilet & Polkow, 1977; Langlois et al., 1991), other experts have included extension of the

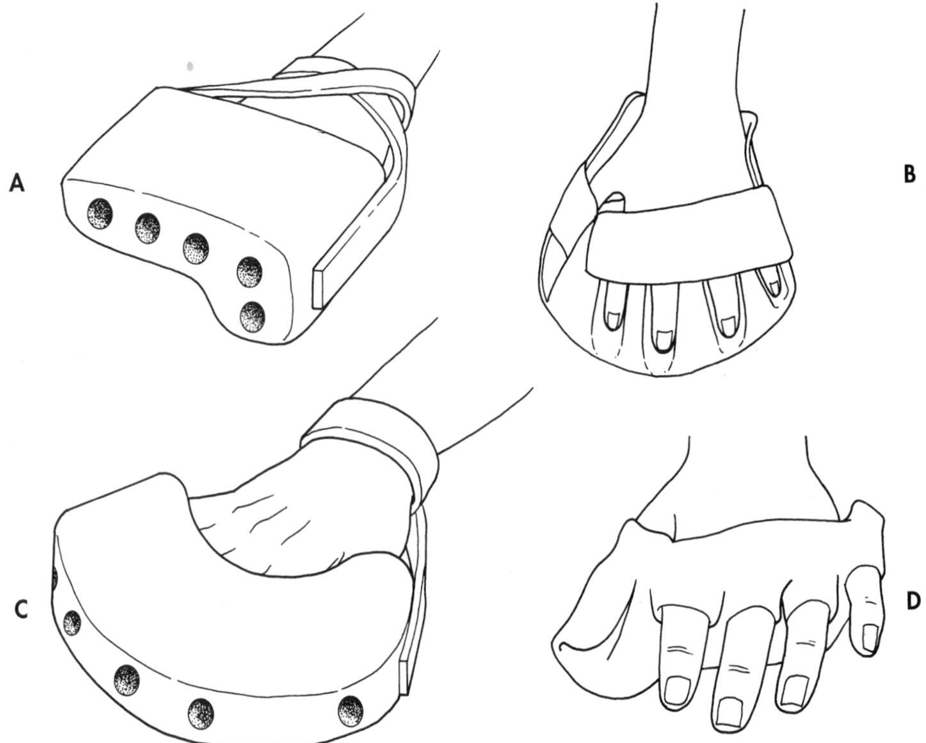

FIGURE 10-2 **Finger spreader designs: A,** thumb extension (Sammons, 1995); **B,** hand based antispasticity ball splint (Rolyan, 1993); **C,** thumb abduction (Sammons, 1995); and **D,** thumb extension (Doubiet & Polkow, 1977)

interphalangeal joints of the fingers, thumb, and wrist (Snook, 1979; McPherson, Becker, & Franszczak, 1985; Scherling & Johnson, 1989). The resulting design provides a continuous chain of stabilizing forces throughout the wrist and digits. This chain is necessary to prevent compensatory patterns that transfer the forces of spasticity to the unsplinted joint.

Cones

Rood (1954) first advocated the inhibition of flexor spasticity by using a firm cone to provide constant pressure over the palmar surface. The device should provide skin contact over the entire palmar surface for maximal effect but should not apply stretch to the wrist and finger flexor muscles. Farber & Huss (1974) observed that the hard cone has an inhibitory effect on flexor muscles because this device places deep tendon pressure on the wrist and finger-flexor insertions at the

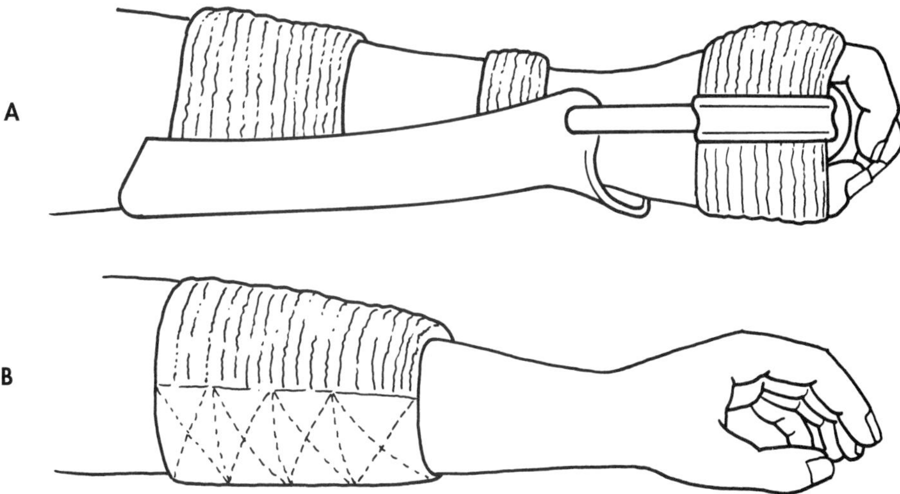

FIGURE 10-3 **Orthokinetic material placement**: **A,** orthokinetic wrist splint (Kiel, 1974); **B,** forearm cuff (Farber, 1974)

base of the palm. Farber (1982) also observed that the total contact from the hard cone provides maintained pressure over the flexor surface of the palm, thus assisting in the desensitization of hypersensitive skin.

Hard cones are typically constructed of cardboard or thermoplastic material (Figure 10-4). This hollow structure is positioned with the smaller end placed radially and the larger end placed ulnarly to provide maximum palmar contact. Kiel (1974, 1982) recommends the provision of a thenar groove to relieve web-space pressure.

Design criteria for hard cones as cited in literature does not include the use of forearm platforms to control wrist position. Although Kiel (1974) uses a volar platform with a hard cone in the orthokinetic wrist splint (Figure 10-3), the movable wrist joint allows free motion to occur in wrist flexion and extension. Hard cones attached to ulnar platforms (Figure 10-1) are commercially available (Sammons-Bissell Health Care Corporation, 1995; Smith & Nephew Rolyan, 1993), but the literature does not appear to discuss the combination of forearm platforms and hard-cone elements designed to control wrist and finger position. When using a firm cone without a forearm platform, the therapist secures the cone to the hand by using a wide (e.g., 2.5 cm) elastic or nonelastic strap over the dorsum of the hand (Figure 10-4) (Dayhoff, 1975; Jamison & Dayhoff, 1980). Dayhoff (1975) reports that contact with soft material on the palmar surface appears to increase flexor tone. This soft stimulus may activate the primitive grasp response (Farber, 1982). Brunnstrom (1970) describes this response as the instinc-

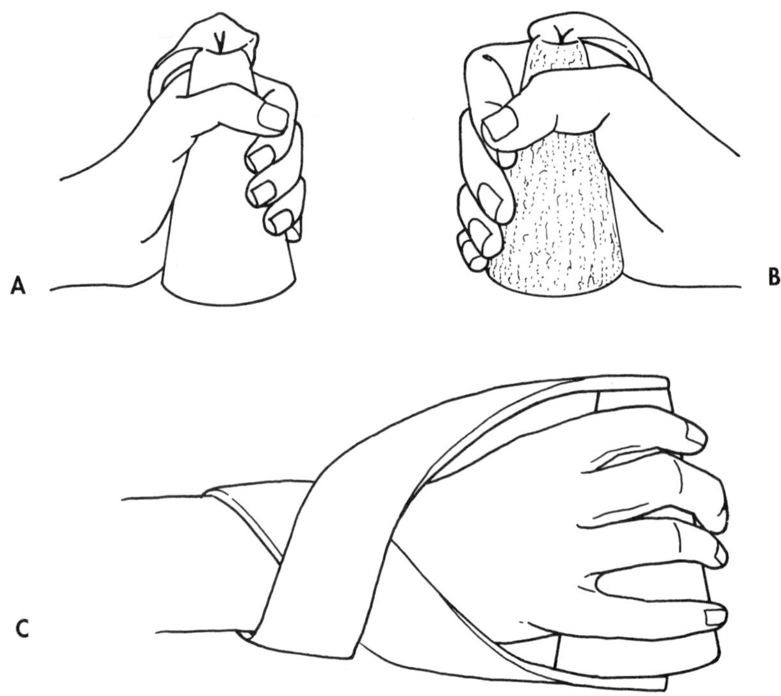

FIGURE 10-4 **Hard-cone designs**: **A,** hand plastic (Sammons, 1995); **B,** terry cloth covering (Sammons, 1995); and **C,** crossover strap system (Contour Fabricator, 1983)

tive grasp reaction. Commercially available soft-palm protectors (Sammons-Bissell Health Care Corporation, 1995; Rolyan, 1993) may be contraindicated for patients who exhibit the primitive grasp reaction.

MacKinnon et al. (1975) adapted the standard hard cone to increase sensory awareness and improve hand function. They altered the design from a 4- to 5-cm diameter hollow cone shape to a 0.3- to 1.3-cm diameter cylindrical shape by using a solid wood dowel. Placement of the dowel is critical to design rationale. Pressure over the palmar aspect of the metacarpal heads may be a key to activating hand intrinsics. In response to increased intrinsic activity, muscle tone is reduced in finger flexors and the thumb adductor. Placement of the dowel more distally shifts the maximum contact area from the palm to the metacarpal heads and exposes a larger palmar surface to sensory feedback, thus enhancing awareness and use of the hand.

The original MacKinnon splint incorporates a dorsal forearm platform consisting of a small rectangle of thermoplastic material attached to the dorsum of

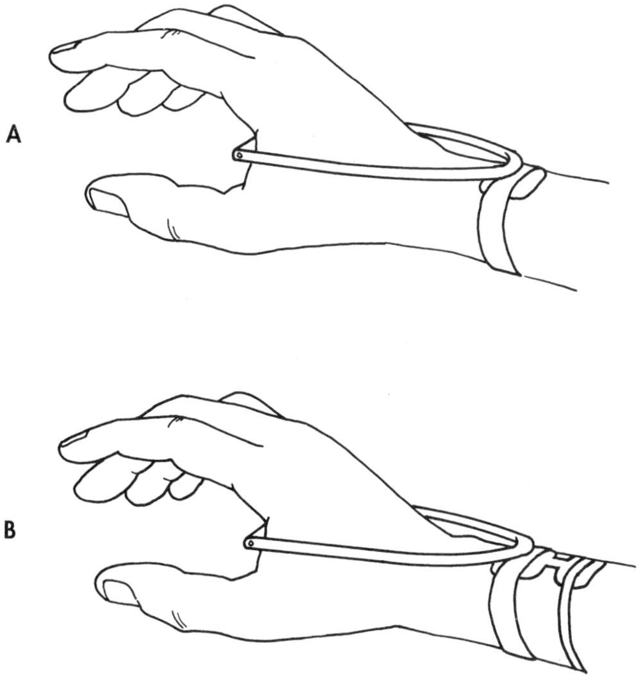

FIGURE 10-5 **Adapted hard-cone designs: A,** MacKinnon (1975); **B,** Exner & Bunder (1983)

the wrist with a volar velcro strap (MacKinnon et al., 1975). This platform serves as the base for plastic tubing that is secured to the palmar dowel. The intention of this platform is not to position the wrist forcefully in extension but to position the dowel to apply maximal pressure to the metacarpal heads. Exner and Bonder (1983) enlarged this dorsal forearm platform because it was insufficient to control the forces of marked wrist flexion spasticity. The design alteration relieves skin pressure, provides increased wrist control, and ensures greater comfort (Figure 10-5).

Hard-Cone Splint Construction for the Wrist and Hand

1. Determine the correct cone size by positioning an acrylic cone in the patient's palm. (Use a small Sammons BK-1500 or large BK-1502 acrylic cone, as shown in Figure 10-6.) The therapist must establish the correct amount of palm pressure that the patient can tolerate without application of stretch to the fingers and thumb. Slide the cone onto the patient's hand to determine the correct position (Figure 10-7).

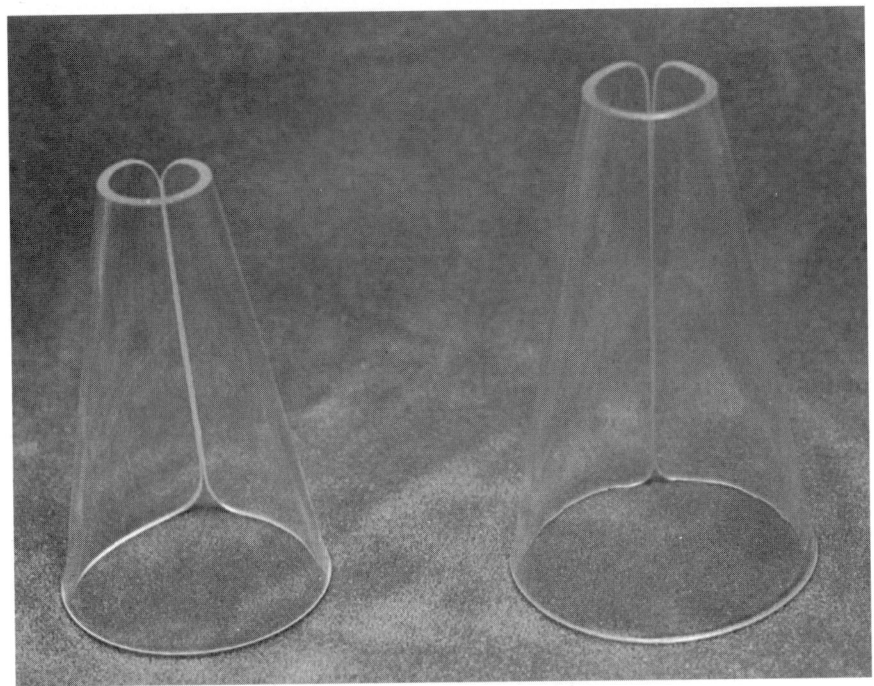

FIGURE 10-6 Small and large acrylic hand cones

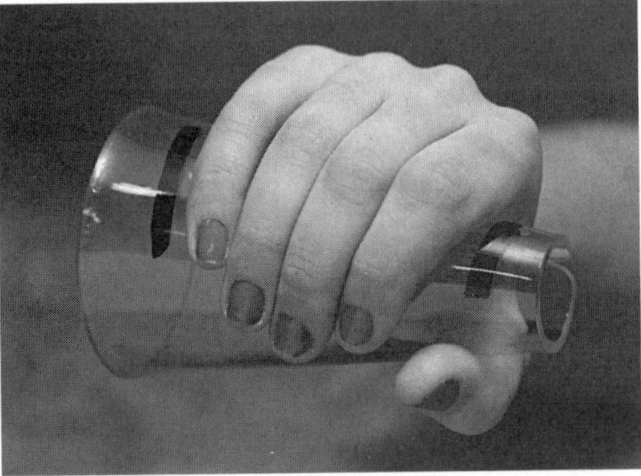

FIGURE 10-7 A hand cone correctly positioned on a patient with medial and lateral borders marked

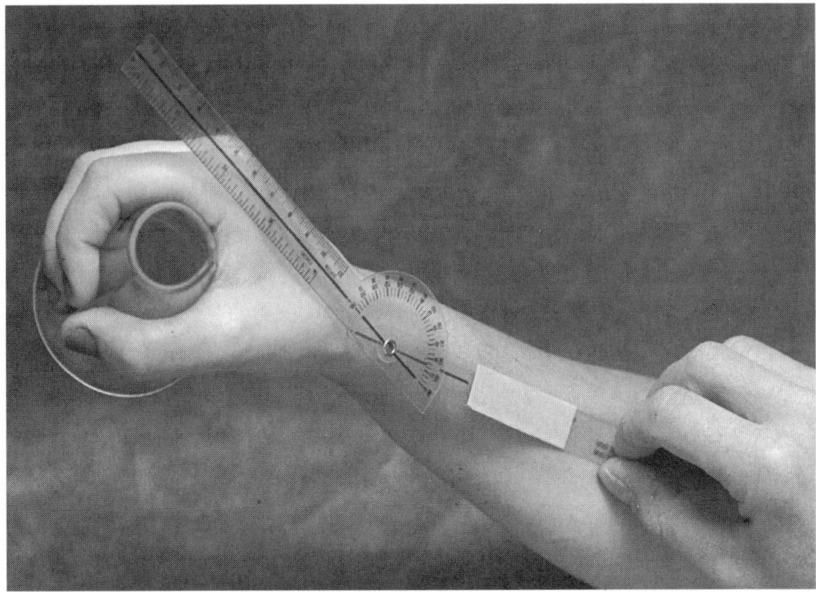

FIGURE 10-8
Use a goniometer to measure the wrist position.

2. Establish the wrist position by using a goniometer to measure the submaximum or maximum amount of wrist extension that the patient can tolerate. This measurement must take place while the patient wears the acrylic cone (Figure 10-8). Mark on the material the medial and lateral borders of the hand while the cone is positioned in the palm (Figure 10-7).
3. Using the template provided (Figure 10-9), trace and cut out the pattern from ⅛-inch thermoplastic material (Figure 10-10).
4. Apply dishwashing liquid to the acrylic cone as a parting agent.
5. Wrap heated thermoplastic material around the cone (Figure 10-11).
6. Using sharp scissors, cut the place where the material meets to create a smooth seam edge (Figure 10-12).
7. Slide the thermoplastic cone off the acrylic cone before the material cools to prevent removal difficulty (Figure 10-13).
8. Fit the thermoplastic cone to the patient's hand (Figure 10-14), and mark the following on the cone:
   a. Medial border
   b. Lateral border
   c. Thumb position
   d. Metacarpal arch support

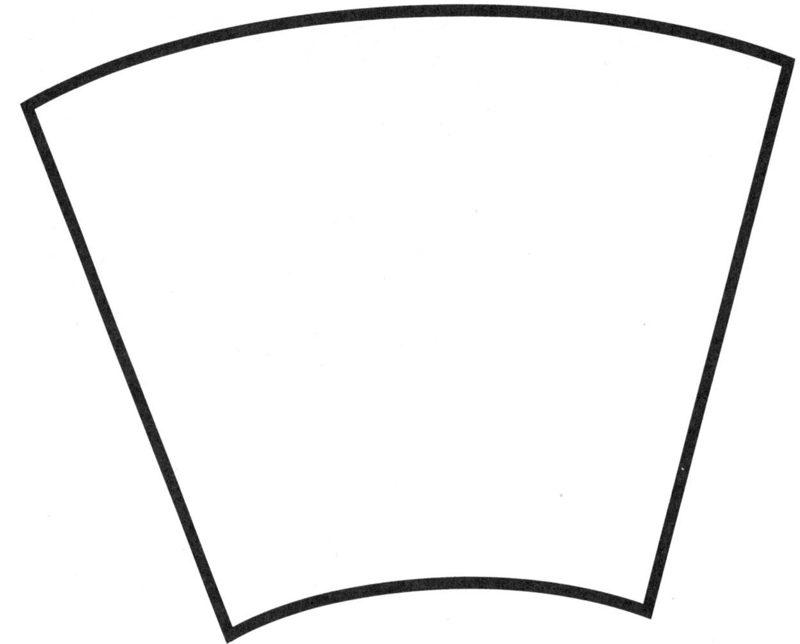

FIGURE 10-9 A template

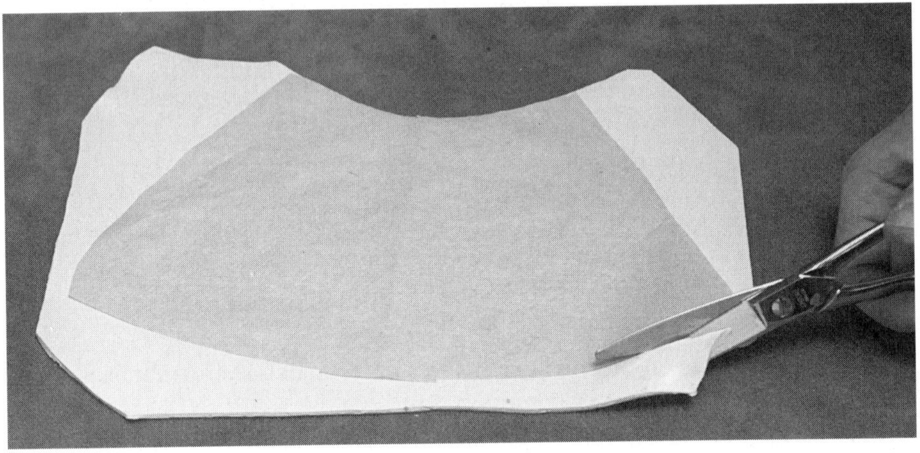

FIGURE 10-10
Use a template to trace and cut out the pattern.

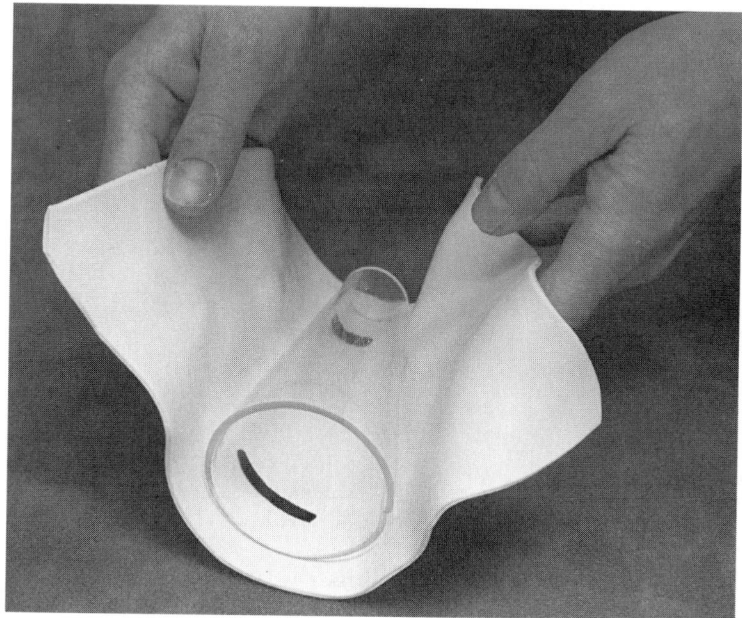

FIGURE 10-11
Wrap the heated material around the cone.

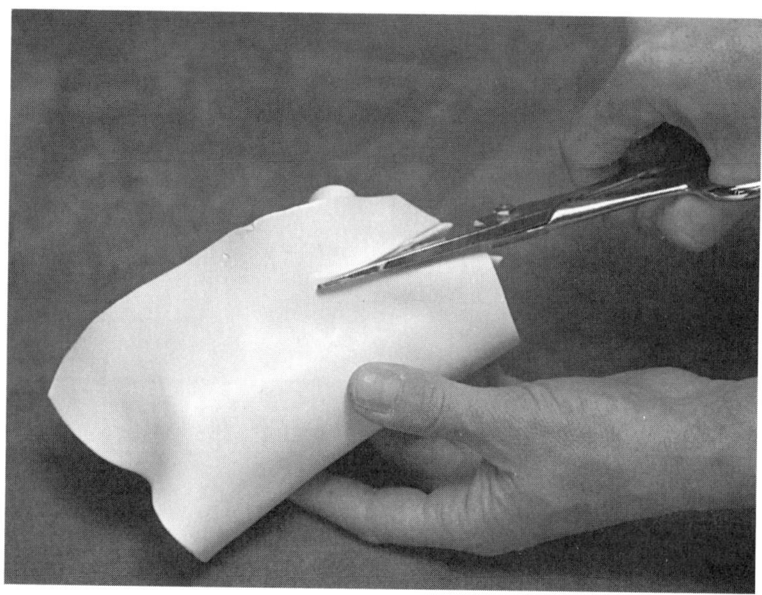

FIGURE 10-12
Use sharp scissors to create a smooth seam.

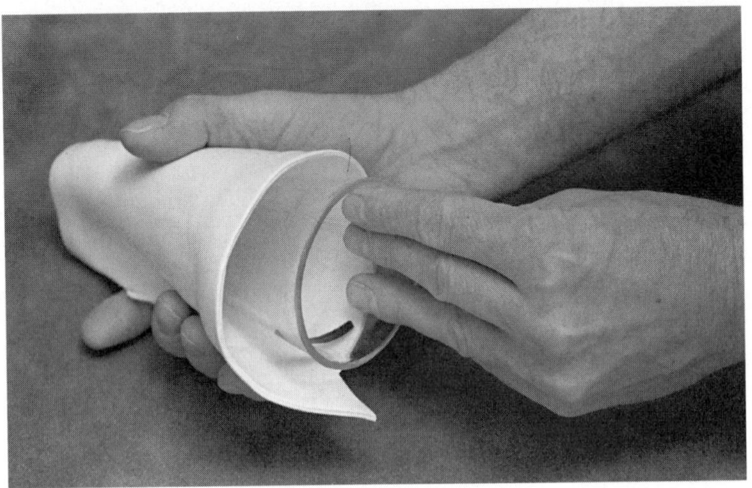

FIGURE 10-13
Slide the thermoplastic cone off the acrylic cone before the material cools.

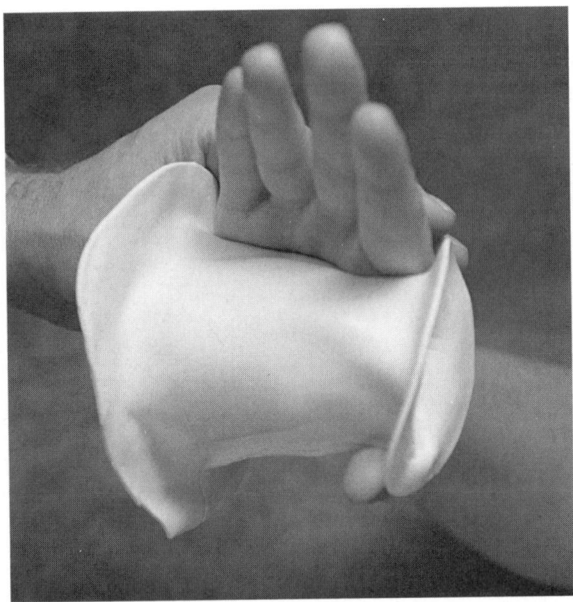

FIGURE 10-14
Fit the cone to the patient's hand.

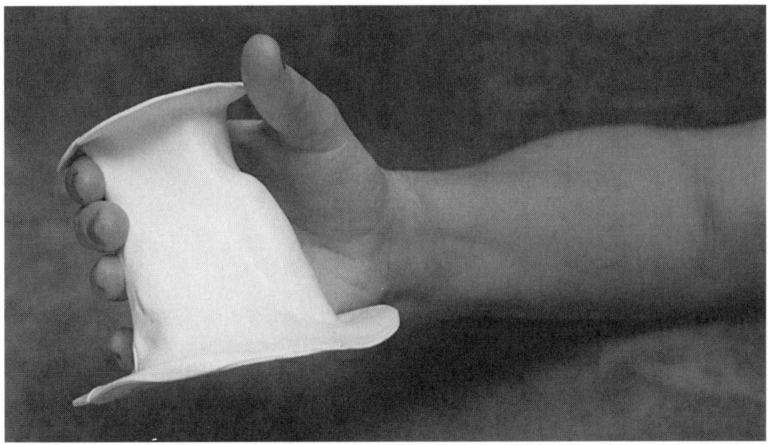

FIGURE 10-15
Spot heat the mold areas A-D separately.

9. Spot heat each of the following areas separately and mold them to the patient (Figure 10-15):
   a. Radial support
   b. Ulnar support
   c. Thumb groove
   d. Metacarpal arch support
10. Using a paper pattern, fabricate a dorsal forearm platform (Figure 10-16) that is one-half the width of the forearm and two-thirds the length of the forearm.
11. Warm two pieces of thermoplastic material that are 2 inches wide and 8 inches long. After doing this, fold and seam the pieces lengthwise to create radial and ulnar supports that connect the forearm platform to the cone (Figure 10-17).
12. Position the completed cone and forearm platform on the patient (Figure 10-18), and maintain the wrist in proper alignment.
13. Apply the radial and ulnar supports (Figure 10-19).
14. After the supports have finished cooling, apply two forearm straps and one strap across the dorsum of the hand in order to complete the splint (Figure 10-20).
15. Next, use a goniometer to measure the patient's wrist position while the patient is secured in the completed orthosis in order to ensure proper wrist position.

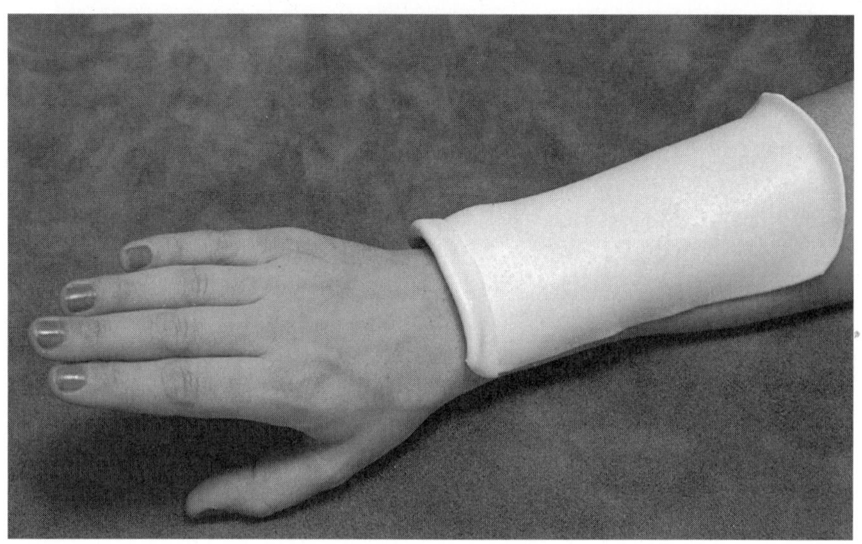

FIGURE 10-16
Fabricate a dorsal platform.

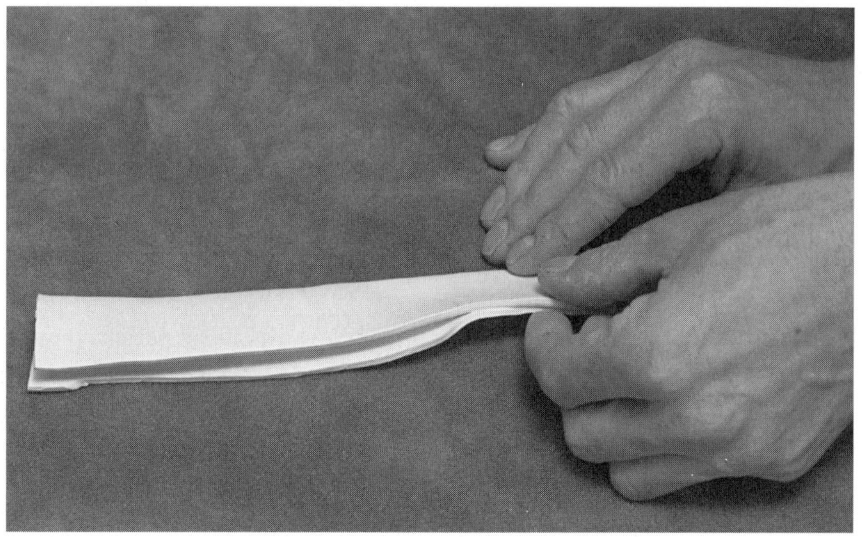

FIGURE 10-17
Fold and seam the material lengthwise.

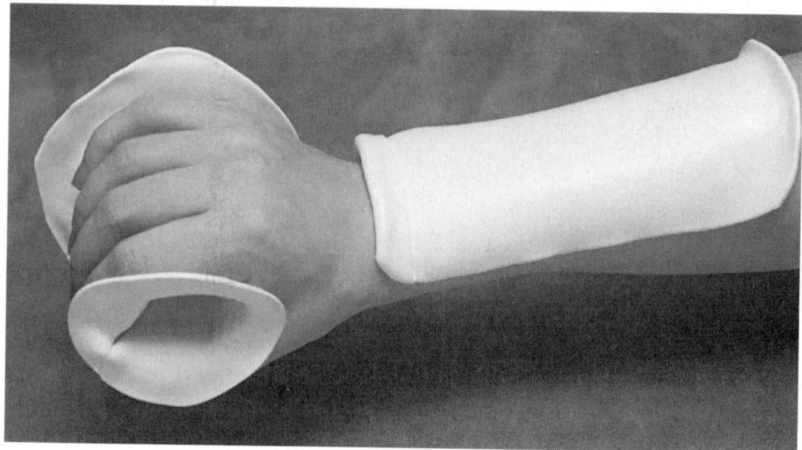

FIGURE 10-18
Position the completed cone and forearm platform on the patient.

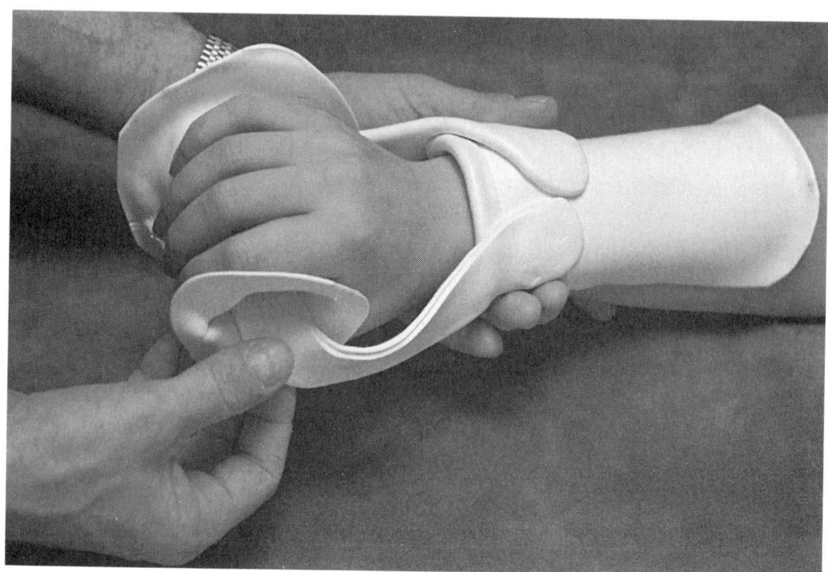

FIGURE 10-19
Apply the radial and ulnar supports.

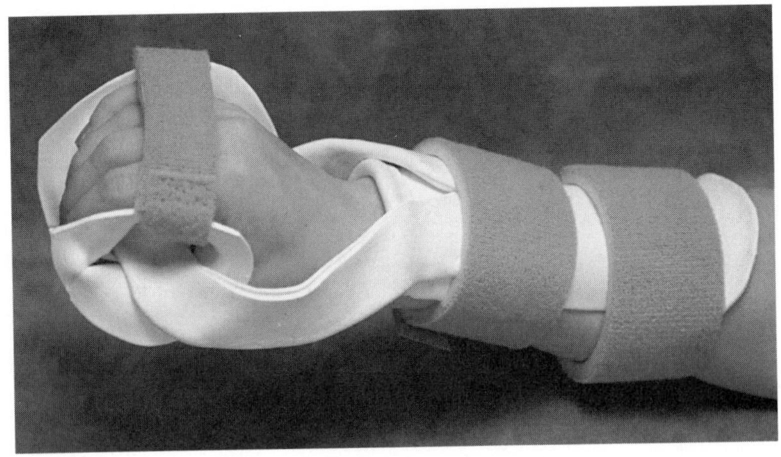

FIGURE 10-20
Apply the straps.

Laboratory Exercise 10-1

1. Practice fabricating a hard-cone wrist and hand splint on a partner. Use a goniometer and acrylic cones to position the hand and wrist correctly.
2. After fitting the cone, use Form 10-1 at the end of the chapter. This is a check-off sheet for self-evaluation of the hard-cone wrist and hand splint. Use Grading Sheet 10-1 at the end of the chapter as a classroom grading sheet.

Static and Dynamic Prolonged Stretch

Spasticity is a positive symptom of UMN lesion damage because it is an exaggeration of normal muscle tone (Tona & Schneck, 1993). Therapists commonly evaluate muscle tone by measuring the amount of resistance a muscle offers to quick-passive stretch or elongation (Trombly & Scott, 1989). Abnormal resistance to passive movement (i.e., stretch reflex) may be a static (i.e., passive) response to the muscle's maintained state of stretch or a dynamic response to the force and velocity of movement during stretching of the muscle. The static component (i.e., the nonreflexive, elastic properties of the muscle) and the dynamic component (i.e., the reflexive or active tension of the muscle during stretch) contribute to exaggerated stretch reflex or spasticity (Jansen, 1962; McPherson, 1981). The stretch reflex can be triggered at any point of the range-of-motion arc,

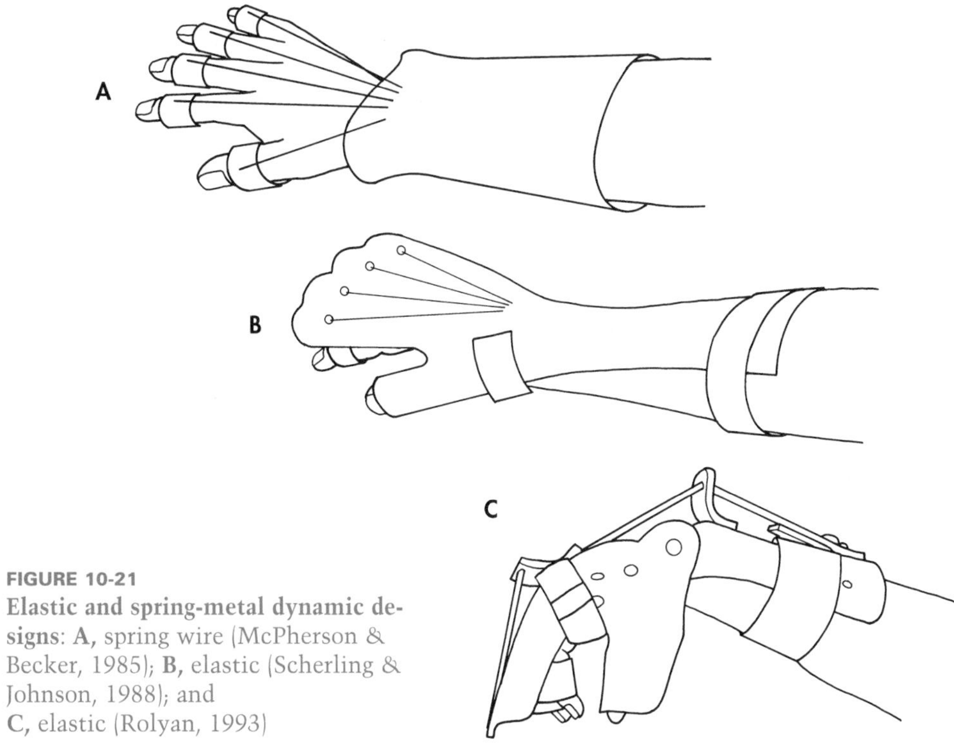

FIGURE 10-21
Elastic and spring-metal dynamic designs: **A,** spring wire (McPherson & Becker, 1985); **B,** elastic (Scherling & Johnson, 1988); and **C,** elastic (Rolyan, 1993)

thus limiting free range of motion. This reflex may also be a significant force to pull the wrist or finger muscles into an abnormal, shortened resting state. This activity creates *hypertonus*, which is defined as a force of spasticity sufficient to move the limb toward an abnormal resting state (McPherson et al., 1985).

Researchers concur that positioning the wrist and finger flexors in gentle, continuous stretch reduces the passive component of spasticity (McPherson, 1981; McPherson et al., 1985; Rose & Shah, 1987; Scherling & Johnson, 1989). Some authors recommend a static thermoplastic splint that positions the spastic flexor muscle in less than maximum available passive range of motion (i.e., submaximum range) but beyond the point the stretch reflex is triggered (Rose & Shah, 1987; Tona & Schneck, 1993). Other authors advocate a static thermoplastic splint that positions the spastic flexor muscle in a fully elongated state (i.e., maximum range) (Farber & Huss, 1974; Snook, 1979).

A dynamic thermoplastic design is also advanced because it provides a more sustained, uniform stretch to the spastic muscle. The use of an elastic or spring-metal force (Figure 10-21) may ensure slow stretch that does not trigger stretch-reflex receptors (McPherson et al., 1985; Scherling & Johnson, 1989).

Material Properties

Orthokinetic Materials

Dr. Julius Fuchs, an orthopedic surgeon, developed orthokinetic (righting-of-motion) principles in 1927. Some experts have described, refined, and adapted these principles (Blashy & Fuchs 1959; Neeman, 1971 & 1973; Neeman & Neeman, 1984; Farber, 1982; Farber & Huss, 1974; Kiel, 1974, 1982). The term *field* refers to material qualities in orthokinetic terminology.

Dr. Fuch's hand-splint design consists of an orthokinetic tube or cuff (Figure 10-2) that uses dynamic forces to increase range of motion rather than a static device that often contributes to pain and immobilization (Farber & Huss, 1974). The cuff is constructed of an active or a facilitatory field that the therapist places over the agonist muscle belly. The therapist places the passive or inhibitory field over the antagonist muscle belly. The elastic bandage-material construction of the active field provides minute pinching motions to the dermatome of the agonist muscle (i.e., exteroproprioceptive stimulation) as the muscle contracts and relaxes (Farber, 1982). The inactive field is constructed of layers of elastic bandage sewn or stitched together and provides continuous, nonchanging input to the antagonist dermatome.

Because the facilitatory effects of the orthokinetic cuff are activated during the contraction and relaxation of the muscle, this device is most effective when active range of motion is present (Farber, 1982).

Other authors recommend alternative materials for construction of inactive fields. Kiel (1974, 1982) uses the unchanging thermoplastic surface of the volar forearm platform in her design of the orthokinetic wrist splint (Figure 10-3). Exner and Bonder (1983) substitute velfoam as the nonelastic material. Kiel (1974, 1982) also suggests that foam lining over a thermoplastic surface transforms that surface from a passive field to an active field as the foam material changes shape to provide facilitatory stimulation.

Inhibition Casting

Orthopedic casting materials include plaster or fiberglass bandaging that is water activated. Both materials require six to eight layers of thickness for adequate strength and harden in 3 to 8 minutes depending on the water temperature. The materials emit heat as a by-product in the curing process. Plaster splints are not water resistant, do not clean easily, may cause allergic reactions, and pose limitations to function because of their heaviness. A plaster bandage is relatively inexpensive and easy to handle. Fiberglass splints are water resistant, cleanable, lightweight, and not prone to allergic reactions. In addition, fiberglass materials are significantly more expensive and difficult to handle than plaster. The therapist typically applies several layers of cotton-cast padding to the extremity before the application of layers of plaster or fiberglass for skin protection.

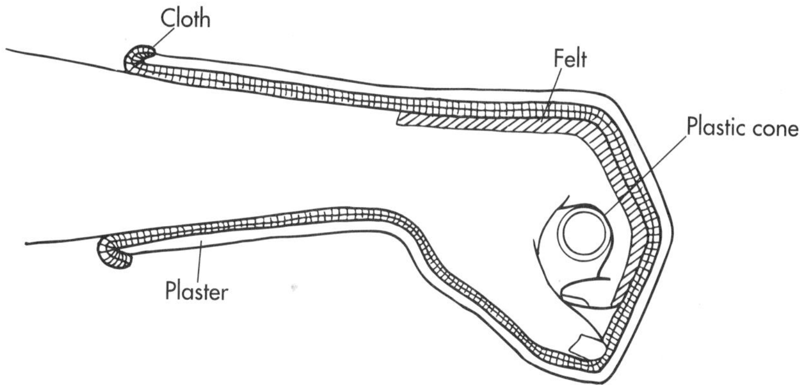

FIGURE 10-22 An inhibitive cast with a hard plastic cone

Therapists routinely use casts to decrease joint contractures. Frequent, periodic cast changes (i.e., serial casting) provide prolonged, continuous pressure to gradually lengthening muscles and soft tissue. A plaster cast is a cost-effective choice if the practitioner desires to gradually increase passive range-of-joint motion by using a series of static splints.

Therapists also use plaster and fiberglass materials for inhibition or tone-reducing casting. The exact mechanism for the inhibitory effect of these materials is not known (Tona & Schneck, 1993). Gentle, passive stretching and the neutral warmth of the underlying cotton padding may serve as primary relaxing agents (King, 1982). Some authors believe that inhibitive casting materials are more effective than thermoplastic materials at providing deep pressure, prolonged immobilization, neutral warmth, and consistent tactile stimulation (Tona & Schneck, 1993). These authors advocate the use of a separate thermoplastic-inhibitive splint (e.g., hard cone) incorporated into an inhibitive cast to enhance the tone-reducing effects of both materials (Figure 10-22). Lower-extremity, tone-reduction orthotic literature includes the use of a separate footboard as an inhibitive element in the plaster-negative-model casting procedure. The end product of this process is a continuous, one-piece thermoplastic orthosis (Hylton, 1990). Current lower-extremity, tone-reduction orthotic literature focuses on the incorporation of various inhibitive and facilitatory design elements into one total-surface-contact thermoplastic splint (Lohman & Goldstein, 1993).

Other Materials

Authors have reported the spasticity-reduction effectiveness of other materials that provide neutral warm and passive stretch. Pneumatic-pressure arm splints that are orally inflatable (Figure 10-23) are especially effective as adjuncts to up-

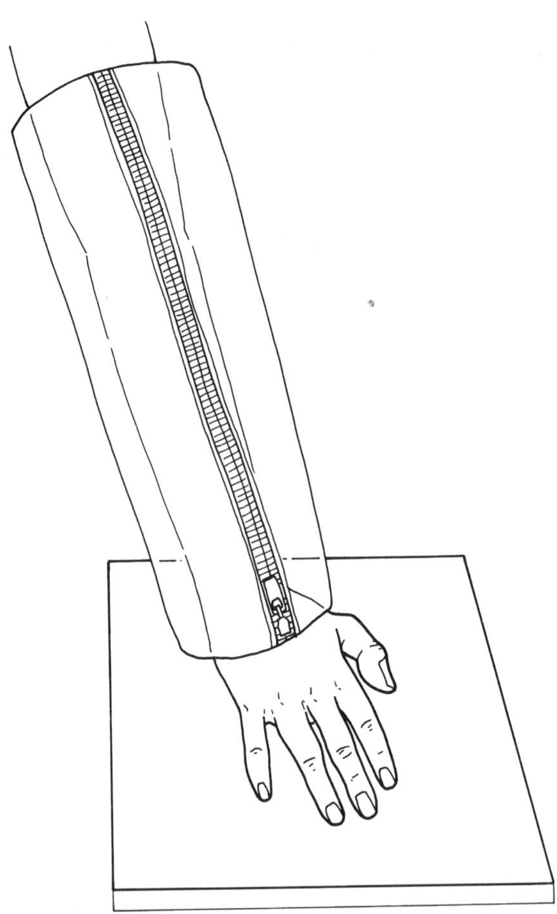

FIGURE 10-23 An orally inflatable, pneumatic-pressure arm splint

per-extremity weight-bearing (Bloch & Evans, 1977; Johnstone, 1981; Poole, Whitney, Hangeland, & Baker, 1990; Poole, Whitney, & Haworth, 1992; Lofy, Pereida, & Spores, 1992). These tubular devices are open at the distal end, thus allowing the therapist to place the patient's wrist and hand into the desired position of extension. Wallen and O'Flaherty (1991) have devised a cylindrical foam splint (Figure 10-24) that reduces the muscle tone of the upper extremity. The foam material reacts dynamically and automatically adjusts to greater degrees of extension.

Elastic tubular bandages have been successful in providing relaxation of upper-extremity hypertonicity through the application of neutral warmth and deep

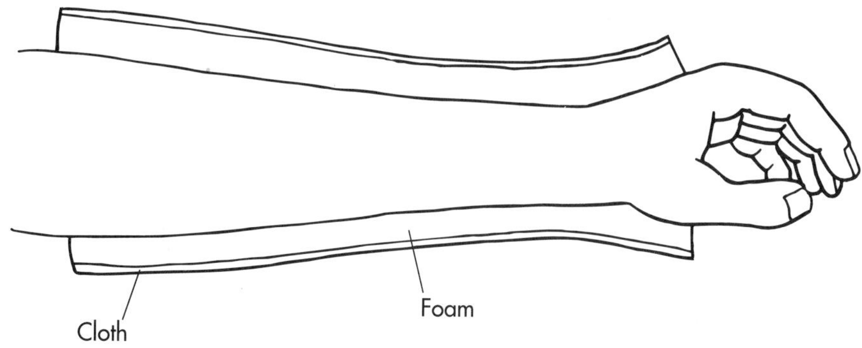

FIGURE 10-24 A cylinder foam splint

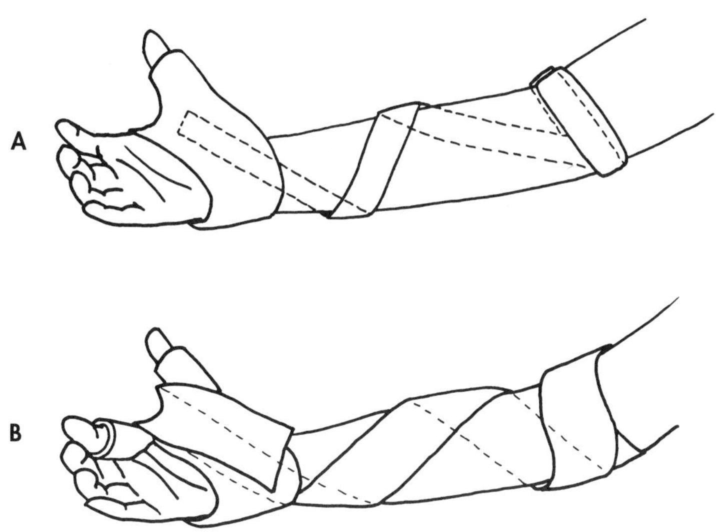

FIGURE 10-25 **Neoprene splint designs**: **A,** tass (Casey & Kratz, 1988); **B,** TAP™ (Rolyan, 1993)

pressure (Johnson & Vernon, 1992). Takami et al. (1992) describe the use of a titanium metal alloy that gradually changes shape in response to room temperature and provides gentle passive stretch to spastic wrist flexors. In addition, neoprene material provides a dynamic force that produces gentle stretch. The neoprene thumb abduction supination splint (TASS) (Figure 10-25) facilitates key-point positioning of the upper extremity, thus reducing spasticity (Casey & Kratz, 1988).

FORM 10-1* Hard-Cone Wrist and Hand Splint

Name: ____________________

Date: ____________________

Type of cone wrist and hand splint:

Volar platform ❍ Dorsal platform ❍

Answer the following questions after the splint has been worn for 30 minutes. (Mark NA for nonapplicable situations.)

Evaluation Areas				Comments
Design				
1. The wrist position is at the correct angle.	Yes ❍	No ❍	NA ❍	
2. The correct cone-diameter size reflects the palm width and web-space size.	Yes ❍	No ❍	NA ❍	
3. The small end of the cone is placed radially and the large end is placed ulnarly.	Yes ❍	No ❍	NA ❍	
4. The thumb is positioned in palmar abduction with the web space preserved.	Yes ❍	No ❍	NA ❍	
5. The splint is two-thirds the length of the forearm.	Yes ❍	No ❍	NA ❍	
6. The splint is half the width of the forearm.	Yes ❍	No ❍	NA ❍	
Function				
1. The wrist is positioned in submaximum or maximum range.	Yes ❍	No ❍	NA ❍	
2. The fingers are positioned to provide firm pressure but not stretch the flexors.	Yes ❍	No ❍	NA ❍	

*See Appendix B for a perforated copy of this form.

FORM 10-1 Hard-Cone Wrist and Hand Splint—cont'd

Evaluation Areas				Comments
Straps				
1. The straps avoid bony prominences.	Yes ❍	No ❍	NA ❍	
2. The straps are secure and rounded.	Yes ❍	No ❍	NA ❍	
3. The active field materials are used over the extensor muscle bellies.	Yes ❍	No ❍	NA ❍	
4. The passive field materials are used over the flexor muscle bellies.	Yes ❍	No ❍	NA ❍	
Comfort				
1. The edges are smooth with rounded corners.	Yes ❍	No ❍	NA ❍	
2. The proximal end is flared.	Yes ❍	No ❍	NA ❍	
3. Impingements or pressure areas are not present. (The ulnar styloid is relieved.)	Yes ❍	No ❍	NA ❍	
Cosmetic Appearance				
1. The splint is free of fingerprints, dirt, and pencil or pen marks.	Yes ❍	No ❍	NA ❍	
2. The splinting material is not buckled.	Yes ❍	No ❍	NA ❍	

Discuss adjustments or changes you would make based on the self-evaluation:

____

____

____

____

____

____

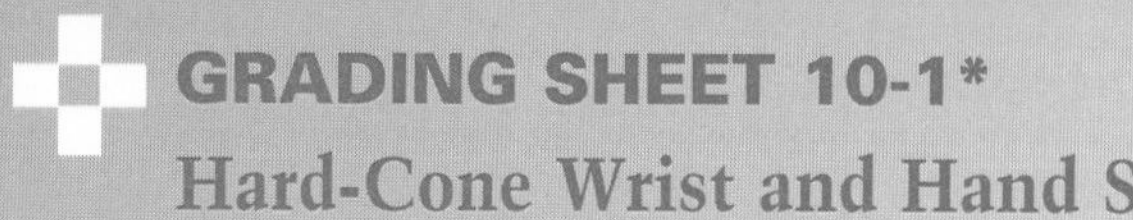

GRADING SHEET 10-1*

Hard-Cone Wrist and Hand Splint

Name: ______________________________

Date: ______________________________

Type of cone wrist and hand splint:

Volar platform ❍ Dorsal platform ❍

Grade: ____________

1 = beyond improvement, not acceptable
2 = requires maximal improvement
3 = requires moderate improvement
4 = requires minimal improvement
5 = requires no improvement

Evaluation Areas		**Comments**
Design		
1. The wrist position is at the correct angle.	1 2 3 4 5	
2. The correct cone diameter size reflects the palm width and web-space size.	1 2 3 4 5	
3. The small end of the cone is placed radially and the large end is placed ulnarly.	1 2 3 4 5	
4. The thumb is positioned in palmar abduction with the web space preserved.	1 2 3 4 5	
5. The splint is two-thirds the length of the forearm.	1 2 3 4 5	
6. The splint is half the width of the forearm.	1 2 3 4 5	
Function		
1. The wrist is positioned in submaximal or maximal range.	1 2 3 4 5	
2. The fingers are positioned to provide firm pressure but not stretch the flexors.	1 2 3 4 5	

*See Appendix C for a perforated copy of this grading sheet.

GRADING SHEET 10-1
Hard-Cone Wrist and Hand Splint—cont'd

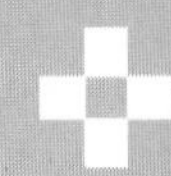

Evaluation Areas		**Comments**
Straps		
1. The straps avoid bony prominences.	1 2 3 4 5	
2. The straps are secure and rounded.	1 2 3 4 5	
3. The active field materials are used over the extensor muscle bellies.	1 2 3 4 5	
4. The passive field materials are used over the flexor muscle bellies.	1 2 3 4 5	
Comfort		
1. The edges are smooth with rounded corners.	1 2 3 4 5	
2. The proximal end is flared.	1 2 3 4 5	
3. Impingements or pressure areas are not present.	1 2 3 4 5	
Cosmetic Appearance		
1. The splint is free of fingerprints, dirt, and pencil or pen marks.	1 2 3 4 5	
2. The splinting material is not buckled.	1 2 3 4 5	

Case Study*

Read the following scenario and answer the questions based on information in this chapter.

ML suffered a CVA 2 months ago. Over a 4-week period of flaccidity, upper-extremity wrist and finger-flexion spasticity has gradually increased. Pain-free range-of-motion is limited to 5° of wrist extension. No active wrist and finger motion is present. A strong stretch reflex is elicited at 10° wrist flexion. The nursing staff is concerned that ML will develop palm maceration because his fingers rest in a tightly clenched position. The patient is using a rolled washcloth positioned in his palm to reduce the likelihood of skin breakdown, but nursing notes indicate that use of this device has increased finger-flexion tightness. The thumb is tightly flexed across the palm, thus causing skin irritation to the thumb-web space.

1. Which of the following orthotic designs is most appropriate for ML? Explain your answer.
   a. A dorsal-based forearm platform and finger spreader that positions the wrist and fingers statically in maximum extension
   b. A volar-based forearm platform and hard cone that positions the wrist and fingers dynamically in submaximum extension
   c. An orthokinetic cuff positioned on the forearm that leaves the wrist and fingers unsplinted
   d. An inhibitive cast that places the wrist in maximum extension and the fingers in a current resting position
   e. A neoprene thumb-abduction splint that leaves the wrist and fingers unsplinted

____

____

____

____

____

____

____

____

____

*See Appendix A for the answer key.

Case Study—cont'd

2. The nursing staff is resistant to discontinuing ML's present soft-hand positioning device. How would you approach the staff members to convince them to change the splint management of this patient?

Three weeks have passed. ML has been wearing the new tone-reduction splint consistently for several hours daily. Nursing reports indicate that tight fist clenching has reduced significantly. Passive range of motion has increased to 30° of wrist extension. Minimum stretch reflex can be felt at 20° of wrist extension. Weak wrist and finger extension is present when the extremity is positioned with gravity eliminated. The thumb, however, remains tightly flexed into the palm.

3. Which of the following orthotic designs is the most appropriate for ML at this time? Explain your answer.
   a. A finger spreader that positions the thumb in radial abduction and leaves the wrist unsplinted
   b. A hard cone that positions the thumb in opposition and leaves the wrist unsplinted
   c. An orthokinetic cuff on the forearm that leaves the fingers and thumb unsplinted
   d. An orally inflatable splint that leaves the wrist, fingers, and thumb in extension
   e. A neoprene thumb-abduction and extension orthoses that leaves the wrist and fingers unsplinted

4. What specific suggestions would you offer to the nursing staff to encourage increased functional hand skills while ML is wearing tone-reduction orthosis?

References

Basmajian, J., Burke, M., Burnett, G., Campbell, C., Cohn, W., Corliss, C., Ferguson, D., & Fraser, J. (1982). Illustrated Stedman's medical dictionary (24th ed.). London: Williams & Wilkins.

Bishop, B. (1977). Spasticity: Its physiology & management part III: Identifying & assessing the mechanisms underlying spasticity. Phys Ther, 57, 385-395.

Blashy, M. R. M., & Fuchs (Neeman), R. I. (1959). Orthokinetics: A new receptor facilitation method. Am J Occup Ther, 13, 226-234.

Blashy, M., Harrison, H. E., & Fuchs, E. M. (1955). Orthokinetics, a preliminary report on recent experiences with a little known rehabilitation therapy. VA Information Bull, 10, 72.

Bloch, R., & Evans, M. (1977). An inflatable splint for the spastic hand. Arch Phys Med Rehabil, 58, 179-180.

Bobath, B. (1970). Adult hemiplegia: Evaluation and treatment. London: William Heinemann, Medical Books, Ltd.

Bobath, B. (1978). Adult hemiplegia: Evaluation and treatment. London: William Heinemann, Medical Books, Ltd.

Brennan, J. (1959). Response to stretch of hypertonic muscle groups in hemiplegia. Br Med J, 1, 1504-1507.

Brunnstrom, S. (1956). Associated reactions of the upper extremity in adult patients with hemiplegia—an approach to training. Phys Ther Rev, 36, 225-236.

Brunnstrom, S. (1970). Movement therapy in hemiplegia. New York, Evanston, and London: Harper & Row, Publishers Inc.

Caldwell, C. B., Wilson, D. J., & Braun, R. M. (1969a). Evaluation and treatment of the upper extremity in the hemiplegic stroke patient. Clin Orthop, 63, 69-93.

Caldwell, C. B., Wilson, D. J., & Braun, R. M. (1969b). Orthopedic management of stroke. Clin Orthop, 63, 80.

Casey, C. A., & Kratz, E. J. (1988). Soft splinting with neoprene: The thumb abduction supinator splint. Am J Occup Ther, 42(6), 395-398.

Charait, S. (1968). A comparison of volar and dorsal splinting of the hemiplegic hand. Am J Occup Ther, 22, 319-321.

Costanzo, D. M., & Neeman, R. L. (1990). A patient's and therapist's experiences with pain treatment by orthokinetic orthoses. Occup Ther Forum, 49, 6-18.

Currie, D. M., & Mendiola, A. (1987). Cortical thumb orthosis for children with spastic hemiplegic cerebral palsy. Arch Phys Med Rehabil, 68, 214-216.

Davies, P. (1985). Steps to follow: A guide to the treatment of hemiplegia. New York: Springer-Verlag New York Inc.

Dayhoff, N. (1975). Re-thinking stroke soft or hard devices to position hands. Am J Nurs, 75(7), 1142-1144.

Doubilet, L., & Polkow, L. (1977). Theory and design of a finger abduction splint for the spastic hand. Am J Occup Ther, 32, 320-322.

Exner, C., & Bonder, B. (1983). Comparative effects of three hand splints on bilateral hand use, grasp, and arm-hand posture in hemiplegic children: A pilot study. Occup Ther J Res, 3, 75-92.

Farber, S. (1982). Neurorehabilitation: A multidisciplinary approach. Toronto: W. B. Saunders Co.

Farber, S. D., & Huss, A. J. (1974). Sensorimotor evaluation and treatment procedures for allied health personnel. Indianapolis: Indiana Univ Foundation.

Feldman, P. A. (1990). Upper extremity casting and splinting. In M. D. Glenn & J. Whyte (Eds.), The practical management of spasticity in children and adults. Malvern, PA: Lea & Febiger.

Fess, E. E., & Philips, C. A. (1987). Hand splinting principles and methods. St. Louis: Mosby.

Fuchs, J. (1927). Technische operationen in der orthopaedie orthokinetik. Berlin: Verlag Julius Springer.

Hylton, N. M. (1990). Postural and functional impact of dynamic AFOs and FOs in a pediatric population. J Prosthet Orthot, 2,(1), 40-53.

Jamison, S., & Dayhoff, N. (1980). A hard hand-positioning device to decrease wrist & finger hypertonicity: A sensorimotor approach for the patient with non-progressive brain damage. Nurs Res, 29, 285-289.

Jansen, J. K. S. (1962). Spasticity: Functional aspects. Acta Neurol Scandinav (Suppl. 3) 38, 41-51.

Johnson, J., & Vernon, D. C. (1992). Elastic tubular bandages: An adjunctive treatment approach to abnormal muscle tone. Gerontology Special Interest Selection Newsletter, 15,(2), 3-4.

Johnstone, M. (1981). Control of muscle tone in the stroke patient. Physiol, 67, 198.

Kaplan, N. (1962). Effect of splinting on reflex inhibition and sensorimotor stimulation in treatment of spasticity. Arch Phys Med Rehabil, 43, 565-569.

Kiel, J. (1974). Dynamic orthokinetic wrist splint: Sensorimotor evaluation and treatment procedures. Indianapolis, Indiana: Indiana-Purdue University.

Kiel, J. (1982). Orthokinetic wrist splint for flexor spasticity: Neurorehilitation. Toronto: W. B. Saunders Co.

King, T. (1982). Plaster splinting as a means of reducing elbow flexor spasticity: A case study. Am J Occup Ther, 36, 671-674.

Langlois, S., MacKinnon, J. R., & Pederson, L. (1989). Hand splints and cerebral spasticity: A review of the literature. CJOT, 56(3), 113-119.

Langlois, S., Pederson, L., & MacKinnon, J. R. (1991). The effects of splinting on the spastic hemiplegic hand: Report of a feasibility study. CJOT, 58(1), 17-25.

Lofy, S., Pereida, L. & Spores, M. (1992). Air splints: Technique propels stroke rehab. OT Week, 6(18), 18-19.

Lohman, M., & Goldstein, H. (1993). Alternative strategies in tone-reducing AFO design. J Prosthet Orthot, 5(1), 21-24.

Louis, W. (1962). Hand splinting effect on the afferent system. Am J Occup Ther, 16, 143-145.

MacKinnon, J., Sanderson, E., & Buchanan, D. (1975). The MacKinnon splint: A functional hand splint. Can J Occup Ther, 42, 157-158.

Mathiowetz, V., Bolding, D., & Trombly, C. (1983). Immediate effects of positioning devices on the normal and spastic hand measured by electromyography. Am J Occup Ther, 37, 247-254.

McPherson, J. (1981). Objective evaluation of a splint designed to reduce hypertonicity. Am J Occup Ther, 35, 189-194.

McPherson, J., Becker, A., & Franszczak, N. (1985). Dynamic splint to reduce the passive component of hypertonicity. Arch Phys Med Rehabil, 66, 249-252.

McPherson, J., Kreimer, D., Aalderks, M., & Gallager, T. (1982). A comparison of dorsal & volar resting hand splints in the reduction of hypertonus. Am J Occup Ther, 36, 664-670.

Mills, V. (1984). Electromyographic results of inhibitory splinting. Phys Ther, 64, 190-193.

Neeman, R. L. (1971). Technique of preparing effective orthokinetic cuffs. Bulletin on Practice (AOTA), 6(1), 1.

Neeman, R. L. (1973). Orthokinetic sensorimotor treatment. Aust Occup Ther J, 20, 122-125.

Neeman, R. L., & Neeman, M. (1984). Comments on orthokinetics. Occup Ther J Res, 4, 316-318.

Neuhaus, B., Ascher, E., Coullon, B., Donohue, M. V., Einbond, A., Glover, J., Goldberg, S. R., & Takai, V. (1981). A survey of rationales for and against hand splinting in hemiplegia. Am J Occup Ther, 35, 83-90.

Peterson, L. T. (1980). Neurological considerations in splinting spastic extremities. Menomonee Fall, WI: Rolyan Orthotics Lab, Inc.

Poole, J. L., Whitney, S. L., Hangeland, N., & Baker, C. (1990). Function in stroke patients. Occup Ther J Res, 10, 360-366.

Poole, J. L., Whitney, S. L., & Haworth, P. R. (1992). Treatment for individuals with stroke. Phys Occup Ther Geriatrics, 11, 17-27.

Rood, M. (1954). Neurophysiological reactions as a basis for physical therapy. Phys Ther Rev, 34, 444-449.

Rood, M. S. (1956). Neurophysiological mechanisms utilized in the treatment of neuromuscular dysfunction. Am J Occup Ther, 10, 220-224.

Rose, V., & Shah, S. (1987). A comparative study on the immediate effects of hand orthoses on reduction of hypertonous. Aust Occup Ther J, 34(2), 59-64.

Sammons-Bissell Health Care Corp. (1995). Catalog. Western Springs, IL.

Scherling, E., & Johnson, H. (1989). A tone-reducing wrist-hand orthosis. Am J Occup Ther, 43(9), 609-611.

Smith & Nephew Rolyan, Inc. (1993). Catalog. Menomonee Falls, WI.
Snook, J. H. (1979). Spasticity reduction splint. Am J Occup Ther, 33, 648-651.
Switzer, S. (1980). The Switzer splint. Br J Occup Ther, 43, 63-64.
Takami, M., Fukui, K., Saitou, S., Sugiyama, I., & Terayama, K. (1992). Application of a shape memory alloy to hand splinting. Prosthet Orthot International, 16, 37-63.
Tona, J. L., & Schneck, C. M. (1993). The efficacy of upper extremity inhibitive casting: A single-subject pilot study. Am Occup Ther, 47(10), 901-910.
Trombly, C., & Scott, A. (1989). Occupational therapy for physical dysfunction (3rd ed.). Baltimore: Williams & Williams.
Wallen, M., & O'Flaherty, S. (1991). The use of soft splint in the management of spasticity of the upper limb. Aust Occup Ther J, 38(15), 227-231.
Wolcott, L. E. (1966). Orthotic management of the spastic hand. South Med J, 59, 971-974.
Zislis, J. (1964). Splinting of hand in a spastic hemiplegic patient. Arch Phys Med Rehabil, 45, 41-43.

CHAPTER ELEVEN

Geriatric Splinting

SERENA M. BERGER, MA, OTR
MAUREEN T. CAVANAUGH, MS, OTR
BRENDA M. COPPARD, MS, OTR/L
HELENE LOHMAN, MA, OTR/L

Chapter Objectives

1. List splint designs that help persons who have the following problems:
   - Edema
   - Ecchymosis
   - Fragile skin
   - Joint contracture
   - Skin ulceration
   - Diminished cognition
   - Sensory loss
   - Decreased motivation
2. List the four purposes of geriatric splints.
3. Explain indications for the use of soft splints for older patients.
4. Identify common lower-extremity splints for older patients.
5. Explain the way an older person's environment, risk for contractures, skin integrity, and compliance affect splint material selection and design.
6. Describe factors that determine splint wear and care and the method of instruction for an older patient and caregiver.
7. Describe splinting approaches for persons who have impaired:
   - Cognition
   - Hearing
   - Vision
   - Mobility
   - Compliance
8. Explain the splint instructions given to the caregiver and patient.

According to the American Association of Retired Persons (AARP) (1994), the number of people over age 65 in the United States is increasing. Although most older persons live independently, approximately 5% are residents in long-term care facilities. Regardless of health status, 50% of older persons have some limitation in function that prevents them from being fully independent in activities of daily living (ADL) (AARP, 1994; Lavizzo-Mourey, Day, Diserens, & Grisso, 1989). Therapists often provide therapeutic interventions to older patients to improve functional status. Interventions include the designing and fabricating of splints. Aging may affect hand mobility and productivity (Lewis, 1989) and may require splinting to maintain function.

Fundamental principles of splint evaluation, design, and fabrication do not change as patients age. Modifications, however, are often necessary to accommodate the special needs of older persons.

When designing a splint for an older patient, the therapist should consider special needs of the patient, the goal of the splint, and the splinting material available. A splint for a geriatric person should (1) prevent undesirable motion while permitting normal motion, (2) provide adequate stability, (3) decrease energy expenditure when worn, (4) provide safe distribution of force, (5) be comfortable, (6) be applied and removed easily, (7) be economical, (8) be durable, (9) be easily modified (Good & Supan, 1992), and (10) be easily cleaned.

Evaluation of an Older Patient

As with any patient, the therapist must complete a comprehensive rehabilitative assessment to determine whether splinting is indicated. All components of a therapy evaluation are essential for determining an effective treatment plan. (See Chapter 3 for a discussion of a hand examination.) The therapist should pay special attention to the cognitive, sensory, physical, and ADL status of the older patient to determine the usefulness of splinting as part of the treatment plan (Table 11-1).

During the initial evaluation, the therapist notes any current use of adaptive devices and techniques. For example, an older patient may already have a splint for a chronic condition such as rheumatoid arthritis. The therapist should evaluate the splint for its functional purpose and proper fit.

Observation during the assessment is vital to determine the purpose of a splint and to select the design. Observing and assessing movement of the extremities in relation to the trunk is important. For example, a patient who has hemiplegia with a spasticity upper extremity may be wearing a hand splint that is resting and applying pressure to the chest.

The patient's living situation (e.g., independence in a community versus dependence in an institution) is important when the therapist decides the type of splinting. For example, an 80-year-old woman who performs her own self-care

TABLE 11-1 Common Problem Etiologies and Applications to Splinting

Possible etiology	Application to splinting
EDEMA Trauma, congestive heart failure, dependent positioning, IV infiltration, and prolonged immobilization	• Reduce the edema before applying the splint. • Design the splint larger to accommodate slight edema. • Consider using soft, stretchy straps.
ECCHYMOSIS (BRUISE) Trauma, anticoagulants, and fractures	• Consider using padding. • Monitor the splint frequently for pressure areas. • Consider using soft straps. • Avoid transverse dorsal straps.
FRAGILE SKIN Dehydration, poor nutrition, diabetes, renal disease, psoriasis, radiation therapy, long-term steroid use, and advanced age	• Consider using padding. • Monitor the splint frequently for pressure areas. • Consider using soft straps.
JOINT CONTRACTURE Fractures or other orthopedic conditions, poor positioning, and prolonged immobility	• Consider using dynamic or static-progressive splints. • Splint to regain a functional position.
SKIN ULCERATION Poor circulation, positioning, immobility, poor nutrition, excessive perspiration, and incontinence	• Bubble out the splint over the ulceration. • Allow for dressing bulk in the splint design. • Consider using a design that avoids pressure over the ulcerated area and allows air flow to the ulcer.
DIMINISHED COGNITION Dementia, Alzheimer's disease, cerebral vascular accident, multi-infarct dementia, over medication, and depression	• Consider using D-ring straps if the patient spontaneously removes the splint. • Provide thorough patient and caregiver instructions on the splint's wear and care. • Establish a structured routine for splint wear and care.
SENSORY LOSS Diabetes, cerebral vascular accident, and peripheral vascular disease	• Teach the patient or caregiver to frequently monitor the splint for pressure areas. • Consider using a design that avoids coverage of the affected area (e.g., dorsal versus volar base).
MOTIVATION Depression	• Educate the patient about responsibility for following the splint schedule. • Identify patient goals and relate the splint use to goal achievement. • Refer the patient for appropriate psychological support.

and homemaking requires the use of her hands throughout the day. Her sister, however, has been a long-term-care resident for years as a consequence of multiple cerebrovascular accidents (CVAs). The nursing staff performs ADLs for the sister, who is unable to move her limbs volitionally and has increased tone on her left side. The woman at home may be a candidate for arthritic splints. A thumb spica splint may increase her daily function, and a night resting hand splint may decrease morning pain and stiffness. Her sister requires splints to maintain sufficient range-of-joint motion (ROM) so that nursing personnel can dress and bathe her. Hand ROM is necessary to prevent skin maceration in the palm caused by sustained full-finger flexion.

Purposes of Splints for Geriatric Patients

Patients who sustain rheumatologic, neurologic, and orthopedic problems commonly use splints. Diagnoses that often require splints are rheumatoid arthritis; CVA; and arm, wrist, and hand fractures. Splints for these diagnoses are not unique to older patients. In the older population, however, an increase in the effects from chronic health problems occurs. Neurologic and orthopedic problems are also more common in this group (Lewis, 1989).

The purposes for geriatric splinting may include but are not limited to the following:

1. Reduction of pain
2. Maintenance of functional use of an extremity
3. Contracture management
4. Prevention and reduction of skin ulceration

Pain Reduction

With acute and chronic conditions, one goal of geriatric splinting is to reduce pain by providing support and rest to the involved joints. For example, in a patient who has rheumatoid arthritis, the purpose of the splint is primarily to reduce pain by stabilizing the involved joints (Ouellette, 1991; Merritt, 1987). The therapist can use different splint designs according to the stage of the arthritis and the joints involved. However, "the use of splints to rest the hands during periods of pain and inflammation is controversial" (Ouellette, 1991, p. 68). Intermittent periods of rest (i.e., 3 weeks or fewer) appear to be beneficial, but prolonged immobilization for longer periods may cause loss of range of motion (Colditz, 1995; Ouellette, 1991).

Functional Maintenance

A splint may improve or maintain an older person's function. Adapting the environment is often more appropriate than restricting the ROM in a hand splint.

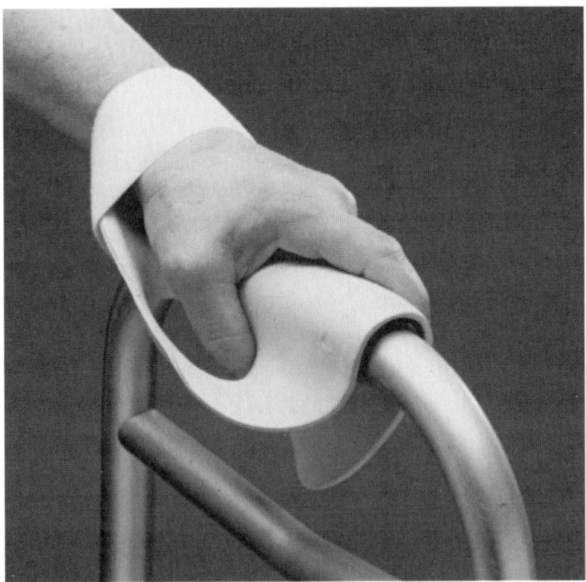

FIGURE 11-1 Walker splint
This splint promotes function. (From Smith and Nephew Rolyan. [1990]. Rehabilitation Products Catalog. Germantown, WI.)

For example, a figure-of-eight finger splint on a patient's pen allows the patient to continue writing. Rather than making a wrist splint for use during shaving, the therapist may make adaptations from thermoplastic material on an electric razor to allow a patient to remain independent. Using hand splints during ADLs is extremely awkward when sensory input is impeded (Redford, 1986). Specially adapted splints that help promote function are available (Figure 11-1). Patients who have severe rheumatoid arthritis (i.e., third stage) may benefit from hand splints that immobilize joints to stabilize rather than mobilize (Fess, Gettle, & Strickland, 1981).

Contracture Management

In an ideal world, proper routine care of passive ROM, positioning, and exercise prevents contractures in long-term care residents. In reality, such prevention is often impossible because of patient cognitive and/or physical incapacity, limited caregiver time, and financial constraints. Furthermore, changes in the older person's connective tissue and cartilage increase the risk of contractures, especially during inactivity (Jackson, 1989). The goal becomes the maintenance of current ROM to enable adequate skin care and functional use. Therapists commonly use resting hand splints to prevent further deformity. Resting hand splints also reduce contractures by serial application. (Serial casting and splinting are more advanced skills and beyond the scope of this book.)

Prevention or Reduction of Skin Ulceration

Patients who hold their hands in a fist position or continually flex their elbows, knees, and hips create an environment conducive to skin breakdown. The accumulation of perspiration within the skin folds allows bacteria growth (Redford, 1986). This constant posturing and the resulting bacteria growth may cause joint contractures, skin maceration, and possible infection. A splint made of molded thermoplastic, a hand roll, or a palm protector positions the involved joints in submaximum extension, thus allowing adequate hygiene of the hand. To accomplish any of these goals, the therapist must obey the following rules:

1. A splint should not impede function unnecessarily. For example, the splint should not prevent a patient from safely grasping an ambulation device or interfere with wheelchair propulsion.

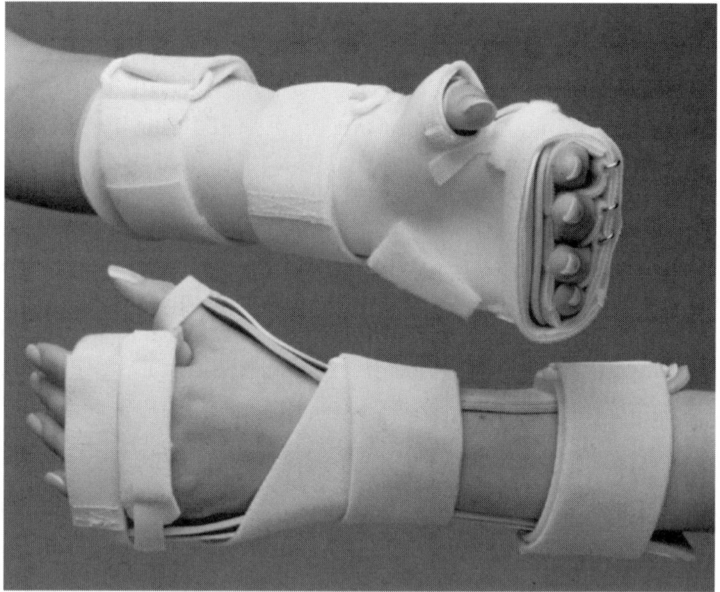

FIGURE 11-2 Arthritis-mitt splint

This splint immobilizes the wrist at 20° of extension, MCPs at 45° of flexion, and allows movement of the PIPs. (From Smith and Nephew Rolyan. [1992]. Rehabilitation Products Catalog. Germantown, WI.)

2. A splint should not exacerbate a preexisting condition. For example, a patient who demonstrates a flexor-synergy pattern may wear a functional position splint at night for pain and contracture management. The patient may also have carpometacarpal osteoarthritis in the thumb. The functional position splint should therefore place the thumb metacarpal (MP) and interphalangeal (IP) joints in extension and the carpometacarpal (CMC) joint in 45° of abduction, midway between radial and palmar abduction. This thumb position differs from that of functional position splints in which the thumb is placed in palmar abduction and opposition to the tips of the index and middle fingers. This midway position may provide more comfort to the thumb CMC joint than palmar abduction (Mallick, 1976).
3. A splint should not limit the use of uninvolved joints. An example is the arthritis mitt splint (Figure 11-2), which immobilizes the wrist in 20° of extension and MCPs in 45° of flexion but allows movement at the proximal interphalangeal (PIP) joints. When wearing these bilateral splints, patients are able to pull up blankets, ring call bells, and hold glasses of water.

Soft Splinting

Soft splints are made from materials such as fabric, flexible plastics, neoprene, foam, and leather (Figure 11-3). Many soft splints are available commercially but may require modification by the therapist at the time of fitting. Often a metal or moldable thermoplastic-material stay is part of the splint to increase support and restrict motion. Most soft splints are hand washable and require air drying.

In institutional settings, soft splints may be more acceptable to the staff because of reduced risk of skin breakdown. Because of the texture, conformity, and less restrictive nature of soft splints, patient compliance with them may be better than with hard splints (Stern, Sines, & Teague, 1994). Soft splints reduce secondary joint stiffness and edema caused by complete immobilization.

Some soft-splinting materials are difficult to sew. Soft splints may be time consuming to custom fabricate, and many clinicians prefer to purchase prefabricated soft splints. The therapist must be careful to accurately assess the size and fit of commercial soft splints. Splints made of rigid thermoplastic material may be more appropriate for tone reduction (see Chapter 10).

Lower-Extremity Splinting

In some practice settings, therapists may need to fabricate lower-extremity splints. Common lower-extremity resting splints are ankle-foot-orthoses (AFOs), also known as *footdrop splints* (Figure 11-4). Therapists use AFOs to maintain 90° of ankle dorsiflexion and may add lateral stabilization bars to decrease external rotation of the hip (Smith & Nephew Rolyan, 1995). This splint positions the foot in 90° of passive ankle dorsiflexion to ensure that functional ankle ROM is

A

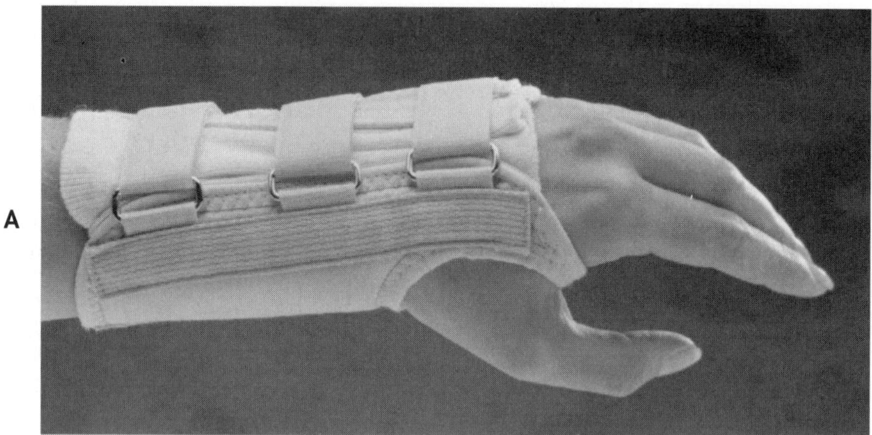

B

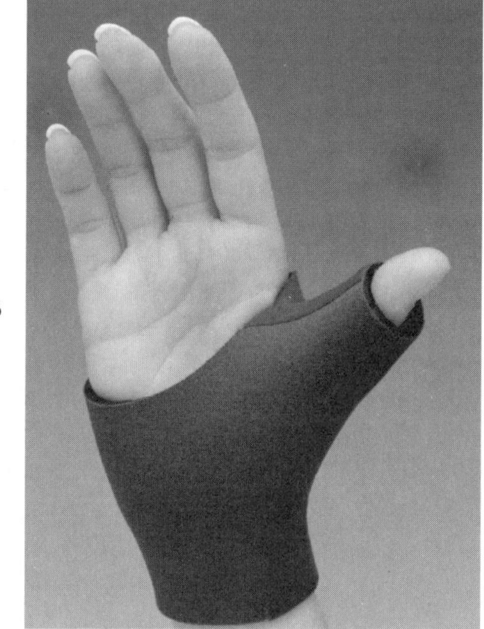

FIGURE 11-3

A, The D-Ring wrist brace for positioning has a circumferential design that holds the splint in place during application. **B,** The neoprene pull-on thumb support provides warmth and compression to reduce pain and prevent overuse while permitting maximal hand function. (From Smith and Nephew Rolyan. [1995]. Rehabilitation Products Catalog. Germantown, WI.)

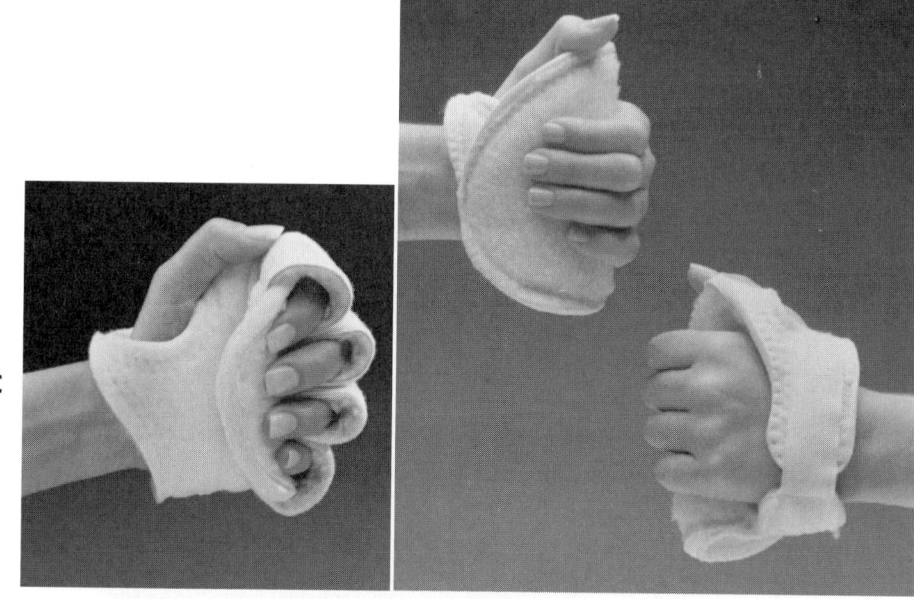

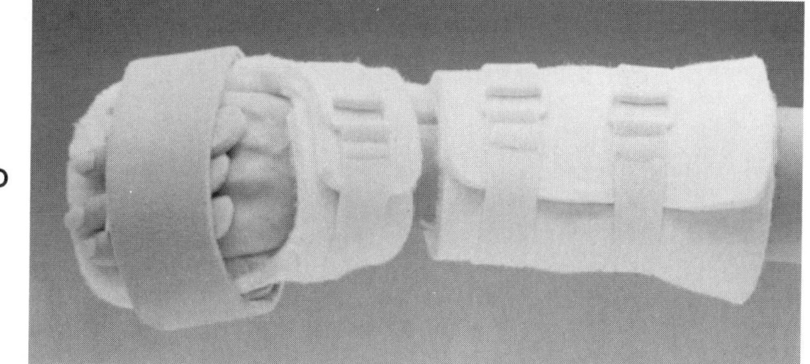

FIGURE 11-3—cont'd

C, The palm protector with (*left*) and without (*right*) finger separators prevents fingers from digging into the palm of the hand. The palm protector is fabricated from closed-cell foam that has pile lining. **D,** The progressive palm protector with a wrist support has a firm foam hand piece and thermoplastic wrist stay that are lined with soft foam in a circumferential design. (From Smith and Nephew Rolyan. [1995]. Rehabilitation Products Catalog. Germantown, WI.)

Continued.

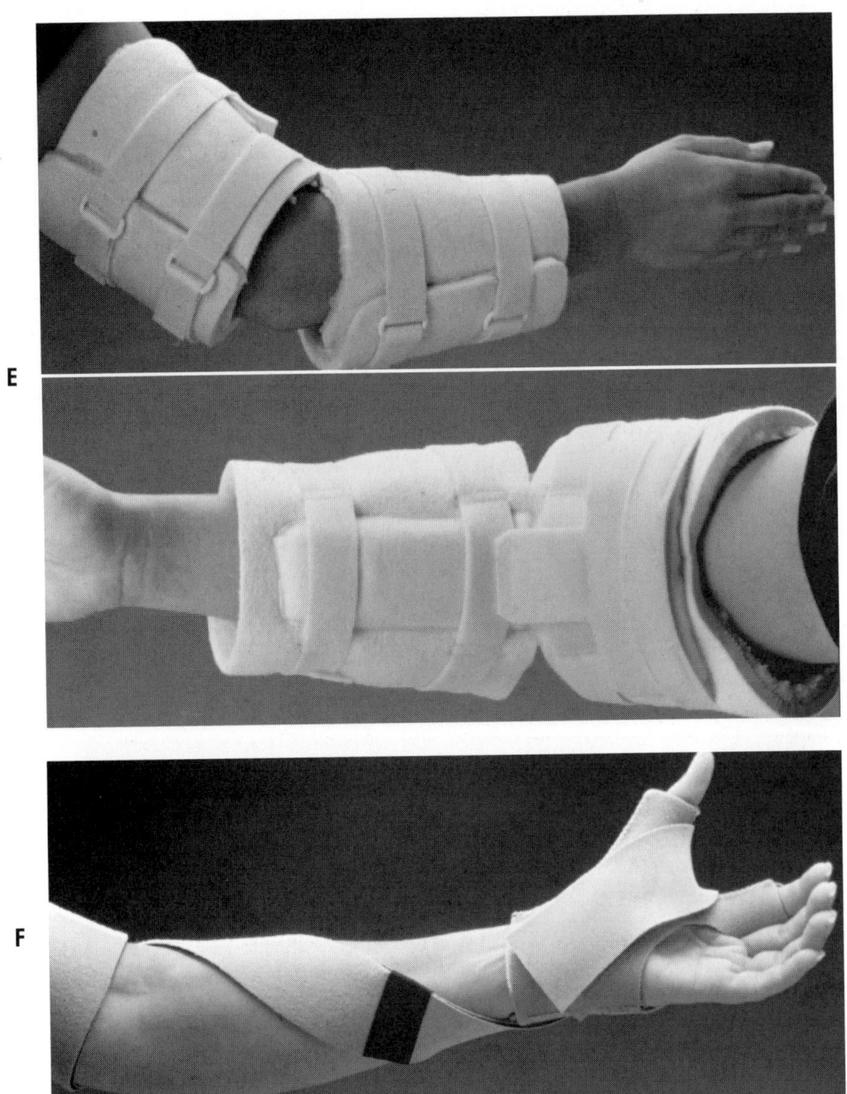

E

F

FIGURE 11-3—cont'd

E, The progressive elbow and knee splints have soft-foam splint bases that decrease the risk of skin breakdown. The therapist uses the base to progressively splint into increased extension by remolding Ezeform thermoplastic stay. **F,** The TAP™ splint is a dynamic splint that a therapist uses for decreased hypertonicity and progressive stretching by providing constant low-level stretch into pronation or supination. Therapists also use this type of splint to dynamically reduce pronation contractures caused by Colle's fractures. (From Smith and Nephew Rolyan. [1995]. Rehabilitation Products Catalog. Germantown, WI.)

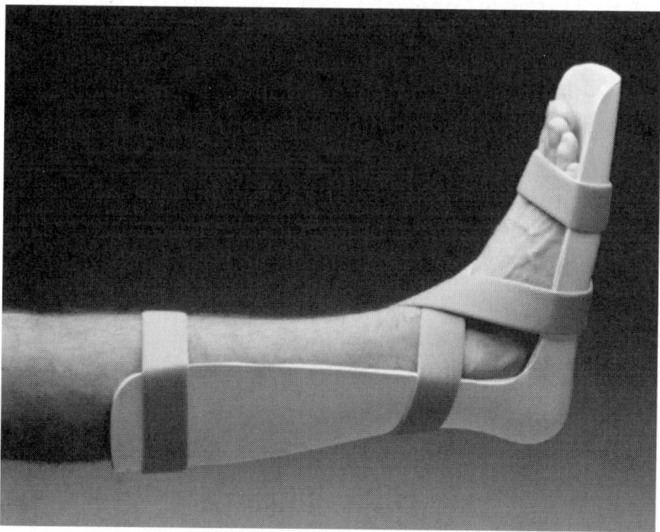

FIGURE 11-4 **Preformed footdrop splint**
The strapping pattern extends across the ankle. (From Smith and Nephew Rolyan. [1995]. Rehabilitation Products Catalog. Germantown, WI.)

maintained for standing and ambulation. Therapists often use these splints to treat persons who have spinal cord injuries, CVAs, and traumatic brain injuries. Increased muscle tone can lead to contractures, and shortened muscles facilitate increased tone. A prolonged stretch by the splint is necessary for lengthening to occur in the collagen of the involved connective tissue and re-form the collagen to an appropriate length (Harbun & Potter, 1993).

A deep peroneal nerve injury is another cause of footdrop, which results in the inability to actively dorsiflex the ankle (Clarkson & Gilewich, 1989). For a patient with footdrop the AFO maintains the passive ankle motion in the absence of active motion. Patients commonly wear AFOs for footdrop during ambulation.

An AFO that supports the ankle while the patient is confined to bed for prolonged periods serves a second purpose. The AFO decreases the risk of heel breakdown because of prolonged pressure and shear forces of the heel moving across the bed.

A patient who has dementia and is confined to bed often assumes a fetal position of hip and knee flexion. Knee extension splints often reduce the risk of knee joint contractures. Therapists also use these splints to prevent knee flexion contractures in patients who have had below-knee amputations.

Material Selection, Instruction, and Follow-Up Care

The choice of thermoplastic splinting material, straps, and padding varies based on the patient's needs. For instruction and follow-up care, many factors influence the patient's needs, including the following:

1. Environment: home, long-term care, hospital settings, assisted-living facilities, sub-acute care, hospice, or adult day care
2. Severity of contractures: mild, moderate, or severe
3. Skin integrity: fragile skin, open wounds, or pressure areas
4. Level of care: home health aide assistance, full- or part-time family/caregiver assistance, or independent functioning
5. Other impairments: cognitive or sensory impairments

Environment

Older patients may reside in a variety of settings, including homes, condomin ums, apartments, or assisted-living facilities. Other older patients may live permanently or temporarily in hospitals or subacute or long-term care facilities. The patient's environment affects the selection of strapping and thermoplastic splinting material properties and follow-through. For example, persons responsible for their own splint follow-through receive complete instructions. For patients in institutional settings the therapist gives instructions to all caregivers responsible for the patients' care.

Contracture Risk

The level of joint-contracture risk affects the splint-wearing schedule. For example, an older person suffering from spasticity has a high risk for joint contractures and may frequently wear a splint. Patients who have a low contracture risk with increasing active ROM may decrease wearing time, thus allowing the affected hand to engage in activities. The therapist uses clinical judgment to determine wearing schedules and completes frequent monitors to adjust wearing schedules according to patients' needs.

Skin Integrity

Skin integrity can influence the choice of splint materials. For example, the therapist may use soft, stretchy strapping for a patient who experiences edema fluctuations. The therapist may use a splint made of soft material for a person who has fragile skin. In addition, the therapist may apply stockinette under a splint to absorb perspiration.

Level of Care/Impairments

Anticipated patient and caregiver compliance affects material choice and splint design. For example, the therapist should use a simple splint design for a patient receiving care from various health care providers in a long-term care facility. The therapist should use a brightly colored thermoplastic material that has contrasting colored straps for a patient who has difficulty with figure-ground discrimination. Older persons who have hearing loss may need written directions. These approaches increase compliance and tolerance to the splint-wearing schedule.

Selection of Thermoplastic Splinting Material

Selection of a low-temperature thermoplastic splinting material is determined by the following: (1) the extent to which a patient's joint can assume and maintain a gravity-assisted position, (2) the size of the splint, (3) the performance requirements of the splint, (4) the padding requirements, (5) the weight of the splinting material, and (6) the therapist's skill level.

If the patient is physically and cognitively able to hold the limb in the desired splinting position, the therapist should use a splinting material that has high drapability and moldability to ensure an intimate fit. The therapist should position the patient's extremity to ensure that gravity assists in the draping of the material over the extremity. Splinting material that has a high degree of conformability allows detailed molding for a precise fit, thus increasing comfort and decreasing the risk of splint migration and friction over bony prominences.

Some patients cannot assume positions that allow gravity to assist in the molding of splints. Older patients may be anxious and may respond to the stretch applied during splinting by exhibiting increased tone and decreased compliance. In such a situation or during the fabrication of large splints, material that has resistance to drape and memory is helpful. A material that lightly sticks to stockinette placed on the patient facilitates antigravity splinting (see Chapter 1). Preshaping techniques are also helpful.

Thinner thermoplastic materials (e.g., $\frac{3}{32}$ inch, $\frac{1}{16}$ inch) are less rigid. The therapist should select the thinnest material that can perform effectively. The more contoured the splint is to the underlying shape, the greater the strength. For example, patients who suffer from rheumatoid arthritis appreciate lightweight splints. Minimizing the weight of a splint increases comfort and enhances compliance.

Strapping Material

Wide, soft, foamlike strapping material distributes pressure over more surface area than thin, firm straps. The softer strapping accommodates slight fluctuations of edema. In addition, fragile skin tolerates soft straps well. For patients who have fragile skin the therapist should always use the velcro loop strap to completely cover the velcro hook on the splint surface. This prevents abrading the patient's skin or catching the splint on clothing and blankets. The use of presewn, self-adhesive velcro straps reduces the loss of the strap.

D-ring straps provide mechanical leverage to effectively tighten the strap. A patient who has diminished dexterity may have difficulty threading the strap through the D-ring. Using D-ring strapping may be an advantage for a patient who has dementia and does not understand the splint's purpose because the patient may experience greater difficulty spontaneously removing the splint.

Padding Selection

The two basic types of padding are open-cell foam (i.e., absorbent) and closed-cell foam (i.e., nonabsorbent). Before molding, the therapist can apply closed-cell foam padding to the thermoplastic splinting material. This ensures a proper fit to accommodate the thickness of the padding. If the therapist adds padding after the molding process, splint modifications must account for the thickness of the padding. The fabrication of a splint with the addition of $\frac{1}{16}$-inch padding results in a splint that is $\frac{1}{16}$-inch too tight.

Closed-cell padding does not hold moisture and is easily washed and towel dried. Open-cell padding absorbs moisture, is more difficult to keep clean, and can become a breeding ground for bacteria. Even in a patient who perspires heavily, open-cell padding may be quite effective if the padding is changed frequently. Therapists should not immerse open-cell foams in heat pans. Multiple layers of stockinette placed over the extremity during the fabrication process mimic the space required for the foam.

Padding may not be required only on the inside of the splint. If the splinted extremity rests against another body part, the therapist should pad the outside of the splint. For example, a patient who has hemiplegia and a flexed upper extremity may rest the splint against the rib cage or a right ankle splint may press against the left leg when the patient is side lying.

Choosing the correct thermoplastic, strapping, and padding material is important. Clinical judgment and the ability to make adaptations are important during the splinting of older patients because the older population is most prone to contractures and pressure sores (Bennett, 1992). The splint should fit well, achieve the clinical goal, and be acceptable to the patient and caregiver.

Technical Tips

Therapists acquire technical skills through practice. During the splinting of an older patient, one or more of the following technical tips may be helpful to the therapist:

1. Choose a splinting material that has a slightly longer working time. For example, when fabricating a resting hand splint (see Chapter 6), preshape the hand portion of the resting pan before applying it to the patient. Complete the preshaping on a hand of similar size.

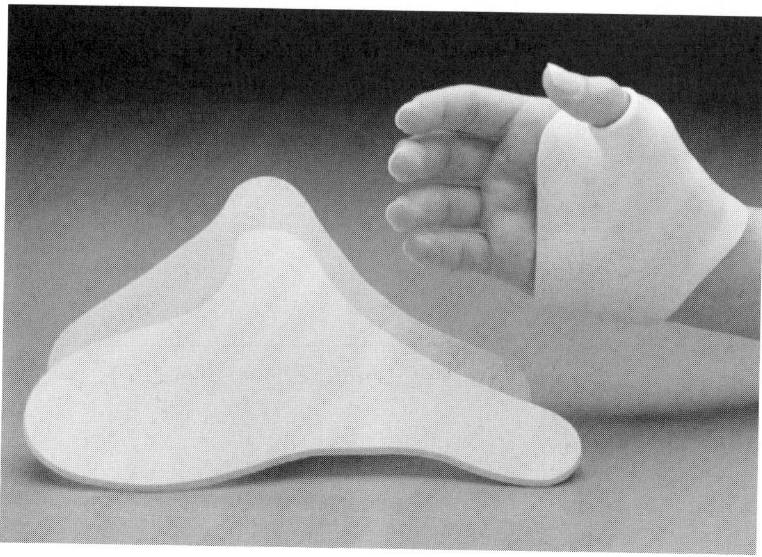

FIGURE 11-5 Hand-based thumb spica splint
This splint is designed for immobilization of the CMC and MCP thumb joints and is prepadded with Polycushion® padding. (From Smith and Nephew Rolyan. [1995]. Rehabilitation Products Catalog. Germantown, WI.)

2. During the molding process, use Theraband or an elastic bandage to temporarily secure the forearm trough. This activity allows attention to be focused on the contouring of the hand and wrist parts of the splint.
3. Prepad bony prominences by using circular pieces of adhesive-backed foam or gel padding. Mold the splint over the padding. When molding the splint, place the foam or gel pad inside the splint to ensure intimate, congruous contact (Figure 11-5).
4. Use tubular stockinette under the splint to maintain skin hygiene and prevent pressure areas. Loss of skin elasticity and adipose tissue make older patients prone to skin breakdown. The stockinette helps to shape the excess soft tissue.
5. Use material that is uncoated and self-bonding for splints if darts or tucks are necessary. Therapists often use this type of design for ankle, knee, and elbow splints.
6. Use a coated material for thumb spica splints. Often the thumb IP joint is enlarged or deformed, thus making application and removal of a closed circumferential splint difficult or impossible. Using a coated material allows cir-

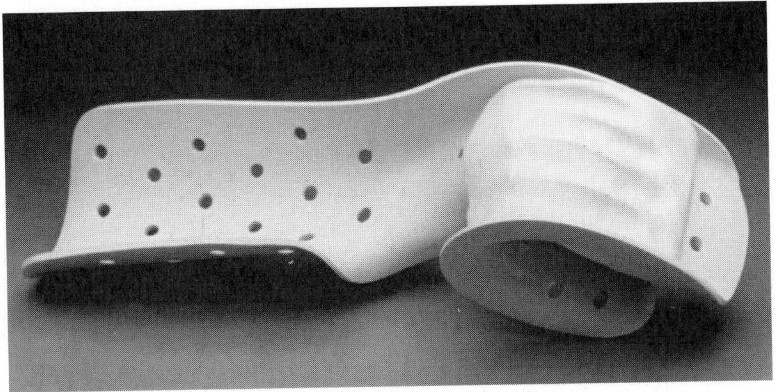

FIGURE 11-6
The therapist uses a putty-elastomer insert on this resting hand splint for finger separators. (From Smith and Nephew Rolyan. [1995]. Rehabilitation Products Catalog. Germantown, WI.)

cumferential wrapping around the thumb proximal phalanx. After hardening, the overlap on the proximal phalanx pops open. If self-bonding materials are preferred, use a wet paper towel between the overlapping surfaces to prevent bonding.

7. During planning of serial repositioning, select a splint material that has memory.
8. Use putty-elastomer inserts as finger separators (Figure 11-6) and to add contour in the hand or foot area if a nondraping material is necessary (Schutt, 1992). A therapist may also use putty elastomer as a palm-protector splint by imbedding a loop strap in an elastomer roll. Do not use elastomer over open wounds.
9. For an extremely deformed extremity, make the splint pattern on the opposite extremity and reverse it. If the patient is uncooperative, draw the pattern while the patient is sleeping.

Patient and Caregiver Instructions and Follow-Through

Clear patient and caregiver instructions and consistent follow-through are of paramount importance in successful splinting. Many factors influence compliance to a splint-wearing schedule. The person who is responsible for the splint's wearing schedule and care is the patient or caregiver. The box on the following page outlines problems that may influence successful splinting for older patients, lists solutions to problems, and indicates the person who is responsible for follow-through.

Splinting Problems, Preventative Solutions, and Persons Responsible for Follow-Through

COGNITION
Patient Responsible

- Evaluate the person's ability to understand the splint's purpose, schedule, and precautions.
- If memory is impaired, develop a routine for the patient that includes splint wear and care.
- Label the splint for easy application.
- If cognition is severely impaired, recommend a caregiver to provide assistance.

Caregiver (Family and Staff) Responsible

- Use D-ring straps to avoid removal by the patient.
- Mark the patient's name and room number on the splint and provide application instructions.

HEARING
Patient Responsible

- Use the guidelines for talking to the hearing impaired that are listed in the box on page 243.
- Provide simple written instructions.
- Use demonstrations as part of the instructions.
- Share the guidelines for talking to the hearing impaired with involved staff, family, and caregivers.

VISION
Patient Responsible

- If vision is impaired, give simple, large-print instructions. Be sure the print is in high contrast to the color of the paper.
- Allow the patient to practice splint application and removal.
- Use magnification devices for reading instructions and performing skin inspection.
- Use contrasting colors for the splint and its straps.
- Recommend that an ophthalmologist examine the patient if the prescription is old and/or vision appears to be impaired.
- If the patient has macular degeneration (central vision deficit), teach scanning and head-turning techniques.

MOBILITY
Patient Responsible

- Keep the splint within reach and/or easy walking distance.
- Maintain a consistent storage location for the splint.
- Keep the splint simple so that the patient can easily apply and remove it.
- Permanently attach one end of each strap to the splint to prevent the straps from falling to the floor.

COMPLIANCE
Patient Responsible

- Explain the purpose and goals of the splint to the patient and caregiver.
- Provide simple written and oral instructions.
- Use positive reinforcement for correct follow-through.
- Listen to the patient's complaints and make splint adjustments.

Continued.

Splinting Problems, Preventative Solutions, and Persons Responsible for Follow-Through—Cont'd

COMPLIANCE
Caregiver (Family and Staff) Responsible
- Provide simple written and oral directions.
- Explain the purpose of the splint.
- Demonstrate proper splint application.
- Encourage the caregiver to demonstrate the correct procedure several times.
- Use pictures to demonstrate correct application.
- In an institution, correlate the patient's splint-wearing schedule with staff work shifts.
- In an institution, ensure that the splint-wearing schedule and hand hygiene are part of the patient's care plan.
- Educate the caregiver about precautions and the way to contact the therapist to report splint problems.
- Label the splint for easy application.

SPASTICITY
Patient and Caregiver Responsible
- Instruct the patient and caregiver about inhibition techniques that assist in splint application.

Cognition

The therapist should assess the cognitive status to determine the patient's ability to follow a splint-wearing schedule and to be aware of splint problems. If the patient has significant cognitive impairments, the therapist should recommend assistance for the person. The therapist must educate any new caregiver about the splint purpose, wearing schedule, care, correct application, and possible problems.

Short- or long-term memory impairment may prevent the patient from recalling the splint's storage location or application procedure. If memory is a problem, the therapist should establish a routine schedule for splint wear and care and label the splint for easy application. If cognitive impairment is so severe that the person is incapable of follow-through, the therapist should recommend a caregiver to provide assistance.

Hearing

Approximately 25% of patients over age 65 are hard of hearing. This percentage rises to 50% for patients over age 85 (AARP, 1994). Hardness of hearing influences verbal explanations and statements. However, the therapist should not rely solely on printed information to relay instructions because some patients may be

Guidelines for Talking to the Hearing Impaired

- Seat or position the hearing-impaired person to see the face of the person speaking.
- Whenever possible, face the hearing-impaired person on the same level during verbal communication.
- Before talking, gain the patient's attention by using a touch, a gesture, and eye contact.
- Use visual aids when possible. Take a photograph or draw a diagram that shows correct splint application.
- Keep hands away from your face while talking.
- If the person misses statements, rephrase the statements rather than repeat the same words.
- Reduce background noises during verbal communication (e.g., turn off television or radio). When possible, work with the person one-on-one in a quiet room.
- Do not shout because doing so distorts voices. Talk in a normal voice but at a close range.
- Avoid chewing gum during verbal communication because doing so makes speech more difficult to understand.
- Be aware that people hear better if they are vertical rather than horizontal. If a person is standing or sitting, sound waves are directed into the ears; if a person is lying bed, sound waves are dispersed over the head.
- Recognize that hearing-impaired persons may not hear as well if they are tired or ill.
- If hearing is better in one ear, direct speech toward that ear. Never shout directly into the ear.

Adapted from Lewis, S. C. (1989). Elder care in occupational therapy. Thorofare, NF: Slack Inc.; Barlowe, E., Siegal, D. L., Edwards F., & Doress, P. B. (1987). Vision, hearing, and other sensory loss associated with aging. In P. B. Doress & D. L. Siegal (Eds.), Ourselves, growing older (pp. 365-379). New York: Simon & Schuster Inc.; & Maguire, G. H. (1985). The changing realm of the senses. In B. B. Lewis, Aging: The health care challenge (2nd ed.). Philadelphia: F. A. Davis Co.

unable to read or have visual impairments that make reading difficult or impossible. When talking to a person who is hard of hearing, the therapist should use the guidelines in the box above.

Vision

Visual impairments rank third among the reasons that individuals over age 70 need assistance with ADLs (Ruben, 1990). Of people over age 65, 5% have severe visual impairments. The percentage increases to 50% for older patients in long-term care facilities (AARP, 1994). Decreased vision can also play a role in non-compliance of splint wear. For example, some older patients may be unable to apply their splints because of poor figure-ground discrimination. Using colored thermoplastic splinting material and contrasting colored straps may assist the patient who has poor visual discrimination. Bright colors may prevent the splint from being easily lost or mistakenly sent to the laundry.

When receiving splint instructions by demonstration, patients who have correctable vision should wear their glasses.* The patient should demonstrate to the therapist proper splint application and removal. The therapist should provide simple, large-print instructions for the patient. A high contrast of the ink and paper is helpful. The use of magnification devices can also help with reading and performing skin inspection.

For patients who have macular degeneration (e.g., blurred or loss of central vision) the therapist must use compensatory techniques during application and removal of the splint and during skin inspections. Compensatory techniques include eye scanning, head turning, and placement of the splint or hand into the field of vision.

Mobility

Many older people become sedentary, which decreases aerobic capacity, muscle strength, ROM, and coordination (Lavizzo-Mourey, Day, Diserens, & Grisso, 1989). For persons over age 65, 75% of injuries occur in the home and are attributed to falls that result in arm, wrist, hand, and hip fractures (Lavizzo-Mourey et al., 1989; Potempa, Carvalho, Hahn, & LeSage, 1990; Daleiden, 1990). If a splint is out of reach, the patient may not reapply the splint because of difficulty with ambulation and reach. Maintaining a consistent splint storage location that is within reach and easy walking distance is important.

The splint design should be simple. The patient may be unable to manipulate multiple straps to apply a splint by using one hand. Riveting one end of the strap to the splint or using adhesive straps prevents their removal and loss. Attached straps reduce the risk of the patient falling while attempting to retrieve a dropped strap.

Instructions to Caregivers

Patients unable to care for themselves need caregiver assistance. Caregivers are family members or staff members from an agency or a facility. When fitting a splint to a patient, the therapist must provide thorough instructions to the caregiver. Instructions should include information regarding (1) the splint's purpose, (2) the wearing schedule, (3) the splint's care, and (4) the splint precautions. The therapist should inform caregivers about a person to contact if a splint problem occurs.

*If the prescription is old and the patient has not had an appointment with an ophthalmologist recently, the therapist should recommend that an appointment be made.

The therapist must give oral and written instructions to the caregiver and demonstrate any procedure the caregiver is to perform. The therapist should ask the caregiver to demonstrate the application of the splint, correct mistakes the caregiver makes, and ask the caregiver to repeat the demonstration until it is mastered.

The therapist should label parts of the splint for easier application (e.g., right/left, thumb/wrist/forearm). When possible, photographs of proper splint position, a written wearing schedule, a list of precautions, and a splint maintenance sheet should be readily available and consistently updated.

When splinting an older patient in a long-term care facility, the therapist should include instructions in the chart to ensure staff follow-through. In addition, the therapist should speak with the immediate caregivers in order to determine a realistic splinting program. If a patient is to wear a splint for a portion of the day, evening, or night shift, all staff members involved with that patient's care must receive instructions about the splint-wearing schedule and precautions. The splint-wearing schedule may require modification to match the staff schedule.

When appropriate, the therapist should instruct caregivers about the use of inhibition techniques to facilitate proper splint application. The therapist should also teach the patient and caregivers about the importance of intermittent-passive ROM and active-assisted ROM to the immobilized joints (Dittmer, MacArthur-Turner, & Jones, 1993).

Skin Care

Maintenance of skin integrity is important for older patients who need long-term splinting. The splint must be clean for application, washed with warm water and soap, rinsed thoroughly, and dried. Chlorine is appropriate for removal of stains. An autoclave cannot be used and a machine is not appropriate for washing the splint. After removal of the splint, the hand requires thorough washing and drying. Stockinette worn under the splint absorbs perspiration, and powder may be helpful with moisture management.

Wearing Schedule

To determine a splint-wearing schedule, the therapist should consider the goals of the splint. Perhaps the purpose of the splint is pain reduction during activity, maintenance of functional activities, prevention of skin ulceration, or prevention of a joint contracture. The goal determines whether a day, night, or intermittent splint-wearing schedule is most beneficial. For example, an intermittent wearing schedule helps the palm or skin to dry and prevents potential skin maceration. A night-wearing schedule is most appropriate if the patient uses the extremity for functional assistance during the day.

SELF-QUIZ 11-1*

Please circle either true (T) or false (F).

1. T F Observing the skin condition is important when deciding the way to splint an older patient.
2. T F The therapist should apply closed-cell foam after the formation of the splint.
3. T F To ensure intimate contour, the therapist should use a drapey splinting material for a patient who has spasticity.
4. T F The therapist should use wide straps on a patient who has fragile skin.
5. T F A functional position splint is always appropriate to position the arthritic hand.
6. T F Older patients are more prone to joint contractures than younger patients who have similar diagnoses.
7. T F After splint completion the patient in a long-term care facility requires little follow-up.
8. T F A younger patient is more prone to skin breakdown than an older person.
9. T F The therapist may use splinting materials to adapt ADL devices.
10. T F The therapist should not use soft splints if complete immobilization is the goal.

*See Appendix A for the answer key.

SELF-QUIZ 11-2*
Critical-Thinking Case Scenarios

1. You are fabricating a volar resting hand splint for a patient who is unable to actively supinate the forearm. You choose a material that has high drapability and moldability. Is this the best choice? Why?

2. You are treating an 86-year-old woman 1 year after a CVA. Since that time she has held her left hand in a fisted position. Gentle finger-passive ROM is painful to her. The palm of her hand perspires, and the palmar skin is macerated. The patient does not have active motion in the left hand and does not use the hand for functional assistance during ADL. Which kind of positioning device should you use?

3. A patient who has rheumatoid arthritis complains of pain in the wrists and MCP joints. The therapist provides resting hand splints to rest all the joints of the wrist and hand at night. What problems can you identify with this splint provision?

***See Appendix A for the answer key.**

Continued.

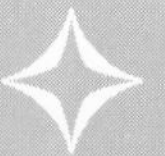

SELF-QUIZ 11-2
Critical-Thinking Case Scenarios—cont'd

4. You fabricate a functional position hand splint for a patient who has spasticity and hemiplegia and is in a flexor-synergy pattern. The patient wears the splint at night for pain relief and contracture management. When the patient is in bed, the splint is positioned against the rib cage. What can you do to relieve the pressure on the rib cage?

____

____

____

____

5. You have fabricated a resting hand splint for a patient who has hemiplegia and congestive heart failure. You are concerned about the fluctuating edema you have noted in the hemiplegic hand. Which type of straps should you use?

____

____

____

____

Case Study*

Read the following scenario and answer the questions based on information in this chapter:

Sadie M. is a frail, 82-year-old, right-handed woman who has osteoarthritis and diabetes mellitus. She is alert and oriented x3. Sadie ambulates independently with a walker, but she has difficulty grasping the walker with her left hand. She is experiencing increasing pain in her left wrist and metacarpophalangeal (MCP) joints because of her arthritis. She states that her hands are "clumsy" when she performs self-care activities. Since the recent death of her sister who assisted Sadie with ADLs (and with whom she shared a first-floor apartment), Sadie realized she can no longer function independently. She has been admitted for outpatient rehabilitation therapy for splinting, ADL training, and functional activities to increase upper-body strength. Now Sadie has a home-health aide 4 hours per day, 3 days per week. The aide assists with bathing, shopping, and housekeeping. Family members live nearby.

1. Which splints do you recommend for night use?
   a. Resting hand splints
   b. Arthritis mitt splints
   c. Wrist immobilization splints
2. What is your splinting rationale?
   a. To rest all hand and wrist joints
   b. To immobilize the wrist and MCPs and allow movement of the proximal interphalangeals (PIPs)
   c. To immobilize the wrist and allow movement of the MCPs and PIPs
3. Which kind of strap should you use?
   a. Velcro loop strapping
   b. Soft, foamlike strapping
   c. D-ring strapping
4. What is the purpose of the strapping?
   a. To accommodate edema
   b. To provide leverage to control tightness and allow easier application
5. What do you recommend to help Sadie grasp her walker?
   a. Building up the handle of the walker by using adhesive foam
   b. Using a walker splint
   c. Using a neoprene thumb support
6. How might the diagnosis of diabetes mellitus affect splinting of this frail, older woman?
   a. She may have impaired sensation.
   b. She may have compromised peripheral circulation.
   c. Diabetes mellitus does not affect the splinting program.

*See Appendix A for the answer key.

Review Questions

1. What are the accommodations a therapist can make for an older person who has problems with edema, ecchymosis, fragile skin, contracture, ulceration, diminished cognition, sensory loss, and motivation?
2. What are four possible goals of splinting an older patient?
3. Why are older patients prone to develop contractures quickly?
4. What are soft splints? When are they indicated?
5. What is the difference between a resting hand (hand immobilization) splint and an arthritis mitt splint?
6. What is the most common lower-extremity geriatric splint? What is its purpose?
7. How do instructions and splint-material selection vary with an individual living independently in the community versus an individual in an institution?
8. What are three specific splint adaptations for older patients who have impaired cognition, sensory systems, and compliance?

References

American Association of Retired Persons. (1994). A profile of older Americans. Washington, DC: Program Resources Department.

Barlowe, E., Siegal, D. L., Edwards, F., & Doress, P. B. (1987). Vision, hearing, and other sensory loss associated with aging. In P. B. Doress & D. L. Siegal (Eds.), Ourselves, growing older (pp. 365-379). New York: Simon & Schuster Inc.

Bennet, G. C. J. (1992). Pressure sores-etiology and prevalence. In J. C. Broklehurst, R. Tallis, & H. Fillit (Eds.), Textbook of geriatric medicine and gerontology (4th ed., pp. 922-926). Edinburgh, NY: Churchill Livingstone Inc.

Casey, A. C., Kratz, E. J. (1988). Soft splinting with neoprene: The thumb abduction supinator splint. Am J Occup Ther, 42(6), 395-398.

Clarkson, H. M. & Gilewich, G. B. (1989). Musculoskeletal assessment joint motion and manual muscle strength. Baltimore: Williams & Wilkins.

Colditz, J. C. (May, 1995). Personal communication.

Daleiden, S. (1990). Prevention of falling: Rehabilitative or compensatory interventions? Top Geriatr Rehabil, 5, 44-53.

Dittmer, D. K., MacArthur-Turner, D. E., & Jones, I. C. (1993). Orthotics in stroke. Phys med rehabil state of the art review, 7(1), 171.

Fess, E. E., Gettle, K. S., & Strickland, J. W. (1981). Hand splinting: Principles and methods. St. Louis: Mosby.

Good, D. C., & Supan, T. J. (1992). Basic principles of orthotics in neurologic disorders. In M. Aisen (Ed.), Orthotics in neurological rehabilitation (pp. 1-23). New York: Demos.

Harbun, K., & Potter, P. (1993). Spasticity and contracture. In R. W. Teasell (Ed.), Physical medicine and rehabilitation: long term consequences of stroke, 7, 113-132.

Jackson, O. L. (1989). Physical therapy of the geriatric patient (2nd ed.). New York: Churchill Livingstone Inc.

Lavizzo-Mourey, R., Day, S. C., Diserens, D., & Grisso, J. A. (1989). Practicing prevention for the elderly. St. Louis: Hanley & Belfus Inc., and Mosby.

Lewis, S. C. (1989). Elder care in occupational therapy. Thorofare, NJ: Slack Inc.

Maguire, G. H. (1985). The changing realm of the senses. In B. B. Lewis (Ed.), Aging: The health care challenge (2nd ed.). Philadelphia: F. A. Davis Co.

Mallick, M. H. (1976). Manual on static hand splinting (3rd ed.). Pittsburg: Harmarville Rehabilitation Center.

Merritt, J. L. (1987). Advances in orthotics for the patient with rheumatoid arthritis. J Rheumatol, 14, 62-67.

Ouellette, E. A. (1991). The rheumatoid hand: Orthotics as preventative. Semin Arthritis Rheum, 21, 65-71.

Potempa, K., Carvalho, A., Hahn, J., & LeSage, J. (1990). Containing the cost of patient falls: A risk management model. Top Geriatr Rehabil, 6, 69-78.

Redford, J. (1986). *Orthotics etcetera.* Baltimore: Williams & Williams.

Ruben, B. (1990). Ophthalmologist looks to OT for vision rehab. OT Week, 4, 10.

Schutt, A. H. (1992). Physical medicine and rehabilitation in the elderly arthritic patient. J Am Geriatr Soc, 25, 80-81.

Smith and Nephew Rolyan. (1995). Rehabilitation Products Catalog. Germantown, WI.

Stern, E., Sines, B., & Teague, R. (1994). Commercial wrist extensor orthoses. J Hand Ther, 7, 237-244.

CHAPTER TWELVE

Splinting Children Who Have Developmental Disabilities

LINDA GABRIEL, MA, OTR/L

Chapter Objectives

1. Identify the characteristics of children who need orthotic intervention.
2. Discuss the purpose of a resting hand, wrist cock-up, and thumb splint for a child who has a developmental disability.
3. Describe the major features of these three types of hand splints.
4. Describe the process for fabricating each of these hand splints.
5. Identify precautions for these three splints.
6. Discuss the way to determine an effective and reasonable wearing schedule.
7. Discuss the way to provide instructions for care providers to maximize correct application and use of the splints.
8. Identify errors in the fit of pediatric hand splints.
9. Apply knowledge of splinting children who have developmental disabilities to a case study.

This chapter presents applications of general splinting principles to the design and fabrication of several basic hand splints that a therapist can use as part of a treatment program for children who have developmental disabilities. As with adults, therapists may use splints for children to prevent deformity and increase function. The resting hand, wrist cock-up, and thumb splints represent basic designs and are discussed in this chapter. In practice the therapist may modify these designs or create entirely new ones to meet the needs of individual children.

Splinting decisions must be consistent with the frame of reference that guides the intervention program. This chapter emphasizes a critical-thinking and problem-solving approach to splinting decisions. Splint designs in this chapter are compatible with a neurodevelopmental treatment (NDT), rehabilitative, and/or biomechanical frames of reference.

Because the purpose is to introduce basic concepts to beginning splinters, many types and variations of pediatric hand splints are not discussed in this chapter. (For readers interested in furthering their knowledge, "Suggested Readings" are included at the end of this chapter.) Some children may respond best to splints designed to reduce spasticity (see Chapter 10). Other children may benefit from the use of plaster or pneumatic splints for elbows and hands, but this type of intervention is beyond the scope of this chapter. Those who desire skills in these areas should explore continuing education courses or arrange advanced study.

"Splinting is often a component of occupational therapy intervention for children with hand function problems" (Exner, 1989, p. 253). However, splinting a child who has a developmental disability may differ from splinting an adult in the following respects:

1. Abnormal muscle tone has been present in the child since birth or infancy and may differ from abnormal muscle tone acquired after the onset of disease or injury.
2. The child experiences the dynamic process of maturational and neurologic development, which has a continuous affect on the acquisition of functional hand skills.
3. The child experiences continued growth of the upper extremities. During a growth spurt the risk for deformity may increase.
4. Many children must rely on adults such as parents or teachers to apply and remove splints. Therefore the level of understanding and cooperation of these adults is also a factor.

Diagnostic Indications

Developmental disabilities include a variety of chronic conditions that are evident at birth or during childhood and that interfere significantly with development and functional abilities (Yamamoto, 1993). Central nervous system dysfunction and abnormal muscle tone accompany many developmental disabilities such as cerebral palsy. Abnormal muscle tone can present many splinting challenges. The therapist makes splinting decisions that are based on the type and severity of abnormal muscle tone, the child's functional level, the child's environment, and the frame of reference guiding therapy rather than on a specific diagnosis.

Assessment

Before fabricating a splint, the therapist must complete an assessment that should include the following factors:

Muscle Tone

The therapist should determine whether muscle tone is increased or decreased. If increased, the therapist should determine whether the amount of tone varies according to the child's mood, physical health, amount of effort exerted, or state of alertness. Some children have greatly increased tone during active movement but minimally increased tone during rest or sleep. If the child's muscle tone is not significantly increased at night, the risk for developing joint contractures may be less. Children who have decreased tone may need splints to stabilize or support joints.

Range of Motion

The therapist should measure active and passive range of motion (ROM) and compare the available measurements with those taken previously to determine whether range is increasing or decreasing. Before moving the joint, the therapist must be sure the child is well positioned and as relaxed as possible. Because tone and sometimes cooperation vary, the therapist should take measurements on several occasions to obtain the most accurate estimate.

Contractures

The therapist should determine whether joint contractures or deformities are present. A *contracture* refers to an abnormal shortening of muscle tissue that limits passive ROM (Yamamoto, 1993). Contractures are most likely to occur in children who have moderately to severely increased muscle tone. Even with an ongoing therapy program, preventing all contractures in children who have severely increased tone can be difficult.

Functional Use of Upper Extremities

The therapist should evaluate components of reach, grasp, manipulation, release, and bilateral hand use and should include the frequency and quality of functional arm and hand movements. Because one of the most important determinants of a successful splint is the improvement of hand function, the therapist should obtain an objective measurement of hand function such as a criterion-referenced assessment tool.

The therapist should also assess the degree of sensory awareness and tactile perception in the hands. In addition, the therapist should obtain information about the child's cognitive level because this level affects the development of functional hand skills.

Integrity of the Skin, Bones, and Circulatory System

The therapist should use extreme caution when splinting a child who has osteoporosis because stress to the bones can cause a fracture. Children who have tightly fisted hands are at risk for developing maceration or skin breakdown in the palms or between the fingers, and maintenance of skin hygiene may become a priority. Some children have extremely sensitive skin or experience pain in certain positions. Other children have poor circulation, which necessitates careful monitoring of the color and temperature of the skin during splint wearing. Finally, some children who have developmental disabilities also have significant feeding problems and may be underweight. Children who have little subcutaneous fat probably have more difficulty tolerating pressure to bony areas, thus affecting the splint's design and wearing schedule.

School and Family Considerations

A child who is young or severely disabled must rely on adults such as parents or teachers to apply the splint correctly and follow the recommended wearing schedule. When developing a splint-wearing schedule, the therapist must be aware that these adults may have multiple and excessive demands placed on them. The therapist must consider splint design and recommendations for wearing in the context of the child's environment, which may include other therapy, educational, and medical interventions.

After an assessment the therapist can establish therapeutic goals and intervention strategies for the child. A splint may be a component of this treatment plan. According to Schoen and Anderson (1993), orthotic devices and adaptive equipment are an important part of intervention. "They [orthotic devices] can reinforce NDT therapeutic goals and aid in the prevention of abnormal patterns and deformities by providing consistent input" (p. 77). The therapist must remember that the provision of a splint is a means to an end and not the end itself.

Resting Hand Splint

The purpose of a resting hand splint is to prevent a contracture or deformity, prevent an existing deformity from becoming worse, or gradually improve or reduce a deformity (deformity-reduction splint). Children who are at the greatest risk for developing contractures are those who have moderately to severely increased tone or those who have severely decreased tone and no active movement. For children who have severely increased muscle tone and tightly fisted hands an additional purpose may be maintenance of skin hygiene.

Features

The components of a resting hand splint for a child are the same as those described in Chapter 6, except for the shape of the thumb trough and C bar. Com-

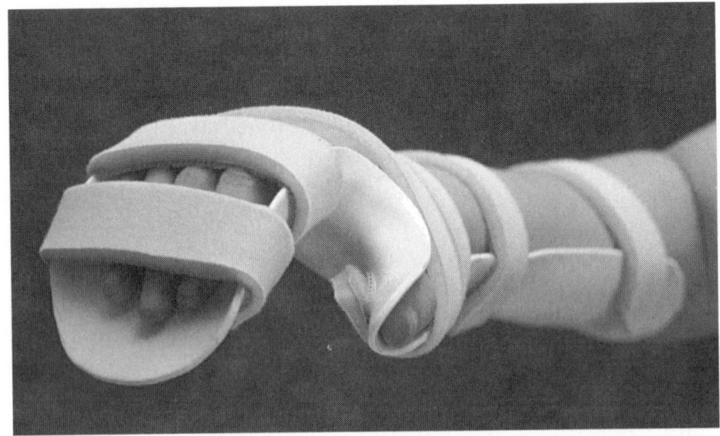

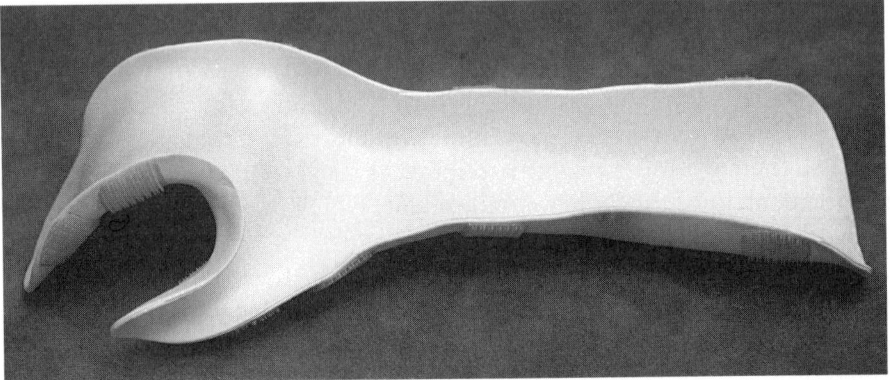

FIGURE 12-1 A resting hand splint

ponents include a forearm trough, pan for the fingers, thumb trough, and a C bar (Figure 12-1). To provide elongation to the opponens muscle, the therapist positions the thumb between radial and palmar abduction rather than in palmar abduction only. When fabricating a resting hand splint for a child who has spasticity, the therapist may consider including finger abduction (see Chapter 10).

For children with moderately to severely increased tone the functional position described in Chapter 6 may not be possible. Because its purpose is to prevent or reduce joint deformity, the splint should provide as much elongation of the tight muscles as possible without causing stress. The child should also be able to tolerate wearing the splint for several hours at a time to obtain the maximal benefit. If the splint places the hand into the maximum range of passive motion, the forces generated may compromise circulation, cause skin breakdown, elicit pain, and reduce the length of time the child can tolerate wearing the splint. Therefore the splint should place the joints in submaximum range (Hill, 1988; Exner, 1989), a position especially important at the wrist to allow extension of the fingers. When flexor spasticity is severe, "serial splinting that gradually raises the wrist from partial flexion to a more extended or neutral position is indicated" (Exner, 1989, p. 254). The therapist can usually determine the best hand position by handling the child's extremity and feeling the amount of passive resistance. After achieving the desired position manually, the therapist should note the amount of flexion and extension and location of the pressure application. This activity determines the optimal position and indicates necessary locations for applying forces during splint fabrication and strap application.

Process to Fabricate a Resting Hand Splint

Thermoplastic Material Selection

When making a splint that counteracts the forces of spasticity, the therapist should select a low-temperature thermoplastic that resists stretch. A considerable amount of pressure is applied against the splinting material while the therapist obtains the desired position of the wrist, thumb, and fingers. This pressure can indent and inadvertently stretch materials that have conformability. Usually a thermoplastic material that contains a high rubber content has the desired working characteristics (see Chapter 1). The choice of plastic also depends on the therapist's experience and preference and the child's needs. If the plastic is available in different colors, the therapist should give the child or family an opportunity to indicate a color preference.

Tools and Materials

Thoughtful preparation before splint fabrication can save considerable time and frustration for the therapist and child. In addition to the thermoplastic material, the therapist should consider the following:

- High-quality, sharp scissors are necessary for the final cuts, and heavy-duty scissors or a utility knife may be necessary to cut cold plastic. Having straight- and curved-blade scissors and smaller scissors may be useful.
- Paper is necessary for patterns. (Paper towels work fairly well.) Pencils, pens, and masking tape to repair torn patterns are also necessary.
- Terry cloth towels keep the counter and working area dry.
- If pressure points are anticipated, several types of padding should be available.
- If a need exists to hasten the hardening process, the therapist may consider a spray coolant. However, if spraying near the child's face, the therapist should use caution. Many children suffer from compromised respiratory systems and cannot understand verbal instructions to look away or hold their breath. An alternative to cooling the splint on the child's hand is to remove the splint and place it into a pan of ice water, which sets the shape.
- An ace wrap can be useful to hold the forearm trough in place while the ther-

apist works on the hand portion of the splint. The therapist should not apply the wrap too tightly and should flare the edges of the forearm trough away from the skin after formation of the splint.

- Strapping material and rivets or adhesive are necessary to attach one end of each strap to the splint.

Assistance

If a child has severely increased muscle tone in the hand or is not able to cooperate, another person can be extremely helpful during splint fabrication. This person can be a teacher, parent, paraprofessional, or therapist. A toy may help occupy the child's attention during this sometimes lengthy process.

Pattern

The pattern should include the measurements and markings of landmarks (see Chapter 6). Because of the different thumb position, the thumb trough and C bar are shaped differently (Figure 12-2). The process may require the holding of the paper under an extremity if the child is unable to lay the hand flat on a surface. After drawing and cutting out the pattern, the therapist fits it to the child and makes further modifications as necessary. While making the pattern and molding the splint, the therapist should position the child to minimize the effects of abnormal tone and postural reflexes on the body and extremities.

Heating and Cutting the Splint

After tracing the pattern on the thermoplastic material, the therapist should soften it in water heated to the appropriate temperature and cut out the splint. The material may require reheating to obtain the desired degree of pliability before the molding process. Before placing plastic on children's extremities, therapists should make sure the plastic is cool enough by placing it against their own skin. Because many children cannot communicate that the plastic is too hot, the therapist should watch the child's face and listen for vocalizations that indicate discomfort.

Forming the Splint

Before placing the plastic on the child's extremity, the therapist should prestretch the edge of the splint that forms the C bar (Figure 12-3). The therapist should then place the soft plastic on the child's upper extremity so that it conforms to the web space of the thumb (Figure 12-4). If available, an assistant can stand beside the child and secure the forearm trough. The therapist should form the splint into the palmar arches and around the wrist and thumb. To obtain the desired contour and fit, the therapist may need to be aggressive when molding into the palm and around the thenar eminence if working against spasticity. The

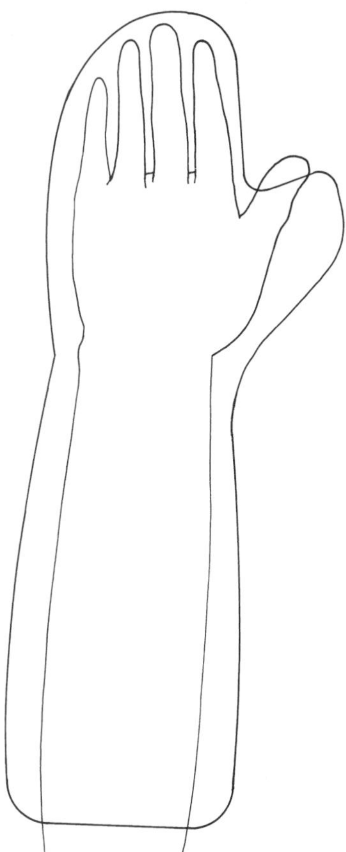

FIGURE 12-2 A pattern for a resting hand splint

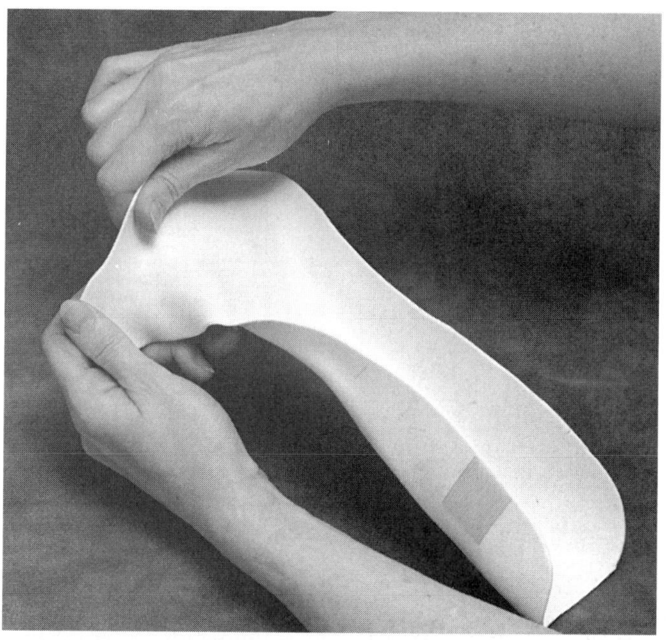

FIGURE 12-3 Prestretching of the C bar

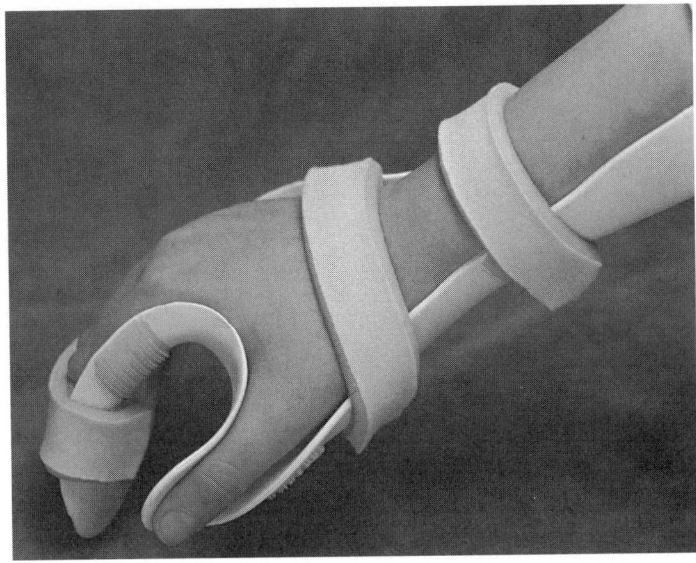

FIGURE 12-4 The fit of the C bar into the web space

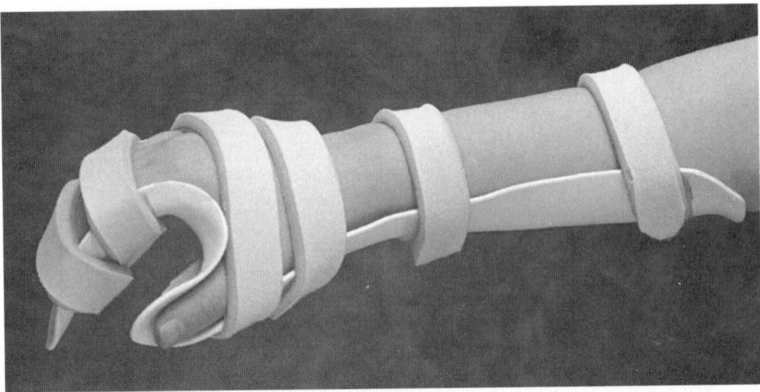

FIGURE 12-5 The contour of the C bar

therapist must form the splint so that the bulk of pressure positioning the thumb is directed below the thumb metacarpal (MP) joint and distributed along the thenar eminence. This formation is necessary to avoid hyperextension and possibly dislocation of the thumb MP joint. The thumb trough should cradle the thumb and extend about ½ inch beyond the end of the thumb. The interphalangeal (IP) joint of the thumb should be slightly flexed, and the C bar should fit snugly into the web space and contour against the radial side of the index finger (Figure 12-5).

Forearm Trough

After completing the wrist, palm, and thumb portions, the therapist can finish forming the forearm trough. (See Chapter 6 for guidelines on securing the forearm in the trough and avoiding pressure points.) If the edges of the trough are too high, the straps bridge (i.e., the straps are raised from the skin's surface and do not follow the contour the forearm). If bridging occurs, keeping the forearm in place is difficult. If not secure, the forearm may rotate in the trough or the splint may shift distally and the position of the wrist, fingers, and thumb are compromised.

Pan

Finally, the therapist can form the pan to position the fingers. The pan may require reheating because controlling all the joints at the same time is often difficult. (See Chapter 6 for the correct width and height of the pan.) In addition, the distal portion of the pan should extend about ½ inch beyond the finger tips to allow growth. When forming the curve of the pan, the therapist should follow the proximal and distal transverse arches.

Padding

The therapist should use padding if the distribution of pressure over a bony area is a concern. Padding does *not* compensate for pressure resulting from a poorly made splint. Padding takes up space, a factor the therapist must take into account before formation of the splint. Otherwise the amount of pressure against the skin may increase. A variety of types of padding exist, including closed- and open-cell foam and gel products. Some new gel products are useful for protecting bony areas for children who have little subcutaneous fat. To ensure a proper fit, the therapist should lay the padding on the child's extremity before molding the plastic or bubble out the areas of the plastic after fabrication.

Straps

The correct placement of straps is as important as correct formation of the splint, especially when the splint is holding against increased muscle tone. If the forearm, palm, fingers, and thumb do not stay in the correct position on the splint, the benefit of the splint is greatly reduced.

A variety of strap materials are available. The therapist should consider strength, durability, elasticity, and texture when the strap is against the skin. In addition, the therapist should determine the best location and angle of each strap in relation to the forces from abnormal muscle tone.

The forearm trough requires two straps. If considerable wrist flexion is present, two straps may be necessary for the hand; one strap should extend across the wrist just distal to the ulnar styloid, and a second strap should be angled from

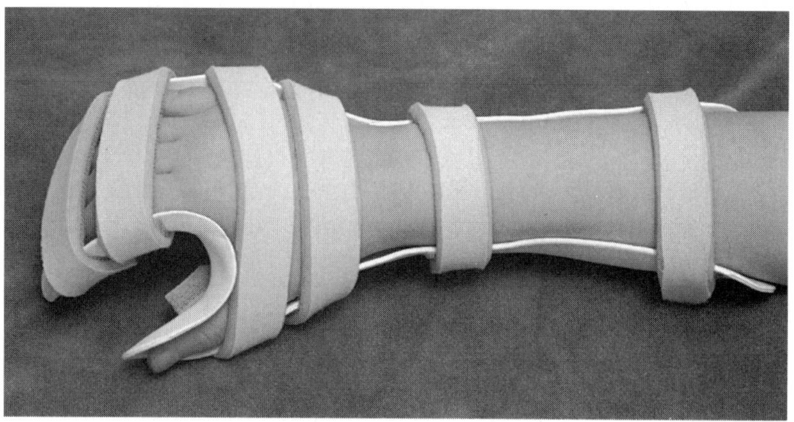

FIGURE 12-6 The placement of straps

the thumb-web space across the dorsum of the hand and secured proximal to the metacarpophalangeal (MCP) joints on the ulnar side. Otherwise one strap across the dorsum of the hand may be sufficient. If considerable finger flexion is present, straps may be necessary across each of the three phalanges. Finally, the therapist should add a strap to support the MP joint of the thumb. When making a small splint for a young child, the therapist should make the straps narrower. (See Figure 12-6 for an illustration of strap placements, although not all of these are necessary on every splint.)

Sometimes attaching one end of each strap to the splint is best because doing so prevents the loss of straps and ensures their correct location and angle for maximal effectiveness. However, straps become soiled and are more difficult to keep clean when attached. The strap can be attached by using a rivet or good contact adhesive. The therapist should also consider comfort and appearance.

Precautions

When splinting against increased muscle tone, the therapist must consider biomechanical principles of force distribution. Precautions are the same as those for any splint. (See Chapter 4 for guidance in determining problems with skin, bone, or muscles.) When applying these precautions to a child who has increased tone, the therapist should shorten the initial wearing time to 15- to 20-minute intervals on the first day. The therapist should then inspect the skin. A distinct red area or generalized redness on the skin that does not disappear within 15 to 20 minutes after splint removal indicates excessive pressure and the need for revisions (Hill, 1988). If no pressure areas are present, the therapist may increase the wearing time to 30-minute intervals. The therapist may then increase the wearing time by adding 15 to 30 minutes until the maximum wearing period for the child is reached. During the day the maximum period is usually not more than 2 hours (Exner, 1989), although therapists make such decisions case by case.

An additional precaution to consider when making a resting hand splint for a child who has moderately to severely increased tone is maintaining the integrity of the MP joint of the thumb. The therapist must direct the pressure below the MP joint to position the thumb. Exner (1989) cautions that distal force to the spastic thumb can result in hyperextension and dislocation of the MP joint.

Wearing Schedule

The wearing schedule is determined individually as are all other aspects of the treatment plan. In general, the more serious the threat of deformity, the more time the patient should wear the splint every 24 hours. However, the wearing time should not be continuous during the day. If tone continues to increase at night, this may be a good time for extended wearing, unless the splint interferes with the child's sleep or presses against another part of the body. During the day, the splint should be removed for periods of passive ranging, active movement, and opportunities for sensory experiences.

To maximize the splint's effectiveness, the child may wear the resting hand splint during weight-bearing activities if appropriate (Hill, 1988). The child may also work on functional activities immediately after removal of the splint to capitalize on increased hand expansion and possible reduction in muscle tone. If developing or improving functional hand skills is a primary goal, splint removal should occur more frequently and for longer periods.

The therapist should document the wearing schedule in the child's records and provide written copies to parents, caregivers, and teachers. The therapist should also provide instructions on correct splint application. These interventions are especially important in a school setting because multiple caregivers are likely involved and the child may change programs, thus resulting in different therapists. As the child's developmental or ROM status changes, the therapist should modify the wearing schedule and possibly the splint itself.

Providing Instruction for Splint Application

Those responsible for applying the child's splint must know the correct procedure. In addition, caregivers should understand the splint's purpose, precautions, risks of incorrect usage, and the way to reach the therapist with questions or concerns. The therapist should provide written instructions and a demonstration of the splint application. The caregiver should then have an opportunity to practice applying the splint while the therapist observes, notes problems, and answers questions. Although the correct wearing procedure may seem obvious, it may not be obvious to many teachers and parents unfamiliar with splints. A photograph showing the proper splint application is often an effective teaching tool if

Laboratory Exercise 12-1*

What problems in splint fabrication are present in the following picture?

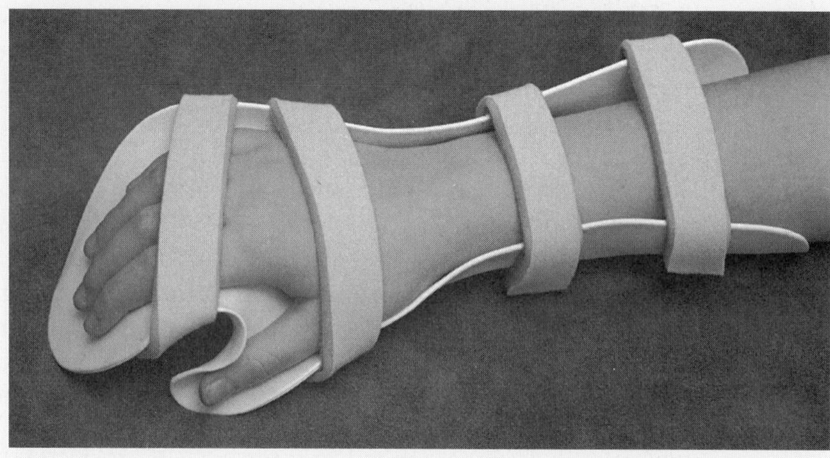

*See Appendix A for the answer key.

Laboratory Exercise 12-2*

What problems in splint fabrication are present in the following picture?

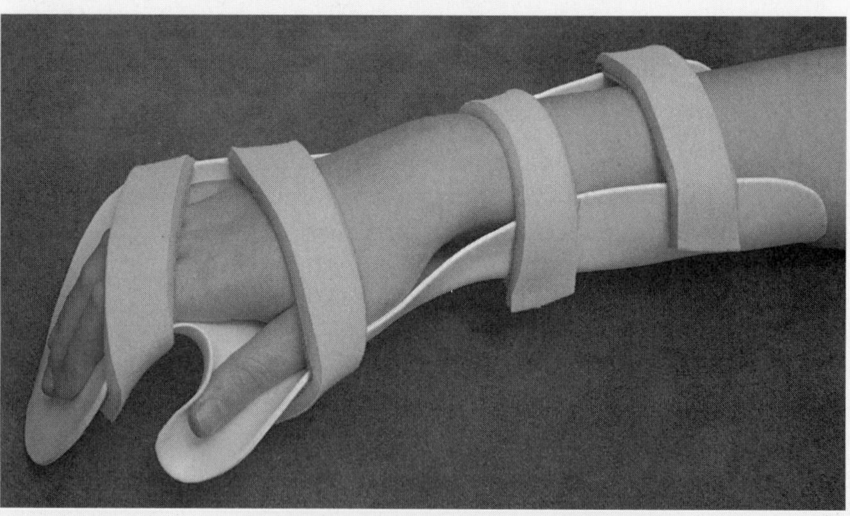

*See Appendix A for the answer key.

it does not conflict with regulations regarding confidentiality. Another strategy to aid the parent or teacher is writing a number or letter on each strap end and a corresponding number on the splint if the straps are not secured to it.

Evaluation of the Splint

The therapist can use the self-evaluation regarding resting hand splints to evaluate the finished splint (see Chapter 6). The therapist should also review the fit of the splint at regular intervals and continuously reevaluate the splint's effectiveness for accomplishing stated goals and outcomes.

Wrist Cock-Up Splint

A therapist usually selects a wrist cock-up splint to improve functional use of the hand rather than to prevent or manage a deformity. For a child who has increased muscle tone, the purpose of the wrist cock-up splint is to place the wrist in a functional position to enable or improve grasp and release. Allowing some wrist flexion in the splint may be necessary when a therapist splints a child who has moderate to severe wrist-flexor tightness. For children who have extreme tightness in the long-finger flexors, however, the cock-up splint may not improve hand use because of the tenodesis effect. If the child has only mild wrist flexion, a soft wrist cock-up splint with a reinforcement for the wrist may be preferable. The therapist can make this splint from materials such as neoprene and leather. If tightness is also present in the opponens muscle, a splint that includes a thumb trough may be indicated.

The therapist may use the wrist cock-up splint alone or alternately with a resting hand splint. This combination is appropriate for a child who has some functional use of the hand but is also at risk for developing contractures.

Features

The features of a wrist-cock up splint for a child are the same as those for an adult (see Chapter 5). Although the design can be dorsal or volar, the volar design is more common for children who have increased tone.

A unique feature of the cock-up splint for some children is the attachment of pointers, crayon holders, and other assistive devices. When designing a pointer, the therapist should angle it to allow good visual contact with the tip of the pointer. When possible, the therapist can make a finger trough to position the index finger for pointing, thus allowing sensory feedback to the tip of the index finger after contact is made with the target (Figure 12-7).

Process to Fabricate a Wrist Cock-Up Splint

Materials

The selection of tools and materials is essentially the same as that described for the resting hand splint previously in this chapter. A thermoplastic material that

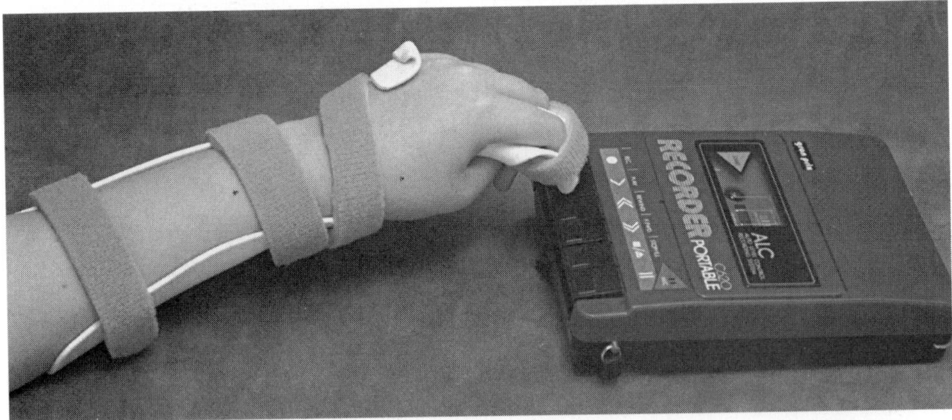

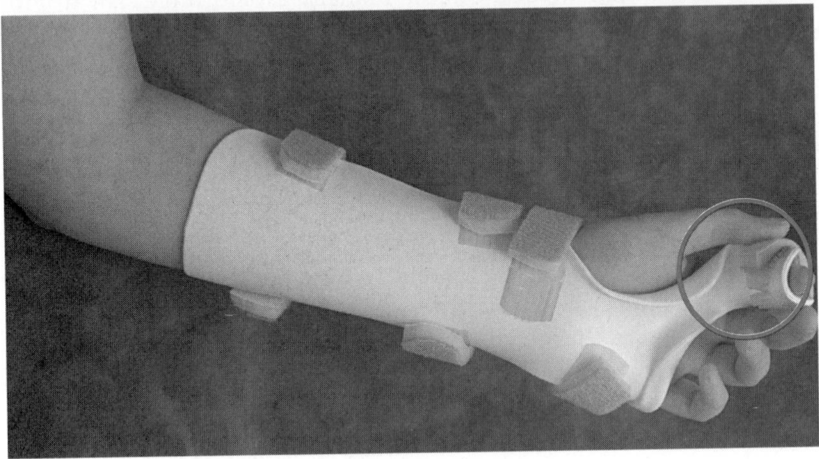

FIGURE 12-7 Wrist cock-up splint with index finger pointer

resists stretch is frequently desirable when the therapist positions the wrist of a child who has spasticity. However, when the purpose of a wrist splint is to serve as a base for the attachment of pointers or holders, a thermoplastic material that has good self-bonding properties is also desirable.

Pattern

After tracing the child's extremity, the therapist makes the splint pattern. The guidelines presented in Chapter 5 can be used to locate landmarks and determine the way the splint should fit in the palm. (See Figure 12-8 for a sample pattern.)

Forming a Splint

The fabrication process is essentially the same as that described in Chapter 5. The splint should follow the contour of the palmar arches configured during

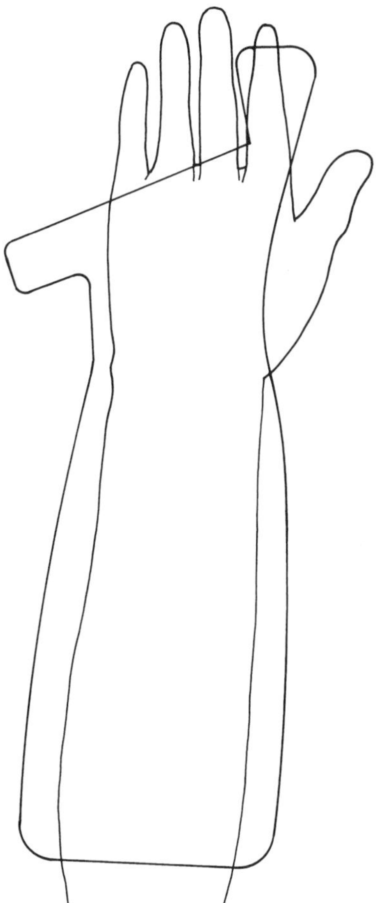

FIGURE 12-8 A pattern for a wrist cock-up splint with a pointer

grasp (Hill, 1988). The splint should not interfere with MP flexion or thumb opposition. The therapist should roll the edges around the thenar eminence and MP bar, and the ulnar side of the splint may require flaring at the ulnar styloid.

Straps

The needs of the child determine the number and angles of straps. Usually two straps secure the forearm trough and one strap secures the hand. The hand strap is angled from the ulnar side of the metacarpal bar to the hypothenar bar.

Precautions

The precautions for the application of the wrist cock-up splint to children are essentially the same as those for the adult (see Chapter 5). The splint should distribute pressure to avoid skin irritation, stabilize the forearm so that the splint does not shift during use, and not interfere with thumb opposition or MCP flexion of the fingers.

Wearing Schedule

Each situation should determine the wearing schedule. The therapist should consider the child's tolerance, therapeutic goals, and the extent of functional hand skills with and without the splint. In general, the splint is worn during activities requiring grasp and release that the patient can do more easily with the splint.

Evaluation of the Splint

The therapist can use a self-evaluation form to determine whether the fabrication of the splint is correct (see Chapter 5). The therapist should also perform frequent, ongoing reevaluation of the splint's effectiveness and the child's functional hand skills.

Thumb Splint

Increased muscle tone frequently pulls the thumb into palmar adduction. The purpose of a thumb splint is to improve functional use of the hand by stabilizing the thumb in a functional position of palmar abduction. The therapist uses this splint for a child who has some active wrist and finger extension but has difficulty actively moving the thumb out of the palm because of increased tone. If tone is moderate to severe, the therapist makes the splint from thermoplastic material. If tone is mild to moderate, the therapist can make the splint from more pliable material such as neoprene or webbing. Thumb splints can be hand or forearm based. This chapter describes hand-based thermoplastic and neoprene thumb splints. (See Chapter 7 for information on forearm-based thumb splints.)

Thermoplastic Thumb Splint

Features

This hand-based thumb splint can be palmar or dorsal. The dorsal design results in less bulk in the palm, but the splint may not apply adequate pressure against spastic thenar muscles. The palmar design includes a metacarpal bar, a thumb trough with a C bar, and a hypothenar bar (Figure 12-9).

Process to Fabricate

Materials

The selection of tools and materials is essentially the same as that described for the resting hand splint.

Pattern

A sample pattern is shown in Figure 12-10.

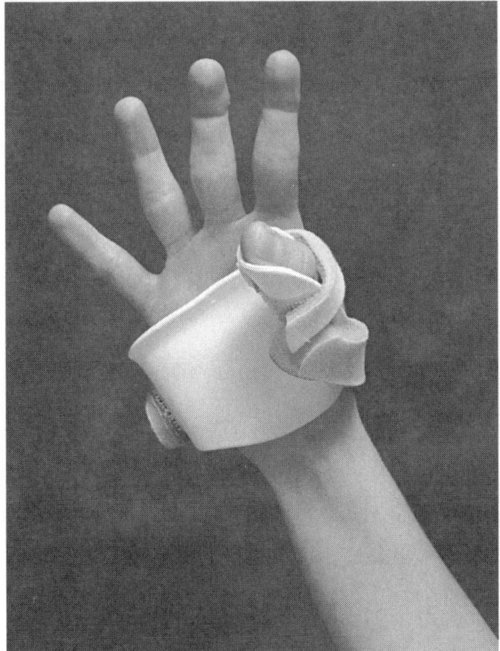

FIGURE 12-9 A thermoplastic thumb splint

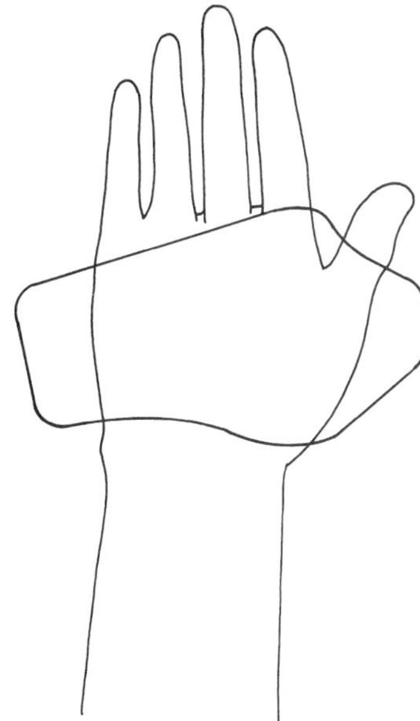

FIGURE 12-10 A pattern for a thermoplastic thumb splint

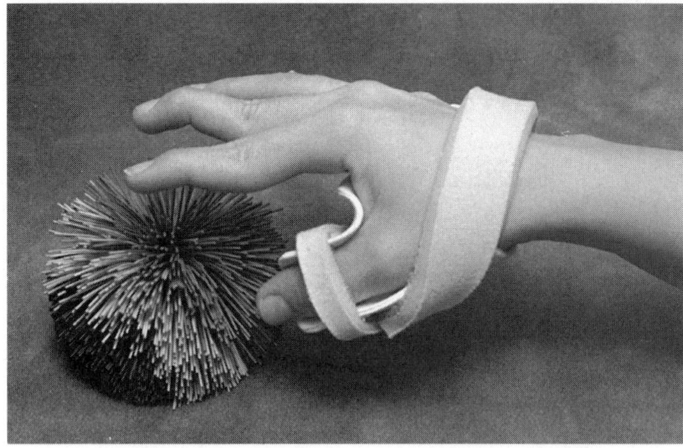

FIGURE 12-11
The thermoplastic thumb splint should allow the index and middle fingers to contact the tip of the thumb during grasp.

Forming the Splint

After cutting out the splint and reheating the material, the therapist places the material on the child's hand and carefully matches the thumb-web space. The hypothenar bar wraps around the ulnar border of the hand far enough to secure the hand, and the metacarpal bar is rolled to allow finger flexion. The body of the splint should conform to the palmar arches as they occur during grasp and should extend proximally far enough to adequately position the carpometacarpal (CMC) joint of the thumb but not so far that it interferes with wrist flexion.

The therapist forms the thumb trough by positioning the thumb in palmar abduction and stretching the plastic to form the C bar. The therapist should distribute pressure to position the thumb along the thenar eminence, thus providing optimal positioning and avoiding hyperextension of the MP joint. The thumb trough should extend just past the IP joint of the thumb but should leave the tip of the thumb free for sensory contact during grasp (Figure 12-11). The finished splint should allow the index and middle fingers to contact the tip of the thumb. The therapist should place a strap across the dorsum of the hand. If necessary, the therapist should also place a strap across the thumb trough.

Precautions

The pressure to position the thumb should be directed below the MP of the thumb to prevent stress and possible dislocation of this joint. The splint should also fit snugly into the thumb-web space. The therapist must watch for signs of

Laboratory Exercise 12-3*

What problems in splint fabrication are present in the following picture?

____

____

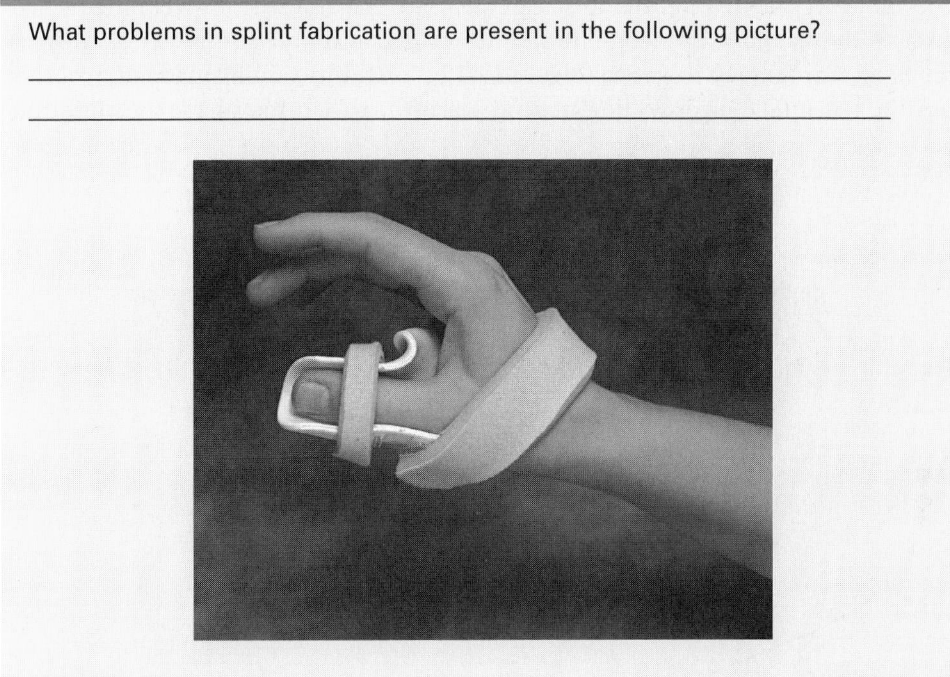

*See Appendix A for the answer key.

skin irritation and pressure, a problem that is most likely to occur in the thumb-web space or at the MCP joints of the fingers.

Wearing Schedule

The patient should wear the thumb splint during functional activities that require grasp and release. Although it is primarily a functional splint, the thumb splint can also be worn during the day to prevent the opponens muscle from remaining in a fully shortened position. If contractures are a concern, the child may also need to wear a resting hand splint to provide further stretch of the thenar muscles. The therapist should give the child opportunities to practice active thumb movement without the splint and should reduce the wearing time as active control increases. Working on activities that require active thumb movement immediately after removal of the thumb splint may be effective.

Soft Thumb Splint

Features

The soft thumb splint allows more movement of the intrinsic muscles of the hand and covers less of the palmar surface than a splint made from thermoplastic material. The soft thumb splint restricts palmar adduction of the thumb but does not prevent it. The therapist can fabricate the splint from webbing or neoprene. Thumb and wrist neoprene splints are also available commercially in sizes ranging from infancy to youth (Figure 12-12).* A thumb splint made of neoprene has the advantage of providing neutral warmth, which may have an inhibitory

*One supplier of such splints is the Benik Corporation, 9465 Provost Road NW, #204, Silverdale, WA 98383 (1-800-442-8910).

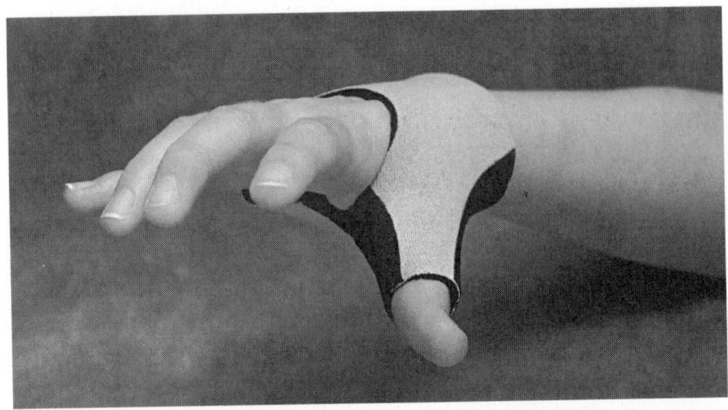

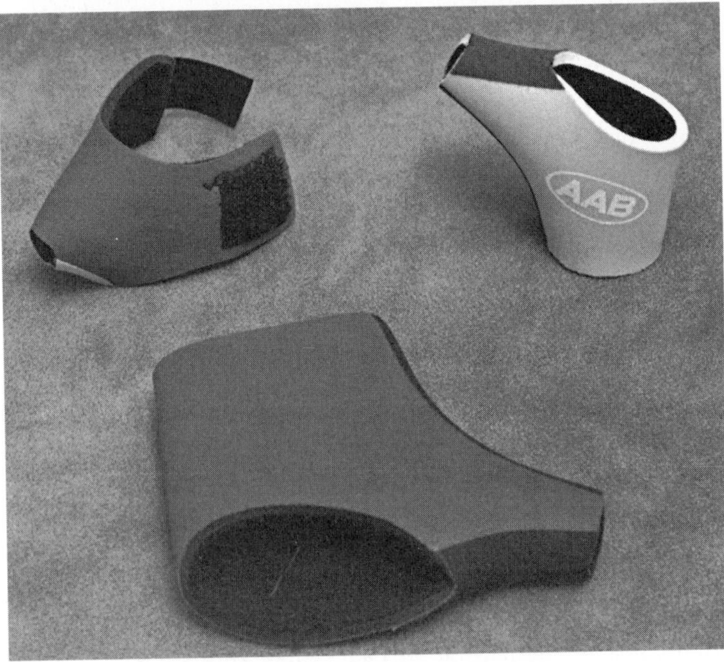

FIGURE 12-12 Neoprene thumb splints

influence on the hypertonicity. If purchasing a neoprene thumb splint, the therapist should consider whether the splint has a velcro closure. A thumb splint that slides over the fingers and thumb may be more difficult to apply. If making a soft thumb splint, the therapist should include a wrist band and thumb loop.

Process to Fabricate a Soft Thumb Splint That Has a Thumb Loop

Materials

The therapist makes the wrist band and thumb loop from a strapping material such as webbing or neoprene. The strapping material should be pliable enough to conform to the web space of the thumb. The strap that forms the thumb loop should be wide enough to support the thumb but not so wide that it buckles or wrinkles in the thumb-web space. The strap that forms the wrist band should be wide enough to secure the thumb loop, remain in place on the wrist, and distribute pressure. This strap should be long enough to form an adequate overlap to secure the velcro. The therapist can determine the specific dimensions by placing the strap material on the child's arm and hand to measure lengths and widths and determine the desired angle of pull.

Pattern

The therapist should make the wrist band to overlap on the volar side of the wrist. The length of the thumb loop should be the distance from the proximal edge of the wrist band, around the thumb, and back around to the point of origin.

Forming the Splint

The therapist should sew one end of the thumb loop on the dorsal portion of the wrist band toward the radial side. The therapist sews the loop velcro to the free end of the thumb loop and sews the hook velcro to the dorsal portion of the wrist band. The thumb loop is directed up across the web space, around the thenar eminence, and pulled diagonally to attach to the dorsal portion of the wrist band (Figure 12-13). The amount of tension on the thumb loop and the attachment location of the free end to the wrist band influences the amount of radial and palmar abduction of the thumb. If the wrist band does not fit snugly, the splint shifts distally on the wrist, thus reducing the amount of tension on the thumb loop.

Precautions and Wearing Schedule

The precautions and wearing schedule are similar to those for the thermoplastic thumb splint, although the soft thumb splint presents less danger of pressure-related problems because of the softer material. Persons applying the splint should be sure the thumb loop fits snugly into the web space. If the child is active and wears it often, the splint is likely to become soiled and worn. The splint then requires washing and eventually replacement.

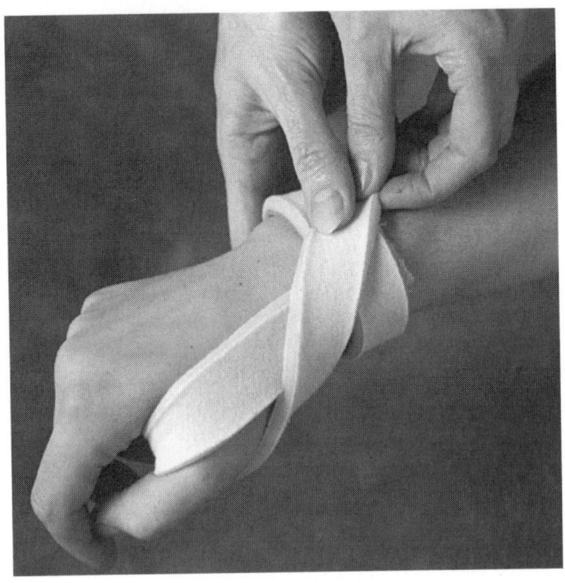

FIGURE 12-13 A soft thumb splint with a thumb loop

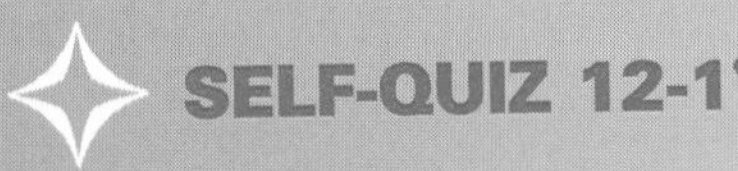

SELF-QUIZ 12-1*

Please circle either true (T) or false (F).

1. T F Many children who have developmental disabilities rely on adults to apply and remove splints.
2. T F Children who have little subcutaneous fat tolerate pressure to bony areas better than children who have ample subcutaneous fat.
3. T F Children who are at the greatest risk for developing contractures are those who have moderately to severely increased tone or those who have severely decreased tone and no active movement.
4. T F A resting hand splint for a child who has spasticity should place the thumb midway between palmar and radial abduction.
5. T F To hasten the hardening process of a child's splint, the therapist should always use coolant spray.

*See Appendix A for the answer key.

SELF-QUIZ 12-1—cont'd

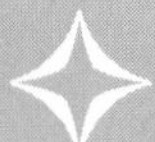

6. T F Distal force to a child's spastic thumb can result in hyperextension and dislocation of the MP joint.
7. T F When a splint is correctly fitted on a child, the therapist should document the wearing schedule in the child's records and provide written copies to parents, caregivers, and teachers.
8. T F Wrist cock-up splints for children should always place the wrist in 30° of extension.
9. T F Children who have moderate to severe tone usually benefit from splints made of neoprene rather than thermoplastic material.
10. T F A soft thumb splint allows more movement of the intrinsic muscles of the hand and covers less of the palmar surface than a splint made from thermoplastic material.

SUMMARY

This chapter describes the use of three types of hand splints in the management of children who have developmental disabilities. Splint designs for children who have abnormal muscle tone differ from many of the adult splint designs. In addition to the dynamics of development, children differ from adults in the types of environments in which they live, learn, work, and play.

Limited resources about splint design and application are available to guide the student or therapist who is working with developmentally disabled children. Most books and texts about hand splinting do not include chapters on children. If included, these chapters usually describe splint designs and applications for children who have orthopedic problems rather than neurological problems.

A review of the literature reveals a paucity of articles describing the use of hand splints with children. Hill (1988) writes "Whereas there is little documentation supporting splinting practices in adults, there is even less research published that demonstrates the efficacy of splinting children with spasticity" (p. 133). Unless therapists submit case studies and research articles more often for publication, many therapists may continue to reinvent wheels. Research studies to examine the effectiveness of pediatric splint designs and applications are also necessary.

Case Study*

Read the following scenario and answer the questions based on information in this chapter:

Mark is a 10-year-old boy who has cerebral palsy and is mentally handicapped. He lives with his mother and younger sister. Mark is in an educational program designed for children who have severe, profound disabilities. He has moderate to severely increased muscle tone in all four extremities and reduced tone in his trunk. Tone in the extremities increases at night and tends to increase further during the day when he is excited, upset, or exerting effort. Mark's functional use of his upper extremities is limited because of increased tone and delayed development.

Mark has been receiving occupational therapy services since he was an infant. His current program consists of a combination of direct and indirect intervention. The latter is carried out in the classroom and at home under the supervision of the occupational therapist.

You have been Mark's therapist for the past 2 years. Therapy goals include increasing speed and accuracy of reach of the right upper extremity, improving functional gross grasp and release of the right hand, and facilitating active movement of the left upper extremity. You have selected neurodevelopmental treatment and biomechanical frames of reference to guide your intervention.

Through the combined efforts of yourself, teachers, and his mother, Mark has maintained nearly full passive ROM of both upper extremities with active and passive ROM activities. Activities are carried out several times daily at school and home.

Splinting has not been a part of his program to date. Over the past year, however, you have noted a decrease in the amount of wrist extension bilaterally with more loss on the left side, which is more involved. Performing passive ROM of the wrist and hands is becoming increasingly difficult. Mark's hands are frequently fisted with the thumbs in the palms. You are concerned about maintaining passive ROM but hesitant to encumber his hands with splints that might interfere with the development of grasp and release on the right side.

1. You are modifying Mark's treatment program to address your concern about increased tightness in the wrist and finger flexors. Which of the following options should you select? Why?

   Option A—Increase the frequency of passive and active ROM activities for both upper extremities.

   Option B—Fabricate resting hand splints for both hands and a thermoplastic thumb splint for the right hand. Recommend that Mark wears both resting hand splints at night and the left splint periodically during the day depending on the status of the ROM. Recommend that he wears the right thumb splint during functional grasp activities. Continue the current program of passive and active ROM activities.

*See Appendix A for the answer key.

Case Study—cont'd

Option C—Fabricate resting hand splints for both upper extremities. Recommend that Mark wear both splints at night and during the day.

Option D—Fabricate resting hand splints for both upper extremities. Because you are not sure that correct application of the splints is likely at home, recommend that Mark wear the splints only during the day at school.

Review Questions

1. What are the components that the therapist should include in an assessment of the child to determine the need for a splint and select the splint design?
2. What are the primary purposes of a resting hand splint for a child who has abnormal muscle tone?
3. What is the correct position of the thumb in a resting hand splint for a child who has increased muscle tone?
4. On what basis does the therapist decide the appropriate angles in which to place the hand joints during fabrication of a resting hand splint for a child who has increased muscle tone?
5. What are the characteristics of thermoplastic material that work best during the splinting of a child who has moderately to severely increased muscle tone?
6. When splinting a hand that has increased muscle tone, the therapist should direct force to position the thumb below which joint?
7. Are the placement and angles of straps on a resting hand splint important? If so, why?
8. What should a therapist consider when deciding on a splint-wearing schedule for a child?
9. What are the types of hand dysfunction that indicate a need for a wrist cock-up splint?
10. Which factors should the therapist consider when selecting a thermoplastic versus a soft thumb splint?
11. What can the therapist do to influence caregiver compliance and correct application of a splint on a child?
12. Should the therapist consider the home and school environments when selecting a splint design? If so, why?

References

Exner, C. E. (1989). Development of hand functions. In P. N. Pratt & A. S. Allen (Eds.), Occupational therapy for children (pp. 235-259). St. Louis: Mosby.

Hill, S. G. (1988). Current trends in upper extremity splinting. In R. Boehme (Ed.), Improving upper body control (pp. 131-164). Tucson: Therapy Skill Builders.

Shoen, S., & Anderson, J. (1993). Neurodevelopmental treatment frame of reference. In P. Kramer & J. Hinojosa (Eds.), Frames of reference for pediatric occupational therapy (pp. 49-86). Baltimore: Williams & Wilkins.

Yamamoto, M. S. (1993). Developmental disabilities. In R. A. Hansen & B. Atchison (Eds.), Conditions in occupational therapy (pp. 52-78). Baltimore, MD: Williams & Wilkins.

Suggested Readings

Bellefeuille-Reid, D. (1984). Ideas Exchange: Aid to independence, hand splint for cerebral palsied children. Can J Occup Ther, 51(1), 37-39.

Casey, C. A., & Kratz, E. J. (1988). Soft splinting with neoprene: the thumb abduction supinator splint. Am J Occup Ther, 42(6), 395-398.

Exner, C. E., & Bonder, B. R. (1983). Comparative effects of three hand splints on bilateral hand use, grasp, and arm-hand posture in hemiplegic children: A pilot study. Occup Ther J Res, 3(2), 75-92.

Flegle, J., & Leibowitz, J. M. (1988). Improvement in grasp skill in children with hemiplegia with the MacKinnon splint. Res Dev Disabil, 9, 145-151.

Goodman, G., & Bazyk, S. (1991). The effects of a short thumb opponens splint on hand function in cerebral palsy: A single subject study. Am J Occup Ther, 45(8), 726-731.

MacKinnon, J., Sanderson, E., & Buchanan, J. (1975). The MacKinnon splint—a functional hand splint. Can J Occup Ther, 42(4), 157-158.

Glossary*

active field an orthokinetic term that describes materials having soft, warm, and texture properties. Also called *facilitatory fields,* these active fields are often placed over the agonist muscle belly.

agonist muscle a contracting muscle; its contraction is opposed by another muscle (i.e., antagonist).

Allen's test a test for the radial and ulnar artery patency. The person is asked to make a fist. The radial and ulnar arteries are then compressed at the wrist while the person opens and closes the hand several times to exsanguinate the hand. Compression of the ulnar artery is continued and compression of the radial artery is alleviated while the fist is opened. If blood perfusion through the radial artery is adequate, the hand should flush and resume normal pink coloration. The ulnar artery is then tested in the same manner.

antagonist muscle a muscle that contends with or is opposed to another muscle.

arthrodesis 1. fixation of a joint, often in an abnormal position and usually resulting from destruction of articular cartilage and subchondral bone, a problem that occurs in rheumatoid arthritis; 2. also called *fusion* and involves surgically induced fixation of a joint to relieve pain or provide support.

arthroplasty the surgical reconstruction or replacement of a painful, degenerated joint to restore mobility to a joint that has osteoarthritis or rheumatoid arthritis or to correct a congenital deformity. The bones of the joint are reshaped and soft tissue or a metal disk is placed between the reshaped ends, or all or part of the joint is replaced with a metal or plastic prosthesis.

*Definitions from Anderson, K. N., Anderson, L. E., & Glanze, W. D. (Eds.). (1994). Mosby's medical, nursing & allied health dictionary (4th ed.). St. Louis: Mosby; Hunter, J. M., Schneider, L. H., Mackin, E. J., & Callahan, A. D. (Eds.). (1990). Rehabilitation of the hand: Surgery and therapy (3rd ed.). St. Louis: Mosby; International dictionary of medicine and biology. New York: John Wiley & Sons Inc, & Pedretti, L. W., & Zoltan B. (Eds.). (1990). Occupational therapy: Practice skills for physical dysfunction (3rd ed.). St. Louis: Mosby.

axonotmesis an interruption of the axon with subsequent wallerian degeneration of the distal nerve segment. Connective tissue of the nerve, including Schwann's cell basement membranes, may remain intact.

biomechanical approach an occupational performance, frame of reference approach that uses principles of kinetics and forces acting on the body.

biomechanics the study of mechanical laws and their application to living organisms, especially the human body and its locomotor system.

blanch test also called a *blanching test* or *capillary refill,* is a test of blood circulation in the fingers or toes. Pressure is applied to the nail over a finger or toe until normal color is lost. The pressure is then removed, and if the circulation is normal, color returns within about 5 seconds.

bonding agent a solvent used for preparing coated thermoplastic material for a strong self-bond.

carpal ganglion 1. a knot or knotlike mass; 2. one of the nerve cells, chiefly collected in groups outside the central nervous system. Individual cells and extremely small groups abound in association with alimentary organs.

carpal tunnel syndrome a common, painful disorder of the wrist and hand induced by compression on the median nerve between the inelastic carpal ligament and other structures in the carpal tunnel.

circumferential splint a splint that fits around the circumference of an extremity.

clawhand deformity an abnormal condition of the hand caused by atrophy of the interosseous muscles and characterized by extreme flexion of the middle and distal phalanges and hyperextension of the metacarpophalangeal joints of the ring and little fingers.

closed-cell padding padding materials that resist absorption of odors, perspiration, and bacteria.

closed-reduction of fractures the manual reduction of a fracture without an incision.

collagen a protein consisting of bundles of tiny reticular fibrils, which continue to form the white, glistening, inelastic fibers of the tendons, ligaments, and fascia.

Colles' fracture a fracture of the radius at the epiphysis within 1 inch of the wrist joint. The fracture causes a dorsal and lateral position of the hand that makes the fracture easily recognizable.

conformability the ability of thermoplastic material to fit intimately into contoured areas.

contracture an abnormal, usually permanent condition of a joint characterized by flexion and fixation and caused by atrophy and shortening of muscle fibers or by loss of the normal elasticity of the skin such as that from the formation of extensive scar tissue over a joint.

creep the adaptation of soft tissue as a result of prolonged force.

criterion-referenced assessment an assessment that uses descriptive standards to measure performance and is judged in terms of a desired outcome.

cumulative trauma injuries musculoskeletal disorders resulting from repetitive motions (usually occupational) that develop over time. Symptoms include pain, inflammation, and function impairment.

cylindrical grasp a grasp pattern in which the cylindrical object rests against the palm of the hand and the fingers flex around the object to maintain a grasp.

Dellon modification of the Moberg Pick-Up test evaluation of hand function when a person grasps specified objects. The test requires a person to have sensory discrimination and prehensive ability.

de Quervain's tenosynovitis tenosynovitis of the abductor pollicis longus and extensor pollicis brevis muscles of the thumb.
discriminatory sensations pertaining to somatic sensations of fast, localized pain; slow, poorly localized pain; and temperature.
dorsal pertaining to the back or posterior.
drapability a handling characteristic of thermoplastic material that allows conformation to an underlying shape.
durability a performance characteristic of thermoplastic material that refers to the length of time the splint plastic will last or endure.
dynamic splint a splint incorporating springs, elastic bands, or other materials that produce a constant active force to counteract deforming forces of an injury.
dynamometer an instrument used to measure grip strength. Test results are compared to norms.
dysesthesia sensations of numbness, tingling, burning, or pain below the level of the lesion.
ecchymosis also called a *bruise,* this is a discoloration of an area of the skin or mucous membrane caused by fragility of the vessel walls or by the extravasation of blood into the subcutaneous tissues as a result of trauma to the underlying blood vessels.
edema the abnormal accumulation of fluid in interstitial spaces of tissues such as the pericardial sac, intrapleural space, peritoneal cavity, and joint capsules.
elasticity a handling characteristic of thermoplastic material that resists stretching and has a tendency to return to its original shape after stretching.
elastomer a liquid or putty-style elastomer that requires the mixing of a base and catalyst to form a compound used over scarred areas. Elastomer provides intimate contour to reduce hypertrophic scar tissue formation.
elongation a state of being lengthened or extended.
fibroblastic phase (or proliferative stage) the second stage of wound healing, in which the fibroblast cells produce closely linked collagen fibers that increase tensile strength.
Finkelstein's test a test for the presence of de Quervain's tenosynovitis. The test is performed by stabilizing the forearm and instructing the patient to clasp the fingers over the flexed thumb. The examiner passively deviates the wrist toward the ulnar side. With this test the patient may complain of pain over the abductor pollicis longus tendon.
flaccid weak, soft, and flabby; lacking normal muscle tone.
flexibility the ability of thermoplastic material to tolerate repeated stresses.
footdrop an abnormal neuromuscular condition of the lower leg and foot characterized by an inability to dorsiflex or evert the foot because of damage to the common peroneal nerve.
frame of reference a conceptual structure that assists in the development and organization of a program, organization, or project.
gamekeeper's thumb an injury to the ulnar collateral ligament of the metacarpal joint of the thumb. This injury is called gamekeeper's thumb because of the gamekeepers who killed birds by twisting their necks, thus constantly stressing this joint.

goniometer an instrument used to measure angles of a joint (particularly range of motion angles).

hard contracture a contracture resulting from osteopathic changes in the joint structure.

high-nerve lesion a peripheral nerve injury that occurs above the elbow level.

hook grasp a grasp pattern in which the DIPs and PIPs flex around the object, and the thumb often remains passive.

hydrocollator a stainless steel container that heats and maintains water temperature between 70° and 212° F. The temperature can be regulated.

hypertonicity excessive tension of the muscles.

hypothenar an eminence or fleshy elevation on the ulnar side of the palm of the hand.

hypotonia diminished tone or tension that may involve any body structure.

inflammatory phase the first phase of wound healing, in which vasoconstriction occurs, thus leading to platelet adhesion of the damaged vessel wall and resulting in clot formation. This phase can last 3 to 6 days.

Jebson-Taylor hand function test a standardized evaluation of functional hand capabilities composed of seven items that are representative of various hand activities. The time of performance is recorded for each test.

lateral prehension contact between the thumb pad to the lateral aspect of the index finger.

low-nerve lesion a peripheral nerve injury that occurs below the level of the elbow.

low-temperature thermoplastic material plastic used to make splints that soften in water heated to 135° to 180° F.

maceration the softening and breaking down of skin from prolonged exposure to moisture.

macular degeneration a progressive deterioration of the maculae of the retina and choroid of the eye.

manual muscle test a procedure for the evaluation of the strength of individual muscles or muscle groups based on relation to the forces of gravity and manual resistance.

maturation phase the final stage of wound healing, which can last up to 1 or 2 years. Tensile strength increases and normal scars may soften and become pliable.

mechanical advantage the ratio of the output force developed by the muscles to the input force applied to the body structures that the muscles move, especially the ratio of these forces associated with the body structures that act as levers. Variations in the sizes of muscles and lengths of bones in individuals partially account for the different mechanical advantages from one body type to another and physical capabilities such as speed and strength.

memory the ability of thermoplastic material to return to its preheated (original) shape and size when reheated.

muscle tone a normal state of balanced muscle tension.

neoprene a soft splinting material that is rubber with nylon lining on one side and pile material on the other, thus making the velcro hook attachment quick. Neoprene retains warmth, has some degree of elasticity, and has contour for a snug fit.

neurapraxia a condition in which a nerve remains in place after a severe injury although it no longer transmits impulses.

neurophysiological approach a theoretical approach that focuses on the effects of sensory feedback provided by the splints in altering muscle tone and promoting normal movement patterns.

neurotmesis a peripheral nerve injury in which laceration or traction completely disrupts the nerve. Neurotmesis requires surgical approximation with unpredictable recovery.

Nine Hole Peg test a standardized test for finger-hand coordination. The examiner times a person to place and remove 9 pegs in a pegboard. Results are compared to norms.

open-cell padding padding that allows absorption.

opponens opposing or placing against; in anatomy, designating those muscles of the thumb and little finger that move these digits to touch each other or other digits.

orthokinetic cuff an elastic covering for a muscle to provide tactile stimulation that induces and restricts contraction of an opposing muscle simultaneously.

orthokinetics therapy for spasticity that includes the use of an orthotic device to enable contraction of one muscle while inhibiting its antagonist.

orthosis a force system designed to control, correct, or compensate for a bond deformity, deforming forces, or forces absent from the body. Orthosis often involves the use of special braces.

osteoporosis a disorder characterized by abnormal rarefaction of bone. Osteoporosis occurs most frequently in postmenopausal women, sedentary or immobilized individuals, and patients undergoing long-term steroid therapy.

outrigger a wire or thermoplastic material component on a dynamic splint that helps guide the direction of traction.

palmar prehension (tripod pinch) the contact of the thumb pads to the pads of the middle and index fingers.

passive field also called an *inhibitory field,* this is an orthokinetic term that describes materials having hard, cool, and smooth properties. A passive field is often placed over the antagonist muscle belly.

pinch gauge an instrument commonly used to measure tip, palmar, and lateral pinch strengths. Test results are compared to norms.

plasty a combining form meaning a molding or shaping, especially by plastic surgery.

pneumatic splint also called an *inflatable splint,* this is a tubular device that is placed around a patient's extremity and inflated with air to maintain rigidity.

prehensile patterns the use of the hands and fingers to grasp or pick up objects.

protocol a written plan specifying the procedures for giving an examination, conducting research, or providing care for a particular condition.

radial pertaining to the radius.

radial nerve palsy a compression or entrapment neuropathy involving the radial nerve. Symptoms of muscle weakness and sensory loss are due to compression of the radial nerve against the humerus.

rehabilitation approach an occupational performance, frame of reference approach that focuses on a person's abilities rather than disabilities.

resting hand posture the posture of a normal hand at rest assumes a position of 10° to 20° of wrist extension, 10° of ulnar deviation, slight flexion and abduction of the thumb, and approximately 15° to 20° of flexion of the metacarpophalangeal (MCP) joints.

rheumatoid arthritis a chronic systemic disease that can affect the lungs, cardiovascular systems, and eyes. Joint involvement resulting from inflammatory disease of the synovium is the primary clinical feature. The disease may range from mild to severe and can result in joint deformity and destruction of varying degrees.

rigidity the ability of low-temperature thermoplastic to be strong and resistant to repeated stress.

self-adherence the degree to which thermoplastic material sticks to itself when properly heated.

self-finishing edges a handling characteristic of thermoplastic material that allows any cut edge to have a smooth texture.

Semmes-Weinstein Monofilament sensory test a sensory test that uses monofilaments. The testing process results in a detailed mapping of the level of functional sensibility.

sensorimotor approach an occupational performance, frame of reference approach for patients who have damaged central nervous systems to inhibit or facilitate normal motor responses.

simian hand deformity a deformity resulting from a median nerve injury in which the thenar eminences atrophies.

soft splints splints fabricated from materials such as fabric, flexible plastics, neoprene, and leather rather than rigid thermoplastic material.

spasticity a form of muscular hypertonicity that has increased resistance to stretch.

spherical grasp a grasp pattern in which spherical objects rest against the palm of the hand and the five abducted fingers flex around the object.

splint an orthopedic device for immobilization, restraint, and support of any part of the body.

static splint a splint that has no moving parts and immobilizes.

stockinette a densely knit tubular bandage that stretches and is commonly used on skin during splinting and cast making.

stretch reflex a reflex muscle contraction after the muscle is stretched because of stimulation of its proprioceptive receptors.

synovitis an inflammatory condition of the synovial membrane of a joint caused by an aseptic wound or a traumatic injury such as a sprain or severe strain. Fluid accumulates around the capsule; the joint is swollen, tender, and painful; and motion is restricted. Usually the inflammation subsides, and the fluid is resorbed without medical or surgical intervention.

tendonitis an inflammatory condition of a tendon, usually resulting from strain. Treatment may include rest, corticosteroid injections, and support.

tenodesis passive tension that produces movements of joints when the muscle is elongated over two or more joints.

tenolysis the surgical release of nongliding adhesions that form along the surface of a tendon after injury or repair. This procedure is useful in the salvage of tendon function.

tenosynovitis also called *tendosynovitis,* this term refers to inflammation of a tendon sheath caused by calcium deposits, repeated strain or trauma, high levels of blood cholesterol, rheumatoid arthritis, gout, or gonorrhea.

tensile strength the amount of force a tendon can withstand.

thenar eminence a raised, rounded area on the palm of the hand near the base of the thumb.

Theraband a stretchable latex rubber available in various thicknesses.

torque the affect that a force has on rotational movement of a point and can be calculated by multiplying the force by the length of the movement arm.

total active motion (TAM) the sum of angles formed by metacarpophalangeal, proximal interphalangeal, and distal interphalangeal joints in maximum active flexion minus the sum of angles of extensor lags on each joint: total flexion−total extensor lag = TAM. TAM is a term applied to one finger.

total passive motion (TPM) the sum of angles formed by metacarpophalangeal, proximal interphalangeal, and distal interphalangeal joints in maximum passive flexion minus the sum of angles of extensor lags in each of these joints: total flexion−total extensor lag = TPM. TPM is a term applied to one finger.

two-point discrimination test a test of the ability of a person to differentiate touch stimuli at two nearby points on the body at the same time.

ulnar pertaining to the long medial bone of the forearm.

universal precautions an approach to infection control designed to prevent transmission of blood-borne diseases. The guidelines for universal precautions include specific recommendations for the use of gloves, masks, and protective eyewear when contact with blood or body secretions containing blood is anticipated.

vasoconstriction a narrowing of the lumen of any blood vessel, especially the arterioles and the veins in the blood reservoirs of the skin and abdominal viscera.

volar also called *palmar,* this term pertains to the palm of the hand or the sole of the foot.

volumeter measurements measurements of composite hand mass by means of water displacement. Volumeters are used to assess changes in hand mass due to atrophy and local edema.

wrist drop a condition caused by paralysis of the extensor muscles of the hand and fingers or by injury of the radial nerve, thus resulting in flexion of the wrist.

Answers to Quizzes, Laboratory Exercises, and Case Studies

Chapter 1
Self-Quiz 1-1 Answers:
1. B, 2. C, 3. A
Case Study Answers:
1. A and B, 2. C, 3. B, 4. B

Chapter 2
Self-Quiz 2-1
Part I Answers:
1. D, 2. A, 3. B, 4. A, 5. C
Part II Answers:
1. distal palmar crease, 2. proximal palmar crease, 3. thenar crease, 4. distal wrist crease, 5. proximal wrist crease
Part III Answers:
1. longitudinal arch, 2. distal transverse arch, 3. proximal transverse arch
Self-Quiz 2-2 Answers:
1. F, 2. F, 3. T, 4. T, 5. F

Chapter 3
Self-Quiz 3-1 Answers:
1. F, 2. T, 3. T, 4. F, 5. F, 6. T, 7. F, 8. T, 9. F

Chapter 4
Self-Quiz 4-1 Answers:
1. F, 2. T, 3. T, 4. T, 5. F, 6. T, 7. F, 8. F, 9. F, 10. T, 11. T
Case Study Answers:
The following are some suggested approaches to these questions. You may have different appropriate answers.
1. Go to the radiology department and view the patient's x-rays. Review the complications of Colles' fracture in an appropriate text.
2. Spend time talking to Pete and his wife before beginning the splint fabrication. Determine their understanding about the diagnosis and the splint order. Clarify concerns and allow time for Pete and his wife to vent their feelings. Explain clearly the medical reasons for the splint. Encourage Pete to formulate a list of questions to present to his physician at the next visit.
3. Never hesitate to call the physician's office. If the physician is not available,

leave your questions with the nurse.
4. A volar-based wrist cock-up splint provides the most support, especially in Pete's line of work.
5. Fabricate the splint out of a thermoplastic material that has some rigidity because the patient is a roofer and does heavy work. Also, choose a thermoplastic material that drapes and conforms to his hand and has some memory qualities because the material may require remolding to help promote wrist extension.
6. Fabricate a good design, and make sure that the splint fits correctly. Use soft, wide straps to hold the splint in place. If fluctuating edema continues to be a problem, consider ace wrapping the extremity. With the splint provision, instruct Pete to elevate the extremity and do active range of motion (AROM) exercises.
7. Keep Pete in the clinic for 20 to 30 minutes to monitor for reddened areas.
8. Educate Pete and his wife about splint precautions such as monitoring for pressure sores and about a splint-wearing schedule. A possible schedule is for Pete to wear the splint during times of right upper extremity pain and inflammation and for work and home activities that require more support. The splint should be removed for exercises and hygiene.

Chapter 5

Self-Quiz 5-1 Answers:
1. T, 2. T, 3. F, 4. F, 5. T, 6. F
Laboratory Exercise 5-2 Answers:
Splint A: 1. The wrist is positioned in extreme ulnar deviation; 2. this extreme position stresses the wrist joint and possibly contributes to the development of other problems such as wrist pain, pressure areas, and de Quervain's tenosynovitis.
Splint B: 1. The wrist is positioned in flexion instead of a functional hand position of extension. Positioning in wrist extension helps with digital flexion. If the wrist is flexed, the patient loses functional grasp.
Splint C: 1. MCP flexion is inhibited because of the splint meta-carpal bar being too high; 2. potential development of skin irritation or pressure areas exists with digital flexion, and the patient does not have a full functional grasp.
Case Study Answers:
1. C, 2. C, 3. A, 4. C, 5. C

Chapter 6

Laboratory Exercise 6-2 Answers:
1. Thumb interphalangeal joint is flexed rather than extended, 2. radial deviation of wrist, 3. poor wrist support and stretched thermoplastic
Case Study Answers:
1. B, 2. A, 3. B, 4. B, 5. B

Chapter 7

Self-Quiz 7-1 Answers:
1. F, 2. F, 3. T, 4. F, 5. T, 6. F, 7. T
Laboratory Exercise 7-1 Answers:
1. Hypothenar bar, 2. metacarpal (palmar) bar, 3. forearm trough
Laboratory Exercise 7-3 Answers:
1. The two problems are the following:
a. The metacarpal bar is too high to allow full finger MCP flexion; b. the thumb interphalangeal joint flexion is limited because of the material around the thumb being too far distal. 2. An irritation might develop at the thumb interphalangeal joint where the thumb opening is too high and at the base of the index finger where the metacarpal bar is too high. The splint limits full finger flexion.
Case Study Answers:
1. A, 2. C, 3. B, 4. A, 5. B, 6. C

Chapter 8

Self-Quiz 8-1 Answers:
1. T, 2. T, 3. F, 4. F, 5. T
Case Study Answers:
1. D, 2. C, 3. B, 4. A, 5. B

Chapter 9

Laboratory Exercise 9-1 Answer:
The following is an example of a S.O.A.P. note: S—The patient reported that he is not experiencing any pain. O—The patient was seen in a follow-up visit for a radial nerve injury to the left forearm for 45 minutes. Manual muscle testing (MMT) results for the extensor digitorum communis, extensor digiti minimi, extensor indicis, abductor pollicis longus, and extensor carpi ulnaris all scored a grade of fair (3). Semmes-Weinstein Monofilaments sensation testing revealed impaired sensation on the dorsum of the index and middle fingers and half of the ring finger to the PIP joint level. A left dynamic MCP extension hand-based splint was fabricated and fitted for the patient. The patient was given verbal and written instructions on the wearing schedule, splint care, and precautions. The pt.'s home program was updated with modifications to be completed 5x/day. Pt. was encouraged to continue with ADL tasks and home program. A—Pt. was receptive to splint and home program. Pt. was able to independently grasp light objects while wearing the splint. Anticipate compliance with wearing schedule and home program. P—Will continue to monitor needs for modification of the splint and home program to improve left hand strength and function.
Self-Quiz 9-1 Answers:
1. T, 2. T, 3. F, 4. F, 5. F, 6. T, 7. T, 8. F, 9. F, 10. T, 11. T, 12. F
Case Study Answers:
1. A, C, D, E, 2. C, 3. A

Chapter 10

Case Study Answers:
1. B. Because limited pain-free passive range of motion (PROM) is available at wrist and fingers, providing comfort offered by submaximum positioning and gentle stretch furnished by dynamic resistance is important. The hard-cone design allows orthotic management to begin even though the fingers are flexed. Because wrist and finger PROM are affected, orthotic design should span all affected joints.
2. Because the soft device has increased flexion tightness, the nursing staff should review literature that addresses this dilemma. After discussion of other options the staff members should be more open to attempt alternative splints.
3. E. Wrist and finger motions, though weak, are now adequate for light functional tasks. The present thumb web space tightness position remains the greatest threat to advanced prehension patterns.
4. With the thumb positioned in opposition the patient may be involved in some self-care activities such as grasping a napkin, assisting in combing hair, and arranging a bed sheet.

Chapter 11

Self-Quiz 11-1 Answers:
1. T, 2. F, 3. F, 4. T, 5. F, 6. T, 7. F, 8. F, 9. T, 10. T
Self-Quiz 11-2 Answers:
1. A material that has high drapability and moldability is not a good choice for antigravity splinting. A material that has resistance to drape and memory is suitable. A slightly tacky splinting material that lightly adheres to underlying stockinette may be helpful. Preshaping techniques assist in molding.
2. A positioning soft splint such as soft roll or palm protector places the involved joints in submaximum extension. This position permits adequate skin hygiene.
3. A splint should not limit the use of uninvolved joints. An arthritis mitt splint immobilizes only the affected joints and positions the thumb in a resting position. The patient can still use the fingers for functional activities at night.
4. Pad the outside of the splint.

5. Wide, soft, foamlike strapping accommodates slight fluctuations in edema.
Case Study Answers:
1. B, 2. B, 3. C, 4. B, 5. B, 6. A and B

Chapter 12

Laboratory Exercise 12-1 Answer:
Two fabrication problems are present in this splint. First, the C bar does not fit into the web space of the thumb and provides inadequate positioning of the thumb between radial and palmar abduction. Second, the sides of the forearm trough are too high, thus resulting in bridging of the straps.
Laboratory Exercise 12-2 Answer:
The straps are not keeping the wrist positioned in the splint. The distal forearm strap should be placed just proximal to the ulnar styloid, and a second strap should be added just distal to the ulnar styloid, thus preventing the flexor action of the wrist from lifting the wrist away from the splint's surface. The splint does not fit snugly into the thumb web space.
Laboratory Exercise 12-3 Answer:
The splint does not fit snugly into the web space. In addition, the thumb trough is slightly too long and does not allow tactile contact of the tip of the thumb with an object being grasped.
Self-Quiz 12-1 Answers:
1. T, 2. F, 3. T, 4. T, 5. F, 6. T, 7. T, 8. F, 9. F, 10. T
Case Study Answers:

Option A is probably not adequate to address concerns of losing range of motion of the wrist and fingers. After its loss, range can be difficult if not impossible to regain. Therefore prevention is paramount. Range-of-motion activities are already being carried out several times daily at home and at school. Increasing this schedule may be difficult. The constant affects of moderately to severely increased tone are difficult to overcome with ROM activities alone.

Option B probably meets Mark's needs at this time. Prolonged stretch to the wrist and finger flexors can occur at night. Active and passive range of motion activities can continue during the day to maximize the potential for movement within available passive range of motion. These activities and other experiences during the day also provide the opportunity for proprioceptive and tactile input. Because the left upper extremity is tighter and less functional, wearing the left resting splint on this hand periodically during the day is prudent. A thermoplastic thumb splint for the right hand controls some of the increased tone in the hand but leaves the wrist and fingers free for active and functional movement. Range of motion measurements are required regularly to determine optimal wearing schedules.

Before implementing the wearing schedule at home, arrange a meeting with Mark's parents. Explain the purpose of the splints, demonstrate the way to apply them, and provide an opportunity for the parents to practice applying and removing them. Also, give the parents written instructions, precautions, and your phone number. Include photographs of the splints on Mark's hands if necessary.

Option C promotes excessive use of resting hand splints. Mark should continue to experience active movement and sensory feedback as much as possible during the day, especially with the right hand. Resting splints should be worn during the day and at night only if a serious threat of deformity is present.

Option D unnecessarily restricts active use of the hands during the day while leaving the wrists and fingers flexors shortened during the night and on weekends. Correct application at home is addressed by meeting with the parents as described under Option B.

APPENDIX B

Forms

FORM 1-1 Hints for Drawing and Fitting a Splint Pattern

- ❍ Explain the pattern-making process to the patient.
- ❍ Ask and/or assist the patient in removing any jewelry from the area that is splinted.
- ❍ Position the affected extremity on a paper towel in a natural, resting position. The wrist should be in a neutral position with a slight ulnar deviation. The fingers should be extended and slightly abducted.
- ❍ To trace the outline of the patient's extremity, keep the pencil at a 90-degree angle to the paper.
- ❍ Mark the landmarks needed to draw the pattern *before* the patient removes the extremity from the paper.
- ❍ For a more accurate pattern, the paper towel can be wet and placed on the area for evaluation of the pattern.
- ❍ Folding the paper towel to mark adjustments in the pattern can help with evaluation of the pattern.
- ❍ When evaluating the pattern fit of a forearm-based splint on the patient, look for the following*:
  1. Half the circumference of the forearm
  2. Two-thirds the length of the forearm
  3. The length and width of metacarpal or palmar bars
  4. The correct use of hand creases for landmarks
  5. The amount of support to the wrist, fingers, and thenar and hypothenar eminencies
- ❍ When tracing the pattern onto the thermoplastic material, do not use an ink pen because the ink may smear when the material is placed in the hot water to soften.

*These biomechanical principles and anatomical structures are discussed in Chapters 2 and 3.

FORM 3-1 Hand Evaluation Check-Off Sheet

- ❍ Patient's history: interview, chart review, and reports
  - ❍ age
  - ❍ occupation
  - ❍ date of injury and surgery
  - ❍ method of injury
  - ❍ hand dominance
  - ❍ vocation
  - ❍ avocational interests
  - ❍ family composition
  - ❍ patient complaints
  - ❍ activities of daily living responsibilities before and after injury
  - ❍ impact of injury on family, economic status, and social well-being
- ❍ Cognition
- ❍ Reimbursement
- ❍ Motivation
- ❍ Hand posture
- ❍ Skin
- ❍ Wound healing
- ❍ Bone
- ❍ Joint
- ❍ Muscle and tendon
- ❍ Nerve
- ❍ Vascular status
- ❍ Range of motion
- ❍ Strength
- ❍ Coordination and dexterity
- ❍ Function

FORM 3-2 Splint Precaution Check-Off Sheet

- ❍ Account for bony prominences such as the following:
  - metacarpophalangeal (MCP), proximal interphalangeal (PIP), and distal interphalangeal (DIP) joints
  - pisiform bone
  - radial and ulnar styloids
  - lateral and medial epicondyles of the elbow
- ❍ Identify fragile skin and select the splinting material carefully. Monitor the temperature of the thermoplastic closely before applying the material to the fragile skin.
- ❍ Identify skin areas having impaired sensation. The splint design should not impinge on these sites.
- ❍ If fluctuating edema is a problem, use a wider splint design.
- ❍ Do not compress the superficial branch of the radial nerve. If the radial edge of a forearm splint impinges beyond the middle of the forearm near the dorsal side of the thumb, the branch of the radial nerve may be compressed.

FORM 3-3 Hints for Splint Provision

- ❍ Give the patient *oral* and *written* instructions regarding the following:
  - ❍ wearing schedule
  - ❍ care of splint
  - ❍ purpose of splint
  - ❍ responsibility in therapy program
  - ❍ phone number of contact person if problems arise
  - ❍ actions to take if skin reactions such as the following occur:
    - rashes
    - numbness
    - reddened areas
    - pain increase because of splint application
- ❍ Evaluate the splint after the patient wears it at least 20 to 30 minutes, and make necessary adjustments.
- ❍ Position all joints incorporated into the splint at the correct therapeutic angle(s).
- ❍ Design the splint to account for bony prominences such as the following:
  - MCP, PIP, and DIP joints
  - pisiform
  - radial and ulnar styloids
  - lateral and medial epicondyles of the elbow
- ❍ If fluctuating edema is a problem, make certain the splint design can accommodate for the problem by using a wider design.
- ❍ Make certain the splint design does not mobilize or immobilize unnecessary joint(s).
- ❍ Make certain the splint does not impede or restrict motions of joints adjacent to the splint.
- ❍ Make certain the splint supports the arches of the hand.
- ❍ Take into consideration the creases of the hand for allowing immobilization or mobilization depending on the purpose of the splint.
- ❍ Make certain the splint does not restrict circulation.
- ❍ Make certain application and removal of the splint is easy.
- ❍ Secure the splint to the patient's extremity using a well-designed strapping mechanism.
- ❍ Make certain the appropriate edges of the splint are flared or rolled.

FORM 5-1 Wrist Cock-Up Splint

Name: ______________________________

Date: ______________________________

Type of wrist cock-up splint:

Volar Dorsal

Wrist position: ____________________

After the person wears the splint for 30 minutes, answer the following questions. (Mark *NA* for nonapplicable situations.)

Evaluation Areas		**Comments**
Design		
1. The wrist position is at the correct angle.	Yes ❍ No ❍ NA ❍	
2. The wrist has adequate support.	Yes ❍ No ❍ NA ❍	
3. The sides of the thenar and hypothenar eminences have support in the correct position.	Yes ❍ No ❍ NA ❍	
4. The thenar and hypothenar eminences are not restricted or flattened.	Yes ❍ No ❍ NA ❍	
5. The splint is two-thirds the length of the forearm.	Yes ❍ No ❍ NA ❍	
6. The splint is one-half the width of the forearm.	Yes ❍ No ❍ NA ❍	
Function		
1. The splint allows full thumb motions.	Yes ❍ No ❍ NA ❍	
2. The splint allows full MCP joint flexion of the fingers.	Yes ❍ No ❍ NA ❍	
3. The splint provides wrist support that allows functional activities.	Yes ❍ No ❍ NA ❍	
Straps		
1. The straps avoid bony prominences.	Yes ❍ No ❍ NA ❍	
2. The straps are secure and rounded.	Yes ❍ No ❍ NA ❍	

Continued.

FORM 5-1 Wrist Cock-Up Splint—cont'd

Evaluation Areas		**Comments**
Comfort		
1. The splint edges are smooth with rounded corners.	Yes ❍ No ❍ NA ❍	
2. The proximal end is flared.	Yes ❍ No ❍ NA ❍	
3. Impingements or pressure areas are not present.	Yes ❍ No ❍ NA ❍	
Cosmetic Appearance		
1. The splint is free of fingerprints, dirt, and pencil or pen marks.	Yes ❍ No ❍ NA ❍	
2. The splinting material is not buckled.	Yes ❍ No ❍ NA ❍	

Discuss possible splint adjustments or changes you should make based on the self-evaluation:

____

____

____

____

____

FORM 6-1 Resting Hand Splint

Name: ______________________________

Date: ______________________________

Position of resting hand splint:

Functional position ❍ (midjoint)

Antideformity position ❍ (intrinsic plus)

Answer the following questions after the patient wears the splint for 30 minutes. (Mark *NA* for nonapplicable situations.)

Evaluation Areas		**Comments**
Design		
1. The wrist position is at the correct angle.	Yes ❍ No ❍ NA ❍	
2. The MCPs are at the correct angle.	Yes ❍ No ❍ NA ❍	
3. The thumb is in the correct position.	Yes ❍ No ❍ NA ❍	
4. The wrist has adequate support.	Yes ❍ No ❍ NA ❍	
5. The pan is wide enough for all the fingers.	Yes ❍ No ❍ NA ❍	
6. The length of the pan and thumb trough are adequate.	Yes ❍ No ❍ NA ❍	
7. The splint is two-thirds the length of the forearm.	Yes ❍ No ❍ NA ❍	
8. The splint is one-half the width of the forearm.	Yes ❍ No ❍ NA ❍	
Function		
1. The splint completely immobilizes the wrist, fingers, and thumb.	Yes ❍ No ❍ NA ❍	
2. The splint is easy to apply and remove.	Yes ❍ No ❍ NA ❍	

Continued.

FORM 6-1 Resting Hand Splint—cont'd

Evaluation Areas		**Comments**
Straps		
1. The straps avoid bony prominences.	Yes ❍ No ❍ NA ❍	
2. The straps are secure and rounded.	Yes ❍ No ❍ NA ❍	
Comfort		
1. The edges are smooth with rounded corners.	Yes ❍ No ❍ NA ❍	
2. The proximal end is flared.	Yes ❍ No ❍ NA ❍	
3. Impingements or pressure areas are not present.	Yes ❍ No ❍ NA ❍	
Cosmetic Appearance		
1. The splint is free of fingerprints, dirt, and pencil or pen marks.	Yes ❍ No ❍ NA ❍	
2. The splinting material is not buckled.	Yes ❍ No ❍ NA ❍	

Discuss adjustments or changes you would make based on the self-evaluation:

____

____

____

____

____

FORM 7-1 Thumb Spica Splint

Name: ______________________________

Date: ______________________________

Type of thumb spica splint:

Volar   Dorsal   Radial gutter   Hand based

Thumb joint positions: ____________

Answer the following questions after the splint is worn for 30 minutes. (Mark *NA* for nonapplicable situations.)

Evaluation Areas		**Comments**
Design		
1. The wrist position is at the correct angle.	Yes ❍ No ❍ NA ❍	
2. The thumb position is at the correct angle.	Yes ❍ No ❍ NA ❍	
3. The thenar eminence is not restricted or flattened.	Yes ❍ No ❍ NA ❍	
4. The thumb post is adequately supported and is not constricted.	Yes ❍ No ❍ NA ❍	
5. The splint is two-thirds the length of the forearm.	Yes ❍ No ❍ NA ❍	
6. The splint is one-half the width of the forearm.	Yes ❍ No ❍ NA ❍	
Function		
1 The splint allows thumb IP flexion.	Yes ❍ No ❍ NA ❍	
2. The splint allows full MCP flexion of the fingers.	Yes ❍ No ❍ NA ❍	
3. The splint provides thumb support that allows functional activities.	Yes ❍ No ❍ NA ❍	
Straps		
1. The straps avoid bony prominences.	Yes ❍ No ❍ NA ❍	
2. The straps are secure and ends are rounded.	Yes ❍ No ❍ NA ❍	

Continued.

FORM 7-1 Thumb Spica Splint—cont'd

Evaluation Areas		**Comments**
Comfort		
1. The edges are smooth with rounded corners.	Yes ❍ No ❍ NA ❍	
2. The proximal end is flared.	Yes ❍ No ❍ NA ❍	
3. Impingements or pressure areas are not present.	Yes ❍ No ❍ NA ❍	
Cosmetic Appearance		
1. The splint is free of fingerprints, dirt, and pencil or pen marks.	Yes ❍ No ❍ NA ❍	
2. The splinting material is not buckled.	Yes ❍ No ❍ NA ❍	

Discuss adjustments or changes you would make based on the self-evaluation:

____

____

____

____

____

FORM 8-1 Radial Nerve Splint

Name: ___________________________________

Date: ___________________________________

Answer the following questions after the splint has been worn for 30 minutes. (Mark *NA* for nonapplicable situations.)

Evaluation Areas **Comments**

Design

1. The forearm trough is the proper length and width. Yes ❍ No ❍ NA ❍
2. The outrigger wire is at the appropriate angles and ½ inch wider than the MCPs at the level of the hand. Yes ❍ No ❍ NA ❍
3. The thermoplastic material on the MCP aspect of the outrigger is secure. Yes ❍ No ❍ NA ❍
4. The line to the outrigger is at a 90° angle from the long axis of the bone when the hand is at rest. Yes ❍ No ❍ NA ❍
5. The anchor hook is secure. Yes ❍ No ❍ NA ❍
6. The thermoplastic patch adequately secures the outrigger. Yes ❍ No ❍ NA ❍

Function

1. The wrist is maintained in neutral when the fingers are in extension. Yes ❍ No ❍ NA ❍
2. The outrigger or lines do not impede composite flexion of the fingers. Yes ❍ No ❍ NA ❍
3. The fit of the trough and straps prevents distal migration of the splint. Yes ❍ No ❍ NA ❍
4. The slings do not migrate distally with finger flexion and extension. Yes ❍ No ❍ NA ❍

Continued.

FORM 8-1 Radial Nerve Splint—cont'd

Evaluation Areas		Comments
Comfort		
1. Excessive pressure is not present on the radial or ulnar styloids.	Yes ❍ No ❍ NA ❍	
2. The edges are smooth with rounded corners.	Yes ❍ No ❍ NA ❍	
3. The proximal and distal ends are flared.	Yes ❍ No ❍ NA ❍	
4. Impingements or pressure areas are not present.	Yes ❍ No ❍ NA ❍	

FORM 9-1 Anticlaw Splint

Name: ______________________________

Date: ______________________________

Answer the following questions after the splint has been worn for 30 minutes. (Mark *NA* for nonapplicable situations.)

Evaluation Areas **Comments**

Design

1. The splint prevents hyperextension of the MCP joints of the ring and little fingers. Yes ❍ No ❍ NA ❍

Function

1. The splint allows full wrist motions. Yes ❍ No ❍ NA ❍
2. The splint allows full function of the middle and index fingers. Yes ❍ No ❍ NA ❍

Straps

1. The straps avoid bony prominences. Yes ❍ No ❍ NA ❍
2. Straps are secure and rounded. Yes ❍ No ❍ NA ❍

Comfort

1. The edges are smooth with rounded corners. Yes ❍ No ❍ NA ❍
2. The proximal end is flared. Yes ❍ No ❍ NA ❍
3. Impingements or pressure areas are not present. Yes ❍ No ❍ NA ❍

Cosmetic Appearance

1. The splint is free of fingerprints, dirt, and pencil or pen marks. Yes ❍ No ❍ NA ❍
2. The splinting material is not buckled. Yes ❍ No ❍ NA ❍

Discuss possible adjustments or changes you would make based on the self-evaluation:

____

____

____

____

____

FORM 10-1 Hard-Cone Wrist and Hand Splint

Name: ______________________________

Date: ______________________________

Type of cone wrist and hand splint:

Volar platform ❍ Dorsal platform ❍

Answer the following questions after the splint has been worn for 30 minutes. (Mark *NA* for nonapplicable situations.)

Evaluation Areas		**Comments**
Design		
1. The wrist position is at the correct angle.	Yes ❍ No ❍ NA ❍	
2. The correct cone-diameter size reflects the palm width and web-space size.	Yes ❍ No ❍ NA ❍	
3. The small end of the cone is placed radially and the large end is placed ulnarly.	Yes ❍ No ❍ NA ❍	
4. The thumb is positioned in palmar abduction with the web space preserved.	Yes ❍ No ❍ NA ❍	
5. The splint is two-thirds the length of the forearm.	Yes ❍ No ❍ NA ❍	
6. The splint is half the width of the forearm.	Yes ❍ No ❍ NA ❍	
Function		
1. The wrist is positioned in submaximum or maximum range.	Yes ❍ No ❍ NA ❍	
2. The fingers are positioned to provide firm pressure but not stretch the flexors.	Yes ❍ No ❍ NA ❍	

Continued.

FORM 10-1 Hard-Cone Wrist and Hand Splint—cont'd

Evaluation Areas **Comments**

Straps

1. The straps avoid bony prominences. Yes ❍ No ❍ NA ❍
2. The straps are secure and rounded. Yes ❍ No ❍ NA ❍
3. The active field materials are used over the extensor muscle bellies. Yes ❍ No ❍ NA ❍
4. The passive field materials are used over the flexor muscle bellies. Yes ❍ No ❍ NA ❍

Comfort

1. The edges are smooth with rounded corners. Yes ❍ No ❍ NA ❍
2. The proximal end is flared. Yes ❍ No ❍ NA ❍
3. Impingements or pressure areas are not present. (The ulnar styloid is relieved.) Yes ❍ No ❍ NA ❍

Cosmetic Appearance

1. The splint is free of fingerprints, dirt, and pencil or pen marks. Yes ❍ No ❍ NA ❍
2. The splinting material is not buckled. Yes ❍ No ❍ NA ❍

Discuss adjustments or changes you would make based on the self-evaluation:

____

____

____

____

____

APPENDIX C

Grading Sheets

GRADING SHEET 5-1
Wrist Cock-Up Splint

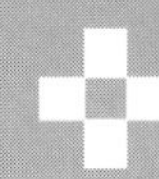

Name: ____________________

Date: ____________________

Type of wrist cock-up splint:

Volar Dorsal

Wrist position: ____________

Grade: ________

1 = beyond improvement, not acceptable
2 = requires maximal improvement
3 = requires moderate improvement
4 = requires minimal improvement
5 = requires no improvement

Evaluation Areas		**Comments**
Design		
1. The wrist position is at the correct angle.	1 2 3 4 5	
2. The wrist has adequate support.	1 2 3 4 5	
3. The sides of the thenar and hypothenar eminences have support in the correct position.	1 2 3 4 5	
4. The thenar and hypothenar eminences are not restricted or flattened.	1 2 3 4 5	
5. The splint is two-thirds the length of the forearm.	1 2 3 4 5	
6. The splint is one-half the width of the forearm.	1 2 3 4 5	
Function		
1. The splint allows full thumb motions.	1 2 3 4 5	
2. The splint allows full MCP joint flexion of the fingers.	1 2 3 4 5	
3. The splint provides wrist support that allows functional activities.	1 2 3 4 5	
Straps		
1. The straps avoid bony prominences.	1 2 3 4 5	
2. The straps are secure and rounded.	1 2 3 4 5	

Continued.

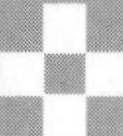

GRADING SHEET 5-1

Wrist Cock-Up Splint—cont'd

Evaluation Areas						Comments
Comfort						
1. The splint edges are smooth with rounded corners.	1	2	3	4	5	
2. The proximal end is flared.	1	2	3	4	5	
3. Impingements or pressure areas are not present.	1	2	3	4	5	
Cosmetic Appearance						
1. The splint is free of fingerprints, dirt, and pencil or pen marks.	1	2	3	4	5	
2. The splinting material is not buckled.	1	2	3	4	5	

Comments:

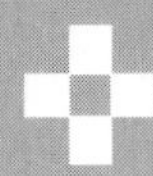

GRADING SHEET 6-1
Resting Hand Splint

Name: ______________________________

Date: ______________________________

Position of resting hand splint:

Functional position ❍ (midjoint) Antideformity position ❍ (intrinsic plus)

Grade: ____________

1 = beyond improvement, not acceptable
2 = requires maximal improvement
3 = requires moderate improvement
4 = requires minimal improvement
5 = requires no improvement

Evaluation Areas		Comments
Design		
1. The wrist position is at the correct angle.	1 2 3 4 5	
2. The MCPs are at the correct angle.	1 2 3 4 5	
3. The thumb is in the correct position.	1 2 3 4 5	
4. The wrist has adequate support.	1 2 3 4 5	
5. The pan is wide enough for all the fingers.	1 2 3 4 5	
6. The length of the pan and thumb trough are adequate.	1 2 3 4 5	
7. The splint is two-thirds the length of the forearm.	1 2 3 4 5	
8. The splint is one-half the width of the forearm.	1 2 3 4 5	
Function		
1. The splint completely immobilizes the wrist, fingers, and thumb.	1 2 3 4 5	
2. The splint is easy to apply and remove.	1 2 3 4 5	
Straps		
1. The straps avoid bony prominences.	1 2 3 4 5	
2. The straps are secure and rounded.	1 2 3 4 5	

Continued.

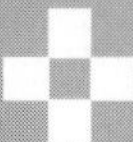

GRADING SHEET 6-1
Resting Hand Splint—cont'd

Evaluation Areas		Comments
Comfort		
1. The edges are smooth with rounded corners.	1 2 3 4 5	
2. The proximal end is flared.	1 2 3 4 5	
3. Impingements or pressure areas are not present.	1 2 3 4 5	
Cosmetic Appearance		
1. The splint is free of fingerprints, dirt, and pencil or pen marks.	1 2 3 4 5	
2. The splinting material is not buckled.	1 2 3 4 5	

Comments:

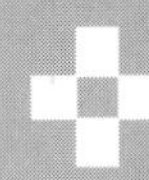

GRADING SHEET 7-1
Thumb Spica Splint

Name: ______________________

Date: ______________________

Type of thumb spica splint:

Volar Dorsal Radial gutter Hand based

Thumb joint positions: ______________

Grade: __________

1 = beyond improvement, not acceptable
2 = requires maximal improvement
3 = requires moderate improvement
4 = requires minimal improvement
5 = requires no improvement

Evaluation Areas		**Comments**
Design		
1. The wrist position is at the correct angle.	1 2 3 4 5	
2. The thumb position is at the correct angle.	1 2 3 4 5	
3. The thenar eminence is not restricted or flattened.	1 2 3 4 5	
4. The thumb is adequately supported and is not constricted.	1 2 3 4 5	
5. The splint is two-thirds the length of the forearm.	1 2 3 4 5	
6. The splint is one-half the width of the forearm.	1 2 3 4 5	
Function		
1. The splint allows thumb IP flexion.	1 2 3 4 5	
2. The splint allows full MCP flexion of the fingers.	1 2 3 4 5	
3. The splint provides thumb support that allows functional activities.	1 2 3 4 5	
Straps		
1. The straps avoid bony prominences.	1 2 3 4 5	
2. The straps are secure and rounded.	1 2 3 4 5	

Continued.

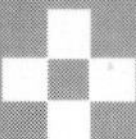

GRADING SHEET 7-1
Thumb Spica Splint—cont'd

Evaluation Areas		**Comments**
Comfort		
1. The edges are smooth with rounded corners.	1 2 3 4 5	
2. The proximal end is flared.	1 2 3 4 5	
3. Impingements or pressure areas are not present.	1 2 3 4 5	
Cosmetic Appearance		
1. The splint is free of fingerprints, dirt, and pencil or pen marks.	1 2 3 4 5	
2. The splinting material is not buckled.	1 2 3 4 5	

Comments:

GRADING SHEET 8-1
Radial Nerve Splint

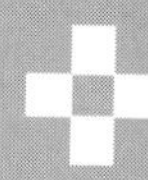

Name: ______________________________

Date: ______________________________

Wrist position at rest:

Grade: ____________

1 = beyond improvement, not acceptable

2 = requires maximal improvement

3 = requires moderate improvement

4 = requires minimal improvement

5 = requires no improvement

Evaluation Areas		**Comments**
Design		
1. The forearm trough is the proper length and width.	1 2 3 4 5	
2. The outrigger wire is at the appropriate angles and ½ inch wider than the MCPs at the level of the hand.	1 2 3 4 5	
3. The thermoplastic on the distal aspect of the outrigger is secure.	1 2 3 4 5	
4. The line to the outrigger is at a 90° angle from the long axis of the bone when the hand is at rest.	1 2 3 4 5	
5. The anchor hook is secure.	1 2 3 4 5	
6. The thermoplastic material patch adequately secures the outrigger.	1 2 3 4 5	
Function		
1. The wrist is maintained in neutral when the fingers are in extension.	1 2 3 4 5	
2. The outrigger or lines do not impede composite flexion of the fingers.	1 2 3 4 5	
3. The fit of the trough and straps prevents distal migration of the splint.	1 2 3 4 5	
4. The slings do not migrate distally with active finger flexion and extension.	1 2 3 4 5	

Continued.

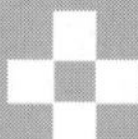

GRADING SHEET 8-1
Radial Nerve Splint—cont'd

Evaluation Areas		**Comments**
Comfort		
1. Excessive pressure is not present on the radial or ulnar styloids.	1 2 3 4 5	
2. The edges are smooth with rounded corners.	1 2 3 4 5	
3. The proximal and distal ends are flared.	1 2 3 4 5	
4. Impingements or pressure areas are not present.	1 2 3 4 5	

Comments:

GRADING SHEET 9-1

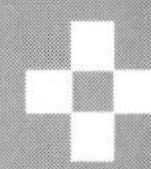

Anticlaw Splint

Name: ______________________________

Date: ______________________________

Grade: ____________

1 = beyond improvement, not acceptable

2 = requires maximal improvement

3 = requires moderate improvement

4 = requires minimal improvement

5 = requires no improvement

Evaluation Areas		**Comments**
Design		
1. The splint prevents hyperextension of the MCP joints of the ring and little fingers.	1 2 3 4 5	
Function		
1. The splint allows full wrist motions.	1 2 3 4 5	
2. The splint allows full function of the middle and index fingers.	1 2 3 4 5	
Straps		
1. The straps avoid bony prominences.	1 2 3 4 5	
2. The straps are secure and rounded.	1 2 3 4 5	
Comfort		
1. The edges are smooth with rounded corners.	1 2 3 4 5	
2. The proximal end is flared.	1 2 3 4 5	
3. Impingements or pressure areas are not present.	1 2 3 4 5	
Cosmetic Appearance		
1. The splint is free of fingerprints, dirt, and pencil or pen marks.	1 2 3 4 5	
2. The splinting material is not buckled.	1 2 3 4 5	

Comments:

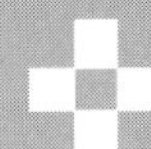

GRADING SHEET 10-1
Hard-Cone Wrist and Hand Splint

Name: ______________________________

Date: ______________________________

Type of cone wrist and hand splint:

Volar platform Dorsal platform

Grade: ____________

1 = beyond improvement, not acceptable
2 = requires maximal improvement
3 = requires moderate improvement
4 = requires minimal improvement
5 = requires no improvement

Evaluation Areas		**Comments**
Design		
1. The wrist position is at the correct angle.	1 2 3 4 5	
2. The correct cone-diameter size reflects the palm width and web-space size.	1 2 3 4 5	
3. The small end of the cone is placed radially and the large end is placed ulnarly.	1 2 3 4 5	
4. The thumb is positioned in palmar abduction with the web space preserved.	1 2 3 4 5	
5. The splint is two-thirds the length of the forearm.	1 2 3 4 5	
6. The splint is half the width of the forearm.	1 2 3 4 5	
Function		
1. The wrist is positioned in submaximal or maximal range.	1 2 3 4 5	
2. The fingers are positioned to provide firm pressure but not stretch the flexors.	1 2 3 4 5	

Continued.

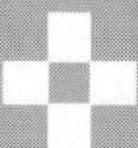

GRADING SHEET 10-1
Hard-Cone Wrist and Hand Splint—cont'd

Evaluation Areas						**Comments**
Straps						
1. The straps avoid bony prominences.	1	2	3	4	5	
2. The straps are secure and rounded.	1	2	3	4	5	
3. The active field materials are used over the extensor muscle bellies.	1	2	3	4	5	
4. The passive field materials are used over the flexor muscle bellies.	1	2	3	4	5	
Comfort						
1. The edges are smooth with rounded corners.	1	2	3	4	5	
2. The proximal end is flared.	1	2	3	4	5	
3. Impingements or pressure areas are not present.	1	2	3	4	5	
Cosmetic Appearance						
1. The splint is free of fingerprints, dirt, and pencil or pen marks.	1	2	3	4	5	
2. The splinting material is not buckled.	1	2	3	4	5	

Comments:

Index